R864 .P44

Person-center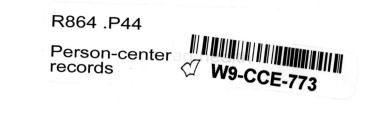
records

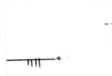

Health Informatics

(*formerly Computers in Health Care*)

Kathryn J. Hannah   Marion J. Ball
Series Editors

Health Informatics Series

(formerly Computers in Health Care)

Series Editors
Kathryn J. Hannah   Marion J. Ball

(continued after index)

James E. Demetriades   Robert M. Kolodner
Gary A. Christopherson
Editors

Person-Centered
Health Records
Toward HealthePeople™

Foreword by Janet M. Corrigan

With 42 Illustrations

SOUTH PLAINS COLLEGE LIBRARY

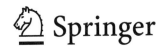 Springer

James E. Demetriades, BS, MS, PE
Chief Health Information Architect
Department of Veterans Affairs
Veterans Health Administration
Albany, NY
USA

Robert M. Kolodner, MD
Chief Information Officer
Department of Veterans Affairs
Veterans Health Administration
Washington, DC
USA

Gary A. Christopherson, MS
Senior Advisor to the Under Secretary for Health
Department of Veterans Affairs
Veterans Health Administration
Washington, DC
USA

Series Editors:
Kathryn J. Hannah, PhD, RN
Adjunct Professor, Department of
    Community Health Science
Faculty of Medicine
The University of Calgary
Calgary, Alberta T2N 4N1
Canada

Marion J. Ball, EdD
Vice President, Clinical Informatics
    Strategies
Healthlink, Inc.
Baltimore, MD 21210
and
Professor
Johns Hopkins University
    School of Nursing
Baltimore, MD 21205
USA

Library of Congress Cataloging-in-Publication Data
Person-Centered Health Records: toward healthepeople / James E. Demetriades,
    Robert M. Kolodner, Gary A. Christopherson, editors.
        p.   cm.
    Includes bibliographical references and index.
    1. Medical care—United States.   2. Medical economics—United States.
    3. Health care reform—United States.   I. Title: Healthy people.   II. Demetriades, James E.
    III. Kolodner, Robert M.   IV. Christopherson, Gary A.
    RA395.A3H432 2005
    362.1'0973—dc22   2004052211

ISBN 0-387-23282-6   Printed on acid-free paper.

Health*e*People is a registered trademark of the Veterans Health Administration, Number 2,732,137 in the U.S. Patent and Trademark Office, effective July 1, 2003. The bold-underscore-italic formatting is standard usage in the Department of Veterans Affairs; the style was simplified to italics only for the purposes of readability in this book.

In recognition of the authors' work undertaken as part of their official duties as U.S. Government employees, reproduction of this work in whole or in part for any purpose of the U.S. Government is permitted.

© 2005 Springer Science+Business Media, Inc.
All rights reserved. This work may not be translated or copied in whole or in part without the written permission of the publisher (Springer Science+Business Media, Inc., 233 Spring Street, New York, NY 10013, USA), except for brief excerpts in connection with reviews or scholarly analysis. Use in connection with any form of information storage and retrieval, electronic adaptation, computer software, or by similar or dissimilar methodology now known or hereafter developed is forbidden.
The use in this publication of trade names, trademarks, service marks, and similar terms, even if they are not identified as such, is not to be taken as an expression of opinion as to whether or not they are subject to proprietary rights.
While the advice and information in this book are believed to be true and accurate at the date of going to press, neither the authors nor the editors nor the publisher can accept any legal responsibility for any errors or omissions that may be made. The publisher makes no warranty, express or implied, with respect to the material contained herein.

Printed in the United States of America.   (BS/SB)

9 8 7 6 5 4 3 2 1   SPIN 10972649

springeronline.com

This book is dedicated to all those around the world committed to transforming health care by

- *Creating systems that are truly person centered*
- *Empowering individuals to participate directly in managing their own health*
- *Making it possible to exchange health records electronically, effortlessly, and securely.*

Foreword

In 2001, the Institute of Medicine released the report, *Crossing the Quality Chasm: A New Health System for the 21st Century*, calling for fundamental change in the American health care delivery system. The IOM report identified six aims for improvement: health care should be safe, effective, patient centered, timely, efficient, and equitable. The IOM report laid out a vision of a future health system that is carefully and consciously designed to respond to the needs, preferences, and values of patients *and* one that ensures that patients are fully informed, retain control, and participate in care delivery, whenever possible.

Person-Centered Health Records: Toward HealthePeople further refines this vision and provides a blueprint for moving forward. Focusing on people—as consumers, patients, enrollees, and members—the report makes a compelling case for the creation of a "virtual health system" that encompasses the full range of services available to assist people in managing their health and health care.

The goal is better health, but the critical enabler is information technology. Building on the extraordinary e-health accomplishments of the Veterans Health Affairs, the editors have brought together contributors from public and private sectors alike. These authors provide an ambitious, but achievable, agenda for establishing an electronic infrastructure that includes personal health records for individuals, electronic health records for providers, and the necessary information standards and supports to enable appropriate health information exchange.

The "virtual health system" will fundamentally alter the interactions among the members of a care team, and the relationships between health care providers and patients. There is little doubt this new health system will open up many opportunities to improve the health of populations and individuals, but the journey will not be an easy one.

The contributors to this book recognize the magnitude and complexity of the change process, and the importance of attending to both technological and human factors. Building a virtual health system will require talented and committed leadership at all levels of the health system. Through their collective knowledge and experience, the editors and authors of *Person-Centered Health Records* provide a wealth of information and excellent guidance to all who are involved in the journey of *Crossing the Quality Chasm*.

Janet M. Corrigan

Series Preface

This series is directed to healthcare professionals who are leading the transformation of health care by using information and knowledge to advance the quality of patient care. Launched in 1988 as Computers in Health Care, the series offers a broad range of titles: some are addressed to specific professions such as nursing, medicine, and health administration; others to special areas of practice such as trauma and radiology. Still other books in the series focus on interdisciplinary issues, such as the computer-based patient record, electronic health records, and networked healthcare systems.

Renamed Health Informatics in 1998 to reflect the rapid evolution in the discipline now known as health informatics, the series continues to add titles that contribute to the evolution of the field. In the series, eminent experts, serving as editors or authors, offer their accounts of innovation in health informatics. Increasingly, these accounts go beyond hardware and software to address the role of information in influencing the transformation of healthcare delivery systems around the world. The series also increasingly focuses on "peopleware" and the organizational, behavioral, and societal changes that accompany the diffusion of information technology in health services environments.

These changes will shape health services in the new millennium. By making full and creative use of the technology to tame data and to transform information, health informatics will foster the development of the knowledge age in health care. As coeditors, we pledge to support our professional colleagues and the series readers as they share the advances in the emerging and exciting field of health informatics.

Kathryn J. Hannah
Marion J. Ball

Preface

Ideas and trends can be as contagious as viruses. Seemingly unrelated, small events can mount to epidemic proportions, and "the slightest push" in "just the right place" will change everything. This is what Malcolm Gladwell (2000) calls the Tipping Point, a unique moment "when everything can change all at once."

After decades of changes, health care is approaching this transforming moment—and we want to be among those who deliver the push in the right place, creating a new system, a "virtual health system," that delivers the greatest good to the greatest number. We believe, as does Gladwell, that "In the end, Tipping Points are a reaffirmation of the potential for change and the power of intelligent action."

This belief has led us to join with colleagues from both public and private sectors to write this book about HealthePeople, to share the concept of a new health system that places the person seeking and receiving care at its center. The concept is framed to solve the monumental problems health care faces with the smallest possible amount of effort, time, and cost—"to make a lot out of a little."

Launched as a tightly focused effort within the Veterans Health Administration, HealthePeople stands ready to serve the hundreds of facilities, thousands of providers, and millions of veterans that make up the nation's largest health system. When deployed, it has worked and will work because it empowers *all* those it serves.

And work it must. Health care is the largest single sector of our economy that has yet to reap the benefits of information technology. In what is arguably the most complex professional service industry, where almost every service is a "custom product" supporting very complex human needs, the stakes are high. We all literally bet our lives that we can access the healthcare services we need—and that those services are affordable, safe, and of high quality.

But are they? In its report, *The Quality Chasm* (2001), the Institute of Medicine says no: "Between the health care we have and the care we could have lies not just a gap, but a chasm." We spend almost one-seventh of our economy in the United States on health care, with insufficient return on our investment. For us all, even those of us who are insured (over 40 million Americans are not), "the care delivered is not, essentially, what we should receive."

What we need, the IOM concluded in 2001, is "a system that uses the best knowledge, that is focused intensely on patients, and that works across health care provides and settings." And what we need to do is create a new virtual health system by "taking advantage of new information technologies" and using them as "an important catalyst to moving beyond where we are today."

The good news is that there has been progress in the few years since then—progress that brings us to the "tipping point." Initiatives in the United States, Canada, Australia, and some countries in Europe are using new technologies and new approaches to develop new systems that place the individual at the center of the healthcare universe. These new person-centered systems forge new partnerships between individuals and clinicians. They support the move from episodic care to "seamless" care for the whole person and, ultimately, the world community.

This new view of the healthcare universe represents a profound and massive change—and stands to offer many new opportunities for public and private sector alike. Health care delivery, we believe, will mirror what happened in genomics when new technologies were used to successfully map the human genome. Only now are we beginning to reap the benefits of this new knowledge and use it to treat and prevent disease.

In the words of Alan Kay, who helped develop object oriented programming and the concept of the laptop, and who architected the modern windowing graphic user interface, "The best way to predict the future is to invent it." We agree. By re-engineering health care to function upon a strong foundation of health information systems, we can better tackle the great issues facing health care.

The contributors to this book represent different disciplines, work in different sectors, and come from different countries. They have joined with us to explain what HealthePeople is and what it can mean for the individual and for health care. Some describe the new tools and approaches (many of which are the result of years of effort) that make HealthePeople and systems like it possible. Others report on efforts to put person-centered systems in place, sharing their insights on making them functional realities.

The signs are clear: We are at the Tipping Point, on the cusp of change. The time has come to "electrify" health care as we "electrified" the world in the last century. With healthcare costs and needs growing throughout the world, HealthePeople can help deliver the promise of better health for all Americans and, potentially, for many others.

James E. Demetriades
Robert M. Kolodner
Gary A. Christopherson

References

Gladwell M. 2000. The Tipping Point: How Little Things Can Make a Big Difference. Boston, MA: Little, Brown and Company.
Institute of Medicine. 2001. Crossing the Quality Chasm: A New Health System for the 21st Century. Washington, DC: National Academy Press.

Acknowledgments

As editors, we are privileged to publish a volume in the Springer Health Informatics Series. It has been a remarkable learning experience to work through the many steps involved in producing a contributed volume. Throughout this process, Judith Douglas expertly and patiently guided us. We are truly grateful for her brilliant ability to work with people, schedules, and, above all, words. Her perseverance through this lengthy and complex task has quite literally made this manuscript possible. This was all done with that wonderfully calming style of hers. We are indebted.

We would also like to recognize and thank Marion J. Ball. Her instant enthusiasm when first asked about the merit of a book propelled us forward. Her thoughtful guidance helped us shape its content. It remains a pleasure to work with her.

Finally, we would like to acknowledge and thank all the individual chapter authors. They showed a remarkable willingness to share their expert knowledge and unselfishly contributed time and talent. To each of them we owe a debt of gratitude.

James E. Demetriades
Robert M. Kolodner
Gary A. Christopherson

Contents

SECTION 1   INVENTING THE FUTURE: ENVISIONING A NEW HEALTH SYSTEM

SECTION 2   BUILDING THE FUTURE: ESSENTIAL TECHNOLOGIES AND METHODOLOGIES

SECTION 3   BEING IN THE FUTURE: CASE STUDIES

Contributors

MARION J. BALL, EdD
Member, Institute of Medicine; Vice President, Clinical Informatics Strategies, Health-link, Inc.; Professor, Johns Hopkins University School of Nursing, Baltimore, MD, USA

THOMAS BEALE, BE, BSc
Chief Technology Officer, Ocean Informatics; Founding Member, Open EHR Foundation; Senior Research Fellow, CHIME, University College London; Mooloolah, Queensland, Australia

JEFFREY S. BLAIR, MBA
Vice President, Medical Records Institute; Member, National Committee on Vital and Health Statistics and Vice Chair, Subcommittee on Standards and Security; Albuquerque, NM, USA

BERND BLOBEL, PhD, MSc
Director, Associate Professor, Otto-von-Guericke University Magdeburg, Institute of Biometry and Medical Informatics, Magdeburg, Germany

STEVEN H. BROWN, MS, MD
Health Information Architect, Veterans Health Administration; Associate Professor of Biomedical Informatics, Vanderbilt University, Nashville, TN, USA

GARY A. CHRISTOPHERSON, MS
Senior Advisor to the Under Secretary for Health, Department of Veterans Affairs, Veterans Health Administration, Senior Fellow, Institute of Medicine, Washington, DC, USA

SIMON COHN, MD, MPH
National Director for Health Information Policy, Kaiser Permanente; Member, National Committee on Vital and Health Statistics and Chair, Subcommittee on Standards and Security, Oakland, CA, USA

JOHN M. DAVIS, BS, MS PHYSICS, BS, MS ELECTRONIC ENGINEERING, CISSP
Security Architect, Science Applications International Corporation, Encinitas, CA, USA

JAMES E. DEMETRIADES, BS, MS, PE
Chief Health Information Architect, Department of Veterans Affairs, Veterans Health Administration, Albany, NY, USA

JUDITH V. DOUGLAS, MA, MHS
Adjunct Faculty, Johns Hopkins University School of Nursing, Reisterstown, MD, USA

SHARI DWORKIN, BA, MES
Senior Consultant, Canadian Institute for Health Information, Toronto, Ontario, Canada

PETER L. ELKIN, MD
Internist, Mayo Clinic, Rochester, MN, USA

J. MICHAEL FITZMAURICE, PhD
Senior Science Advisor for Information Technology, Agency for Healthcare Research and Quality, Rockville, MD, USA

DAVID FORSLUND, BS, MA, PhD
Laboratory Fellow, Los Alamos National Laboratory, Los Alamos, NM, USA

GERARD FRERIKS, MD
Convenor, Working Group 1, CEN/TC 251; Member, Eurorec Institute; TNO-PG, Leiden, The Netherlands

THOMAS L. GARTHWAITE, MD
Director and Chief Medical Officer, Department of Health Services, County of Los Angeles, Los Angeles, CA, USA

NANCY GILL, BSc
Intern, Canadian Institute for Health Information, Toronto, Ontario, Canada

DIPAK KALRA, PhD, FRCGP
Clinical Senior Lecturer in Health Informatics, Centre for Health Informatics and Multiprofessional Education (CHIME), University College London, London, UK

ROBERT M. KOLODNER, MD
Chief Information Officer, Department of Veterans Affairs, Veterans Health Administration, Washington, DC, USA

MICHAEL J. LINCOLN, MD
Associate Professor, Department of Veterans Affairs, Veterans Administration, CIO Field Office, Salt Lake City, UT, USA

BLACKFORD MIDDLETON, MD, MPH, MSc
Corporate Director, Clinical Informatics Research and Development, Partners Health-Care System; Assistant Professor of Medicine, Brigham and Women's Hospital, Harvard Medical School, Boston, MA, USA

Tom Munnecke, BS
Vice President and Chief Scientist, SAIC (retired); Visiting Scholar, Stanford University Digital Visions Program; Founder, GivingSpace.org, Encinitas, CA, USA

Jonathan B. Perlin, MD, PhD, MSHA, FACP
Deputy Under Secretary for Health, Department of Veterans Affairs, Washington, DC, USA

Julie Richards, BSc, MHSc
Senior Consultant, Canadian Institute for Health Information, at time of writing; currently Director Standards, Canadian Institute for Health Information, Toronto, Ontario, Canada

Angelo Rossi Mori, MS
National Research Council, Institute of Biomedical Technology; President, PROREC Italy; Secretary, HL7 Italy; Member, Eurorec Institute, Rome, Italy

David Rowlands, BEc (Hons), GDBA, FACHI
Director, National InfoStructure Development, Australian Government, Department of Health and Ageing, Bowen Hills, Queensland, Australia

Kenneth S. Rubin, BS
Senior Systems Architect, Electronic Data Systems, Inc., Bowie, MD, USA

Steven Wagner, BA, MBA
Deputy Chief and Health Information Architect, Department of Veterans Affairs, Veterans Health Administration, Office of Information, Manchester, NH, USA

Acronyms

AA	Attribute Authority
ACHI	Advisory Council on Health Infostructure (Canada)
ACI	Access Control Information
ADF	Access Decision Function
ADI	Access Decision Information
AEF	Access Enforcement Function
ACMI	American College of Medical Informatics
AHRQ	Agency for Health Research and Quality
AMA	American Medical Association
ANSI	American National Standards Institute
API	Application Program Interface
ASC	Accredited Standards Committee
ASTM	American Society for Testing and Materials
ATM	Automated Teller Machine
CAC/TC	Canadian Advisory Committee/Technical Committee
CAP	College of American Pathologists
CBOC	Community Based Outpatient Clinic
CCAC	Community Care Access Center
CCOW	Clinical Context Object Workgroup
CCR	Continuity of Care Record
CDA	Clinical Document Architecture
CDMS	Chronic Disease Management System (Australia)
CDT	Current Dental Terminology
CEN	European Committee for Standardization (Comité Européen de Normalisation)
CEN/TC 251	European Technical Committee for the Standardization of Health Informatics
CEO	Chief Executive Officer
CHCS	Composite Health Care System
CHDM	Conceptual Health Data Model (Canada)
CHI	Consolidated Health Informatics
CHIN	Child Health Information Network (Australia)
CHIPP	Canada Health Infostructure Partnership Program
CIHI	Canadian Institute for Health Information
CITL	Center for Information Technology Leadership
CM	Clinical Modification

CMS	Centers for Medicare and Medicaid Services
CORBA	Common Object Request Broker Architecture
CPOE	Computerized Physician Order Entry; alternately, Computerized Provider Order Entry
CPT	Current Procedural Terminology
CPRI	Computed-based Patient Record Institute
CPRS	Computerized Patient Record System
CSA	Canadian Standards Association
CT	Clinical Terminology
CTS	Central Terminology Services
CVS	Concurrent Versions Systems
DBC	Diagnosis Treatment Groups (Netherlands)
DHCP	Decentralized Hospital Computer
DICOM	Digital Imaging and Communications in Medicine
DoD	Department of Defense
DRG	Diagnosis Related Groups
DSM	Diagnostic and Statistical Manual of Mental Disorders
DSTU	HL7 EHR Functional Draft Standard for Trial Use
DTD	Document Type Definition
eCHN	Electronic Child Health Network (Canada)
EDDS	Electronic Decision Support Systems
EDI	Electronic Data Interchange
EFMI	European Federation for Medical Informatics
EHCR-SupA	Electronic Healthcare Record Support Action
eHI	eHealth Initiative
EHR	Electronic Health Record
EHRC	Electronic Health Record Collaborative
EHRi	Electronic Health Record Infostructure
EHRS	Electronic Health Record Solution (Canada)
EHRS	Electronic Health Record System
EHTEL	European Health Telematics Association
EIN	Employer Identification Number
EPRP	External Peer Review Program
ER	Emergency Room
FDA	Food and Drug Administration
FGH	Florida General Hospital (fictional)
GCPR	Government Computerized Patient Record
GDP	Gross Domestic Product
GEHR	Good European Health Record
GNU	GNU's Not Unix (pronounced "guh-noo")
GP	General Practitioner
GPL	General Public License
GPRA	Government Performance and Results Act
GTA	Greater Toronto Area
HCPCS	Healthcare Common Procedure Coding System
HEDIS	Health Plan Employer Data and Information Set
HDTF	Healthcare Domain Task Force
HHS	Health and Human Services, Department of
HIAL	Health Information Access Layer
HIBCC	Health Industry Communications Council
HIMSS	Health Information Management and Systems Society

HIPAA	Health Insurance Portability and Accountability Act
HISA	Health Information Systems Architecture
HISB	Healthcare Informatics Standards Board
HL7	Health Level Seven
HSC	Hospital for Sick Children (Toronto, Canada)
HTML	Hypertext Markup Language
HTTP	Hypertext Transport Protocol
ICD9	International Classification of Diseases Ninth Edition
ICD10	International Classification of Diseases Tenth Edition
ICT	Information and Communication Technology
IDE	Integrated Development Environment
IDL	Interface Definition Language
IE	Information Exchange
IEEE 1073	Institute of Electrical and Electronics Engineers, Medical Device Communication
IHE	Integrating the Healthcare Enterprise
IHS	Indian Health Service
IMIA	International Medical Informatics Association
IOM	Institute of Medicine
ISBT	International Society of Blood Transfusion
ISO	International Organization for Standardization
IST	Information Society Technologies (European Union)
IT	Information Technology
ITS	Implementation Technology Specification
JCAHO	Joint Commission on Accreditation of Healthcare Organizations
LOINC	Logical Observations Identifiers Names and Codes
MBS	Medicare Benefits Scheme (Australia)
MDA	Model Driven Architecture
MeSH	Medical Subject Headings
NACC	North American Collaborating Center
NCG	National Guideline Clearinghouse
NCPDP	National Council for Prescription Drug Programs
NCQA	National Committee for Quality Assurance
NCVHS	National Committee on Vital and Health Statistics
NDC	National Drug Codes
NDFRT	National Drug File Reference Terminology
NEC	Not Elsewhere Classified
NeCST	National e-Claims Standard Initiative (Canada)
NEDSS	National Electronic Disease Surveillance System
NHII	National Health Information Infrastructure
NHS	National Health Service (United Kingdom)
NICTIZ	National Information and Technology Institute in Healthcare (Netherlands)
NLM	National Library of Medicine
NPI	National Provider Identifier
NPRM	Notice of Proposed Rule Making
OASIS	Organization for the Advancement of Structure Information Standards
OECD	Organization for Economic Cooperation and Development
OHIH	Office of Health and Information Highway (Canada)
OMB	Office of Management and Budget

OMG	Object Management Group
OTC	Over The Counter
PACS	Picture Archiving and Communications System
PCS	Procedure Classification System
PFI	Private Finance Initiative
PHR	Personal Health Record
PIDS	Person Identification Services
PIM	Platform Independent Model
PKI	Public Key Infrastructure (Australia)
PMI	Privilege Management Infrastructure
PMRI	Patient Medical Record Information
POMA	Patient Oriented Management Architecture
PSM	Platform Specific Model
QUERI	Quality Enhancement Research Initiatives
RAD	Resource Access Decision
RIM	Reference Information Model
RM-ODP	Reference Model for Open Distributed Processing
SAML	Security Assertion Markup Language
SCC	Standards Council of Canada
SDO	Standards Development Organization
SHEP	Survey of Health Experiences of Patients
SIG	Special Interest Group
SNOMED	Systematized Nomenclature of Medicine
SNOMED-CT	Standardized Nomenclature in Medicine-Clinical Terms
SQL	Structured Query Language
TATRC	Telemedicine and Advanced Technology Research Center
TC251	ISO Technical Committee on Health Informatics
TQS	Terminology Query Services
TS	Technical Specification
UCL	University College London
UML	Unified Modeling Language
UMLS	Unified Medical Language System
UPI	Unique Patient Identifier
UPIN	Unique Physician Identifier Number
URL	Uniform Resource Locator
VA	Veterans Administration, also Veterans Health Administration
VERA	Veterans Equitable Resource Allocation Act
VISN	Veterans Integrated Service Network
VistA	Veterans Health Information Systems and Technology Architecture
VISTA	Veterans Health Information Systems and Technology Architecture
WEDI	Workgroup for Electronic Data Interchange
WHIC	Western Health Information Collaborative (Canada)
WHO	World Health Organization
WS	Web Service
WSDL	Web Service Definition Language
XACML	eXtensible Access Control Markup Language
XMI	XML Metadata Interchange
XML	eXtensible Markup Language
XP	Extreme Programming

Section 1
Inventing the Future:
Envisioning a New Health System

1
Inverted Perspectives: Triggering Change

Tom Munnecke and Robert M. Kolodner

Albert Einstein imagined riding a beam of light and discovered relativity. Jonas Salk imagined being a polio virus and discovered a vaccine. Nobel Laureate Richard Feynman discovered new ways of thinking about physics by imagining himself immersed in a messy fog of electrons. In each instance, an inverted perspective triggered a great discovery.

Now invert the traditional healthcare universe, and put the individual at the center instead of the enterprise. The result is a universe where enterprises compete by personalizing the services they offer their customers, not by integrating their internal operations. In this universe, individuals have and control their own health information in a radically person-centered health record that

- is designed around the individual, not the healthcare provider;
- assumes that, over the life of the individual, there will be a large number of providers, suppliers, and other associations involved with the individual's health that will not be physically co-located;
- assumes that information formats will be constantly changing, and that there will not be any static "one correct way" to record health information;
- brings issues of trust, confidentiality, ownership, and access to health information to the forefront, making them critical success factors, rather than side effects of enterprise transaction processing;
- treats health care as only one extreme of the health spectrum—the normal state of the individual is assumed to not be engaged in disease-based activities, but rather, participating in positive, life-affirming activities of society which use and amplify basic character strengths and virtues (Peterson and Seligman 2004);
- supports and enhances the role of communications within a trusted community of interest as a key contributor to the health of the individual.

The record belongs to a person, not a patient. The word *patient* implies a disease state being treated by a provider in a healthcare setting. The new record belongs to the person who ideally is not in a disease state. The goal of the system is to keep the person from becoming a patient, and for that person to live a healthy life independent of disease processes as long as possible. Similarly, it uses the term *health* rather than *health care* to shift the focus on the health process of the individual. Health care is but one portion of the health process.

For the past three decades, informaticians have tried to integrate divergent sources of information into meaningful collections within the confines of the enterprise perspective. During the same time, explosive changes have occurred in biomedicine,

TABLE 1.1. Comparison of enterprise-centric and person-centric systems.

Issue	Enterprise-centric system	Person-centric system
Purpose	Survival of the enterprise	Survival of the individual
Context	What is necessary for the survival and growth of the organization within its stated goals?	What improves the health of the individual?
Trust	Individual must trust entire system	Individual builds trust in community of interest, trusted third party for holding databases
Organization	Integrated around operating units/functions within the organization	Associated with many different and constantly changing set of providers and sources of information
Typical activity	Episodes of intervention	Adopting healthy behavior, adjusting to injury, self-management, recovery, fitness, compliance with providers of health care
Continuity of care	Management policies and workflow	Concerned people and agents acting on behalf of the individual
Information system	Tied to organization chart	Tied to context of person's needs, computer literacy, and virtual community
Authority	Single and management chain within the organization	The individual
Control	Policies, regulations, management chains	The individual, within constraints provided by regulation; community and social standards

healthcare services, and information technology, in areas from nomenclatures and coding schemes, to government regulations and payer needs. The resulting complexity is incomprehensible to anyone dealing with only part of the problem. Single components appear relatively simple, and constraints seem due to the lack of integration with the rest of the system.

Yet this integration crunch is the core of the problem, not a path to the solution. The end to the search for a viable health information system lies in accepting the divergent and constantly changing nature of health information, rather than attempting to force an enterprise-centric perspective on the field.

The alternative—the inverted perspective—is to design the information system from the point of view of the individual. There are many differences between enterprise- and person-centric health information systems, as Table 1.1 shows. The enterprise sees the person as an object to be acted upon, whereas the person sees the healthcare enterprise as only one piece of a larger puzzle. Simply put, the enterprise is solving one problem while the patient perceives another:

Health care providers typically define problems related to diagnosis, poor compliance with treatment regimens or continuing unhealthy behaviors, such as smoking or lack of exercise. Patients, however, are more likely to define problems of pain and other symptoms, their inability to function as they once did, emotional distress, difficulty carrying out prescribed regimens or lifestyle changes or fear of unpredictable consequences of the illness. (Gruman and Von Korff 1999)

The healthcare industry is driven by the survival needs of the organizations that comprise it. Stakeholders may be threatened by the person-centered model because it displaces them from the center of the healthcare universe. A trillion dollar industry does not change easily. The patient-centric model may appear today to be too simplistic and not powerful enough to compete with the established industry. But appearances can be deceiving. In the 1980s, Digital Equipment Corporation dominated the minicomputer industry with their computer systems. They saw little reason to change. Their chief executive officer (CEO), Ken Olsen, denounced personal computers as toys. A decade later, his company was purchased by Compaq, one of those "toy" computer manufacturers.

What appears to be simple and toy-like in its early stages of development can hide tremendous power as it matures. Established models are changing dramatically, industry after industry, as the Internet and the World Wide Web mature. And these changes come from the young upstart attackers rather than the established defenders of the current model. The upstart Amazon.com, not the venerable Barnes & Noble, created the online book sales market.

Recent advances in information technology and complexity theory give new ways to deal with complexity. In what is known as the chaordic model,[1] complex adaptive systems grow organically from simple beginnings, increasing in complexity as a result of interaction with their environment. Complexity grows evolutionarily rather than being built mechanically.

Systems at this level of complexity constantly change and evolve. They are in a state of perpetual novelty, and thus not predictable. As Demetriades explains in Chapter 7, we cannot understand these systems according to traditional mechanical or engineering terms, but must rather seek to understand and shape the environment in which they operate.

Consider the World Wide Web, a major transformational force in the world today. It emerged from a simple "primordial soup" consisting of three simple definitions: the Uniform Resource Locator (URL), Hypertext Markup Language (HTML), and Hypertext Transport Protocol (HTTP). It grew within constraints; the Internet Protocol (IP) delineated the boundaries beyond which the web could not stray. One simple selection criterion controlled its evolution: Web pages to which people paid attention survived, while those that were ignored withered.

At first, complex adaptive systems appear somewhat chaotic and disordered. Over time, order appears from seemingly chaotic "primordial soup." Features come forth as *emergent properties* of the system; they were not designed into it by a body of authoritative experts. Today, the World Wide Web offers search engines, virtual communities, and electronic commerce of far greater sophistication than we could have imagined. Authoritative strategic planning does not control the future growth of the Internet; an evolutionary process drives it.

Evidence of self-organization exists throughout nature. A cut finger heals itself, the body maintains homeostasis, and predator/prey populations adjust to their environment. We also find self-organization in man-made systems, such as the World Wide Web and many of the companies it has spawned. The greatest threats to Microsoft's dominance in the software market may come from self-organizing groups, such as the programmers creating the Linux operating system and the developers collaborating on the open source approach Kalra and Forslund discuss in Chapter 11.

Before we consider how self-organization may be used in the field of health and health care, however, we have to address two questions:

---

[1] For more on this model, see The Trillion Dollar Vision of Dee Hock at http://www.fastcompany.com/magazine/05/deehock.html.

- What is the self that does the organizing? What is the entity that properly serves as the core around which health organizes?
- What is the scale at which this self-organization takes place? Is it the individual, the family, the nation, the world?

Traditionally, we have focused on the interaction between the healthcare provider and the patient, and measured this interaction in the form of transactions. This approach does not deal well with interaction within the family, community, self-help groups, or with other forms of health assistance. Someone who benefits from attending Alcoholics Anonymous generates no transactions to be measured. Alcoholics Anonymous is a self-organizing group that benefits many people around the world, yet it is "invisible" to the world of transaction processing.

There is no single "self" that should drive self-organization in health, nor is there a single scale that can be exclusively used. We must envision an approach that deals with an arbitrarily large number of "selves," involving from a single individual to large aggregations of people, or "ensembles." And for these ensembles in health, the goal is a transformation, a purposeful flow of activities and information.

It is not a transaction, a single moment in time. Transactions and transactional thinking are ubiquitous in modern society and work very well for certain classes of activities. For example, we insert a card into an automated teller machine (ATM) and get cash with ease and accuracy. Complex problems, like health, are different. When interactions are transactionalized in one context and then analyzed in the context of the aggregate, the context of the individual is often lost. The interaction has many dimensions, yet the transaction measures only one.

A transformation, however, deals with the longer-term flow of activities in the context of the individual. It sees the river as a flow, not a series of snapshots. Transformations are specific to the context of the community where they occur. Ion (1993) describes such transformations in a clinical setting:

What takes place as the patient and the physician interact. . . . ? One exchange is that of perceptions of reality, what each knows about the problem. Another exchange is that of trust: the physician trusts that the patient both wants to change or solve the problem and is willing to take action to do so; the patient trusts that physician has the appropriate skills to repair damage or advise on the changes necessary to resolution. These are the interactions of healing, older than Hippocrates and consistent still wherever healing is practiced. The exchange is *transformative* in nature, not *transactional*. The patient, and hopefully, the physician both learn and become different consequent to the interaction. Commerce, the purchase of products, is transactional—neither side of the interaction changes in function or ability to function. (Ion 1993, p 118)

In *Knowledge Coupling*, an earlier book in this Springer-Verlag series (1991), Larry Weed related an interview with a hospital patient about to be discharged:

Dr. Weed: "Do you have a copy of your own medical record?"
Patient: "No."
Dr. Weed: "Are all your medications in the bedside stand, and does the nurse come around at regular intervals to see if you are taking the right ones at the right time?"
Patient: "No. The nurse just comes with little paper cups with pills in them, and I swallow whatever is there."
Dr. Weed: "Do you know what a flowsheet is? What parameters are we trying to follow? What endpoints we are trying to reach?"
Patient: "No."

(At this point, Dr. Weed met with the medical staff to relate what he had found):

Staff: "We never give patients their records."
Staff: "We do not have the time to give the medicines that way. It would not be safe to leave her with them unattended. She is on many powerful drugs."
Staff: "The patient is not very well educated, and I do not think she could do all the things your questions imply."
Dr. Weed: "But, she is going home this afternoon. She lives alone. At 2PM you will put her in a wheelchair, give her a paper bag full of drugs, and send her out the door. Are you going home with her?"
Staff: "No. Is her management at home our problem?"
Dr. Weed: "You just said she could not handle it. Who will do it? The patient may not seem well educated or very bright to you, but what could be more unintelligent that what you are doing?" (Weed 1991, p 13)

Larry Weed advocated developing a system in which "all individuals are nurturers of their own health care and have available to them the guidance of an information system and the skills of providers who have demonstrated competence in performing specific tasks that patients who cannot perform for themselves" (Weed 1991, p 19). In his view, health care could not improve unless a system of this sort was in place. It could only grow worse.

According to Weed,

We must consider the whole information system and not just infinitely elaborate on the parts that interest us or fit into a given specialty. Patients do not specialize, and they or their families are in charge of all the relevant variables 24 hours a day, every day. They must be given the right tools to work with . . . After all,

• They are highly motivated, and if they are not, nothing works in the long run anyway,
• They do not charge.
• They even pay for help.
• There is at least one "caregiver" for every member of the population.

(Weed 1993, p 13)

Larry Weed was ahead of his time. As the father of the problem-oriented medical record, he had already changed medical education and practice. But we are only now beginning to act on his answer to what he called "the voltage drop" in medicine—the gap between medical knowledge and medical practice.

The solution for ending much of the discontinuity and isolation of the kind he described is a patient-centered approach, with health providers helping the patient work toward a transformational goal—in other words, joining in an ensemble to help the patient manage her care and her medications at the hospital and at home. The ensemble provides a "home base" for relationships and associations, past, present, and future. It is more than a record of the transactions that have occurred to a given patient; it is a collaborative approach that supports dialogue:

The real value in the sciences, the arts, commerce, and indeed, one's personal and professional lives, comes largely from the process of collaboration. What's more, the quality and quantity of meaningful collaboration often depends upon the tools used to create it. (Schrage 1990, p 27)

Thinking of health as transformations occurring within ensembles allows us to rethink health and how it is supported.[2] The concept is a fertile foundation for innovative thinking about health:

---

[2] For an in-depth discussion by the author, visit www.munnecke.com/papers/D16.doc.

- It introduces new notions of scale to health. World Wide Web technology provides an infrastructure for connectivity and mass personalization unthinkable just a decade ago. Systems can be designed to support massive numbers of participants at a relatively low cost.
- It makes self-organization feasible. People can discover their own resources for managing their own health transformation. Providers can direct patients to ensembles and resources as appropriate.
- Things that can be reduced to bits of information can be replicated and communicated at very low cost. One expert's advice can be captured once and communicated many times.
- It puts a new emphasis on patient self-efficacy. Patients will find themselves more responsible for their own health.
- It introduces new notions of management and control. No entity can be expected to manage 100 million things simultaneously. Rather, the transformations must become self-organizing.

This concept raises other issues. It creates new problems of information overload, access, and ability of healthcare organizations to understand and communicate in the information era. This requires innovation to allow access, train assistants and family members, and publicize the process. It also requires answering difficult questions about transformations and the interactions involved in them:

- How are these transformations infused with appropriate clinical expertise and medical knowledge?
- What are the constraints limiting these transformations? How do we protect against fraud and quackery?
- How do we ensure that transformations occur are as safe as possible?
- How do we configure medical knowledge and research to maximize its benefit to this massive number of transformations?

The communications revolution has created new interactive media. People's interaction in this medium can be both positive and negative. When the "I Love You" virus appeared, it caused $10 billion in damages to computers around the world. This form of information virus is a new phenomenon; only in recent years have computers been connected densely enough to allow such rapid spread. In this new environment, a small initial condition can cascade to become a massive global phenomenon—witness the changes brought about by the World Wide Web in just 10 years. Today, our healthcare system is poised for dramatic changes by these forces. Whether it "tips" for the better or worse is a critical issue facing society. If it does tip in a positive direction, the assumptions underlying our health system will flip from transactional to transformational, as shown in Table 1.2.

Whereas the enterprise sees patients flowing through it and seeks to provide the best care at lowest cost, people see a multitude of providers flowing past them. They have a longer perspective, extending out as long as their lives. They see a maze of health information, sometimes reliable and sometimes sensationalized by the media or advertisers. From this perspective, as Dr. Donald Berwick states, "doctors are guests in the lives of patients" (Wysocki 2002).

This inversion has radical implications regarding information, authority, and responsibility in the healthcare process. Speaking in 1997 about a trend that has continued to accelerate, Dr. Kenneta said,

TABLE 1.2. Comparison of transactional and transformation assumptions.

Transactional assumptions	Transformational assumptions
Health can be purchased.	Health is natural and creative process that is based on common human values shared by all.
Financial incentives drive health care.	Transformational energy drives health.
Health care is a matter of a "system" doing things to a "patient."	Health is found from within, supported by the system.
Health care can be understood as the supply and demand of a scarce commodity.	Health and transformation are unlimited in their scope and potential.
We are dealing with an "industry" in which producers "provide" health and people "consume" it.	We are dealing with transformational ensembles; health can grow without bounds, improving everyone's lives.
Patients are only consumers of health, not also producers.	The fundamental source of health is within individuals. Health is contagious.
Decompositional analysis is a way of understanding the healthcare system.	We have little language to express the generative, transformational power of health
The process of analysis does not change the system being understood.	If we look for problems, we will find and create more problems. If we look for solutions, we will find and create more solutions.
The system is linear.	Health is based on a web of interactions; the more healthy associations available to an individual, the healthier the individual.
Inputs don't interact.	Everyone's health is interconnected; the health improvement of any one of us is the health improvement of all of us.
It is possible to define health meaningfully across a whole population.	Health is as unique as the individual experiencing it.
This definition can be used to drive an aggregation of activities.	Health can be improved by aggregating stories of success, replicating them in the context of other individuals and communities.
It is possible to maximize health through coordination, planning, and management.	Health is a self-propelling, self-generating process which can be triggered by the proper conditions.
The patient's sense of self is not a factor in the efficacy of the intervention.	The role and identity of the self is a major factor in our notion of health.
Greater measurement with greater precision will converge on greater understanding of the phenomenon being studied.	The true benefits of health cannot be measured.
Categorized transactions can be "rolled up."	Health is an associative web of interaction. The value of this web is measured by its richness of interaction, not through arbitrary categorizations.
There is specific scale and "yardstick" with which we can measure health care.	As personal as health is, so are its yardsticks.
We can manage the system by understanding and defining its problems.	We can enhance our health by understanding our strengths and creating new ones.
The placebo effect, mind–body interaction, racial, cultural and ethnic backgrounds, personal belief system, and family factors relating to a person's health process are outside of "normal" medicine.	These effects allow health to be "one thought away." The individual's perceptions are the basis upon which the healthcare system can be based.
The system can look ahead and understand future consequences of today's activities.	The system must be grounded in the fundamental human intrinsics of love, peace, wisdom, truth, balance, power, happiness, and purity. An approach based on these intrinsics will generate and reward those who enhance these intrinsics.
The "law of increasing return" is not evident in health.	The intrinsics of health can be magnified arbitrarily without limits, and in so doing, create additional magnification.

As a result of the availability of information on the Web, patients have ready access to research findings. Indeed, it is not unheard of today, and in fact, it is becoming increasingly common for our patients to know more about a given condition or the latest in treatment options than does the physician or other healthcare provider. Instead of being the source of information, or the fount of all wisdom, clinicians now a have a new job of interpreting information and helping patients make up their mind as to what treatment options or what diagnostic modality they want to utilize. This will, again, require a different mind set as we provide these services in the future . . . as professionals, we have had a monopoly on the information about the diagnostic and treatment options of our patients. Now, all that has changed . . . largely as a result of the Internet." (Kizer 1997)

Is There a Free Lunch?

The inversion Kizer described is a result of the networked economy, which has made many goods and services that used to be the source of market superiority available at low cost—or even "for free." Self-emergent, they do not require conscious creation and specification. This goes against conventional wisdom. Our management structures, accounting mechanisms, and legislative processes are all based on controlling complexity by adding specificity. We have been taught that, as things become more complex, they require more control, categorization, and measurement.

The Encyclopedia Britannica has made its content available on the web: content for free. American auto manufacturers used to think of quality as something to be added on after assembly, until Japanese competitors discovered that they could build quality in at a lower cost: quality for free. Stock brokerage houses offer free information and research, as well as drastically discounted trading services: information for free. The World Wide Web has exploded on the scene: connectivity for free. It is growing explosively with no management committees, interdisciplinary teams, or CEO: *organization for free*. Complexity scientists have discovered that with sufficient diversity and interactivity, systems can organize themselves: *order for free*.

These inversions are revolutionary in each of their industries, yet they contain a common thread:

If goods and services become more valuable as they become more plentiful, and if they become cheaper as they become valuable, then the natural extension of this logic says that the most valuable things of all should be those that are ubiquitous and free.

Ubiquity drives increasing returns in the network economy. The question becomes, What is the most cost-effective way to achieve ubiquity? And the answer is: give things away. Make them free. (Kelly 1998, p 51)

Health is one of the most valuable things an individual, family, or society can possess. Will health and health care follow the logic of network economics? Should they be ubiquitous and "free"?

In living systems, "Astonishingly simple rules, or constraints, suffice to ensure that unexpected and profound dynamical order emerges spontaneously" (Kauffman 1995, p 207). Consider the World Wide Web, whose inventor, Tim Berners-Lee said:

What was often difficult for people to understand about the design [of the web] was that there was nothing else beyond URIs [his name for URLs], HTTP, and HTML. There was no central computer "controlling" the web, no single network on which these protocols worked, not even an organization anywhere that "ran" the Web. The web was not a physical "thing" that existed in a certain "place." It was a "space" in which information could exist. (Berners-Lee 1999, p 36)

The World Wide Web is growing daily in its complexity, with new companies and information sources continuously emerging. This is an example of "order for free." The World Wide Web did not, and could not have, come from an "expensive" managed approach with blue ribbon panels, interdisciplinary groups of experts, and a CEO to make sure that the web operated correctly.

Our notions of correctness and predictability are based on the notion of imposed control. We expect to use expensive processes, management processes, to create policies, procedures, and policing mechanisms to make a system do what we expect. However, self-organizing systems can be found everywhere in nature and in human social structures, and are able to adapt well without these artificial control structures.

In order for these principles of organization to take hold, it is critical that our primary point of focus be on the individual, not the system. This is a major inversion of our perspective within the industry. And it is necessary.

References

Berners-Lee T. 1999. Weaving the web: the original design and ultimate destiny of the World Wide Web. San Francisco: Harper.

Gruman JC, Von Korff M. 1999. Living with chronic illness: when doctors and patients work together. Center for Advancement of Health. Washington, DC.

Ion HW. 1993. Ethical dilemmas in managed care. In: Ott R, Tannes T, Henderson B, editors. Managed care and the cardiac patient. Philadelphia: Hanley & Belfus. p 118.

Kauffman S. 1995. At home in the universe: the search for laws of organization and complexity. New York: Oxford University Press.

Kelly K. 1998. New rules for the new economy. New York: Viking.

Kizer K. 1997. Forms in the fog: information management in the new VA. Speech to the VA Information Technology Conference, 1997 May 19.

Peterson C, Seligman M. 2004. Character strengths and virtues: a handbook and classification. New York: Oxford University Press.

Schrage M. 1990. No more teams: mastering the dynamics of creative collaboration. New York: Doubleday.

Weed LL. 1991. Knowledge coupling: new premises and new tools for medical care and education. New York: Springer-Verlag.

Wysocki B. 2002. Doctor leads crusade to replace office visits as standard procedure. Wall Street Journal 2002 May 20. http://online.wsj.com/article/0..SBI0227211684781360.dim.00.html. Accessed 11/8/2004.

2
A Window of Opportunity

ROBERT M. KOLODNER

Major changes occur in fits and starts, not in a smooth, even flow. Periodically, circumstances, events, and momentum align to provide an opportunity for affecting and influencing such changes. Today, four factors in health informatics are combining to bring us to a window of opportunity, one that offers us a chance to transform health care. The central focus of health and care is poised to shift squarely onto the individual, a move of seismic proportions that can be catalyzed by successfully converging the rapid advances in electronic health records, health information standards, health information exchange capabilities, and personal health records.

To date, despite estimates that only 15% of an individual's health is related to the provision of health care, the vast majority of the activities have been concentrated in the healthcare sector, consuming resources allocated by the economy for health. Moving the focus of health and care from institutions to individuals is a key step in aligning activities and resources to maximize the health status of individuals and communities.

This can change, and for the better, if we act now.

1. To Inpatient and Back: The Evolution of Health Care in the United States

Often described as a cottage industry, much of health care is still delivered in physician offices or small clinics. Yet health care in the United States has changed considerably over the last 40 years. For the first half of the 20th century, the primary emphasis was on the doctor–patient relationship. Other staff were present to support the doctor, and patients came when they were sick or injured to be taken care of by the doctor. Surgery was performed in hospitals, and acute illnesses were usually treated with extended hospital stays. Patients with severe chronic conditions might be cared for at institutions, occasionally little more than warehouses, where they received food and shelter until they recovered or died.

As health care began to have more effective procedures, pharmaceuticals, and technologies for diagnosing and treating medical conditions, the more elaborate treatments were provided in hospitals and medical centers. Medical and surgical specialties sprang up and were formalized as more specific and intense diagnostic and therapeutic procedures were developed.

In the 1960s, the United States government began to cover healthcare costs for the poor and the elderly and to invest more heavily in medical research. Increased revenues fueled a spiraling growth of research, leading to even more high-cost interventions. In order to pay for increasing costs, insurance and federal health programs became more important components of the healthcare industry. As they took on a more prominent role in health care, these entities influenced and eventually altered the traditional doctor–patient relationship. To reduce costs and extend access, nurse practitioners and physician assistants were trained to become less expensive primary providers of health care (under physician supervision), further redefining the provider–patient relationship. At the same time, chronic conditions became more treatable, decreasing the need for chronic care institutions. Unfortunately, the de-institutionalization of care tended to occur more rapidly than the development of community resources to provide adequate alternative care. This was especially true for patients with chronic psychiatric conditions.

Attempts to control the ever-escalating costs led payers to make more decisions regarding eligibility for specific treatments and interventions. These moved the focus further away from the provider–patient relationship and involved the payers to a much greater degree. Not surprisingly, most information systems were developed with the aim of facilitating payment.

Technology continued to advance, offering more pharmaceutical alternatives for treatment and increasing the ability to perform procedures in an ambulatory setting. Combined with restrictions placed by payers and managed care organizations on higher-cost inpatient treatments, the trend toward inpatient care was reversed, often to the benefit of the patient. A rapidly increasing portion of therapeutic and interventional care was provided in clinics and outpatient settings, while more routine care was still provided at the doctor's office or small clinics.

In more recent developments, aided by technology enhancements in computers and telecommunications, telehealth is laying the foundation for further profound changes in health care. While not yet integrated into the routine process of care delivery, telehealth continues to mature. Telehealth offers the chance not just to move from inpatient to ambulatory care settings but to go beyond the walls of the institution and allow care to be provided at home, at work, or wherever a person happens to be.

At the same time, the numbers of the under- and uninsured have grown, creating a multi-tiered population in the United States. Today, a significant portion of the population is without healthcare insurance, including some of those most in need of ongoing preventive care and treatment. Even the plight of the partially insured has been exacerbated by advances in medicine for conditions previously treated using surgery and procedures that required sometimes expensive inpatient episodes of care. New medications have been developed to treat these conditions much more effectively, extending life and turning debilitating and sometimes fatal conditions into controlled and manageable chronic disorders. New problems arose for patients when the cost of these medications was not covered by third-party payers late in life the way hospitalizations were previously. This was particularly true for conditions that tend to have their onset during the years when someone is usually employed and insured, because medication expenses then extend into the retirement years, which are often associated with fixed or more limited incomes and insurance coverage.

2. Beyond Traditional Health Care

While these changes were occurring in health care, there was also an increasing awareness of general health issues across the population. Starting with the Surgeon General's first report on smoking in 1964, the detrimental effects of smoking on health gradually became part of the public dialogue. In like manner, awareness grew of the importance of exercise to health and the risks of heart attack associated with diet and cholesterol and triglyceride levels.

Outside the healthcare industry, a multi-billion dollar industry related to herbs, vitamins, and other food supplements emerged, with the vast majority of these dollars coming from discretionary spending by consumers. Many Americans, shielded by insurance from significant healthcare costs and resistant to paying a higher proportion of those costs, spend large sums of money on health-related items that often have weak or absent evidence of effectiveness in treating the variety of ailments for which they are used. (In contrast, the uninsured often must choose between paying for basic food and shelter or medications proven efficacious in treating or curing their medical conditions.) This trend in discretionary spending suggested that a growing proportion of the population was paying attention to aspects of their health beyond health care itself and was willing to invest considerable time and resources into improving their health.

Still, changes in behavior lag significantly behind changes in awareness. Consider the long delay between the Surgeon General's report and the decrease in the number of Americans smoking cigarettes, or the plethora of diet books and fast food items for dieters flooding the marketplace at a time when an increasing percentage of Americans are overweight and obese. Despite such lags, the broadening interest in health itself among a growing proportion of the population provides another core element for a major change opportunity in health.

3. A Change in Culture

The role that individuals choose in making decisions about their health care is also undergoing a transformation. The traditional model in the not-too-distant past was that patients trusted their doctors completely and did not question any diagnosis or treatment provided. Patients often had a long-standing relationship with their doctor, holding him (or more rarely, her) in high esteem. Patients trusted their doctor to get them well or to provide comfort when their condition could not be treated or cured. They believed their doctor had all the knowledge and judgment necessary to make correct treatment decisions and that their doctor cared about them as a person.

Now the explosive increase of medical knowledge challenges healthcare providers to keep up with the latest findings. By some estimates, half of what a health provider knows will be shown to be incomplete or incorrect every 10 years (Pickering 1956), and medical knowledge has been increasing at an exponential rate (Chassin et al. 1998). A significant medical finding takes, on average, between 15 and 20 years to become routine practice (Balas and Boren 2000). The resulting gaps between medical knowledge and medical practice are described as a crisis in the quality of health care by the Institute of Medicine in its reports, *To Err Is Human* (Kohn et al. 1999) and *Crossing The Quality Chasm* (Committee on Quality Health Care in America 2001).

There have been multiple attempts to change the processes of care and to formalize medical knowledge so that practitioners can have the latest information at their fingertips. Notable efforts include LATCH (Sowell 1978), the National Library of Medicine's Disease databases (Bernstein et al. 1980), and, more recently, Clinical Practice Guidelines (Shiffman et al. 2003) and evidence-based medicine (Victoria et al. 2004). Other efforts involving computers and electronic health records are addressed later in this chapter.

Today, the role of the individual is changing. "Baby boomers" are more likely than earlier generations to question authority. Many tell horror stories about the care they or their relatives and friends received (see Chapter 5 by Garthwaite), despite the fact that the United States spends a higher proportion of its gross national product on health care than any other country in the world (Huber and Orosz 2003). Increasingly, the media have published news articles and aired television exposés about the incompleteness and inaccuracy of medical knowledge, the prevalence of medical errors, and the poor quality of health care.

Recent reports from The Institute of Medicine have raised public awareness to the current circumstances as the first step in moving toward their goal of improved quality and safety of health care. In addition, the Internet has ignited an explosion in the ease of access and scope of medical information over the past decade. As a result, more Americans want a more complete understanding of their illnesses and conditions and a more active role in their healthcare decisions. With an estimated 66% of adult Internet users looking online for health or medical information (Fox and Fallows 2003), it appears that people themselves are taking steps on their own to learn how to improve their health and to become better educated about their medical conditions.

4. Information Age Advances

Four healthcare information management activities have set the stage for a quantum advance in how information can be used to improve the health and care, not only for the individual but for entire communities. Three of these are electronic health records, standards, and information exchange; the fourth is the personal health record.

4.1. Electronic Health Records Systems

For over 30 years, reminders and alerts for healthcare providers using electronic health record (EHR) systems have been shown to improve the quality of care by helping providers consistently apply medical knowledge at the point of care (McDonald 1976; Gardner et al. 1999; Weiner et al. 2003). Today's robust EHR systems make possible safer, high-quality health care by improving legibility, eliminating transcription errors in orders, enabling immediate feedback to providers regarding allergies, drug interactions, and contraindications, and preventing the administration of the wrong medication to patients through human error. In the United States, EHR systems are more widespread in inpatient settings, and multiple efforts are underway to provide the necessary products and incentives for their use in office and small clinic settings where the majority of health care is delivered.

Given the explosion of medical knowledge, the existing manual process for delivering care is inadequate to support practitioners as they struggle to provide high-quality, up-to-date health care. The resulting variation in the quality of care received by individuals across the country is huge and is the source of unnecessary suffering and death, despite the availability of information to prevent them. The continuing medical education required by many states and most medical organizations has not had a significant impact on this knowledge gap.

The evidence is growing, however, that EHR systems provide an effective method for improving the quality of care. As processes are implemented to identify and incorporate medical knowledge into electronic reminders and alerts, EHR systems can narrow the gap between the time new medical knowledge is published and the time it is practiced.

4.2. Health Data and Communications Standards

After almost two decades, there has been meaningful progress in the identification, creation, approval, and use of data and communication standards in health care. It is still unclear whether these standards will be adopted worldwide or whether different continents will adopt different standards, delaying the ability to exchange health information anywhere in the world. In either eventuality, the use of a common set of standards across healthcare entities in a society forms a solid base on which to advance healthcare quality and safety while cutting costs.

Progress in the United States is the result of several different national activities. At the foundation of this progress is the work done by standards development organizations operating in the healthcare arena, which provides the actual standards that can be used. The administrative simplification portion of the Health Insurance Portability and Accountability Act of 1996 (HIPAA) provided a strong impetus to standards. This law set deadlines for the adoption of standards in a number of areas related to healthcare transactions, some national identifiers, and privacy and security, and also required the National Committee on Vital and Health Statistics (NCVHS) to "...study the issues related to the adoption of uniform data standards for patient medical record information and the electronic exchange of such information ..." (Public Law 104–191, 1996). As a result, NCVHS, the statutory public advisory body to the Secretary of Health and Human Services in the area of health data and statistics, submitted recommendations in 2003 and 2004 regarding standards that are ready for adoption and implementation throughout health care in the United States.

In addition, since 2001, 23 federal agencies/departments have partnered to form the Consolidated Health Informatics (CHI) *e*Government initiative. Through this initiative and in consultation with industry through an arrangement with the NCVHS to ensure that its selections were compatible with the private sector, CHI identified and adopted health data and messaging standards for internal use by the federal government. Finally, the National Library of Medicine reached agreement with the College of American Pathologists (CAP) to license English and Spanish language editions of SNOMED Clinical Terms® for use throughout the United States starting in January 2004, complementing similar widespread access to SNOMED Clinical Terms® in the United Kingdom.

Standards facilitate the exchange of information among providers. In the future, a person will be assured that her complete, lifelong health record can be made available to her healthcare providers. Her allergies will always be known, and her response to past treatments will be readily available to inform and guide present and future care. The net result, for her and others like her, will be an unprecedented level of continuity of care.

4.3. Health Information Exchange

Early efforts in exchanging health information have involved a range of health-related organizations and settings. Some were based within communities, such as those in Indianapolis (Overhage et al. 2002) and Santa Barbara (Brailer 2001). Others involved large health provider organizations, for example, the Department of Defense and the Department of Veterans Affairs (Brown et al. 2003). These systems used different architectures and strategies, and taught valuable lessons about moving health information among participants. Recently, more projects were launched amid growing interest in establishing a National Health Information Infrastructure (NHII). Creation of such an infrastructure will make it possible for health organizations and persons to exchange information nationwide.

4.4. Personal Health Records

The newest realm of healthcare information activity involves the electronic personal health record (PHR). In the United States, individuals rarely receive all their care from a single source throughout their lifetime. Most often, a person has multiple providers over time, due to the high degree of mobility in society and, more recently, to the changing landscape of health organizations.

Today, as has been the practice for decades, individuals request and receive paper copies of their records from organizations, hospitals, and practitioners, often so that they can provide copies to their next healthcare provider. As part of disease management, patients may be asked to keep a record of specific measurements such as blood or urine glucose levels, blood pressure, and mood and to bring it to their healthcare provider at the next appointment. Such records provide a broader base of observations to assess the management of chronic illnesses.

New products on the market allow individuals to record their health information electronically. Some devices connect directly to personal computers or the Internet to upload measurements such as blood sugar levels or blood pressure without having to transcribe them. For the most part, these products have achieved only a moderate level of success because there was little or no value added by recording the information in a computer compared to writing it on paper in a table or graph.

In the past few years, the concept of a robust PHR has gone from an idea to early variations being fielded by healthcare information vendors such as Epic's MyChart® and Cerner's IQHealth®, by healthcare organizations such as CareGroup's PatientSite and the Department of Veterans Affairs' My HealtheVet, and in various EHR products. In its more ambitious form, the lifelong PHR is multifaceted and incorporates information directly from EHRs in addition to that entered by the individual who owns the PHR. Its components include a secure personal health database enriched with general health information and services that are personally tailored to each person based on his own unique health data.

The personal health database includes health information entered directly by the person and/or a significant other (with permission), automatically from measurement devices, or by importing from outside sources. These outside sources may include hospital and provider EHRs, commercial pharmacies and laboratories, and even machines in a health club linked to record information at the time of exercise. Each person can then decide, individually, to share as much or as little personal health information with whomever he chooses, for as long or as short a time as he chooses. Recipients of this information may be other healthcare providers, health-related organizations, and family members. The PHR owner can even identify and authorize trusted others to serve as surrogates on his or her behalf.

A robust PHR enables its owner to "instruct" the contents of her personal health database to select specific topics and sections from general health information sources and present her with the most relevant portions on how she can prevent and manage specific diseases—and maintain wellness. The PHR can also be instructed to trigger a variety of reminders, using both computer-based and non–computer-based alerting methods, to help play a more active role in the management of health and care. For example, the list of active medications in the PHR database could generate a call home or to a cell phone for medications reminders. The owner can even indicate how she is alerted initially and what should be done if she does not acknowledge a reminder. Such a system makes more complex reminders possible, including notifications to seek specific follow-up care or preventive interventions, such as immunizations, given the individual's risk factors.

A new service industry may develop to provide individuals with assistance that is custom-tailored to their needs based on the contents of their personal health database. Services could be specific to single organizations or span across a multitude of them. Organization-specific services might include the ability to make a new appointment, check upcoming ones, ask a doctor for a medication renewal, ask a pharmacy for a refill, or communicate securely with a healthcare provider. Cross-organizational services could include identifying potential research projects in a person's area for which he is eligible, registering for disease-specific updates on the latest research findings published on his illness or the illnesses for which he is at high risk, receiving invitations to join specific "conversations" in relevant support groups, and locating groups in his community that offer exercise and diet services or homeopathic treatments along with their documented outcomes data. Potentially, individuals could review the health status of the community in which they live, receiving early alerts of influenza outbreaks and tracking public health statistics, along with recommendations for behavioral or short-term lifestyle changes that might decrease their chances of being affected.

5. The Tipping Point

Health care has been changing, slowly and profoundly. Increasingly, individuals receive intense care outside the inpatient setting, look beyond traditional sources of care in their quest for health, and question their physician rather than assume that "doctor knows best". In addition to these changes in settings, services, and culture, health care has experienced changes brought about by technology. While changes in medical technology have been stunning, advances in information technology can produce equal or greater change by making possible the ability to access, store, and share information that is both meaningful and useful.

Together, this myriad of changes sets the stage for a fundamental shift in health care to center on the person and that person's health, not on the hospital, or the physician, or the disease. But this unique opportunity to establish interrelated information technologies that are exceptionally configured to support and promote person-centered care is limited. The convergence of the four informatics areas—EHRs, standards, information exchange, and PHRs—needs to occur before they become too well formed, independent of each other, and gain widespread use. This window of opportunity will last for only a relatively short period of time. Some offer the example of Central Park, built at a time when New York City was prospering and expanding. It could never be built now, they say: land costs and ownership would make it too expensive and politically impracticable. Clearly, the complexities of health and care far exceed those involved in the development of New York City.

Change is a constant, but the forms it takes and the opportunity to direct it are variable. Today we are approaching a time when monumental change can occur, when one small push will tilt the balance. In short, we are at the tipping point. Once the healthcare system has "tipped," the moment will be gone.

The challenge we face is not primarily one of technology, but rather of agreeing upon the simple rules of governance that will foster extensive and growing collaboration. Health care is too diverse, with too many players, to be controlled by any one of them, yet every one of them must play a part. This necessitates a fundamental shift among the individuals and institutions that contribute to the health and care of individuals and communities. The traditional healthcare structure, while contributing to only a small portion of the health of an individual, now accounts for over 15% of the United States economy. As the pressures of the healthcare marketplace have intensified, the industry has become increasingly competitive, and its members will no doubt continue to compete for market share.

Yet competition can be simultaneously present with collaboration. Witness the development of VISA, which brought together the banking industry to collaborate on a mechanism to help with consumer credit challenges they were facing in the late 1960s. Once they began to work together, these competitors began to explore and implement the technological solutions that fostered their mutual success. The net result is a company that no one bank owns, yet all can join as equal partners. The banks cooperate together, govern together worldwide, and exchange currency over a network that functions as a shared utility, while simultaneously competing vigorously with one another for consumers and retailers from whom they each gain profits.

How successful has this governance model been? Its success can be measured in financial terms. In a week, VISA processes more money than the Federal Reserve does in a year; in a year, VISA processes over US$1.3 trillion, at less than $0.01 per transaction. Using this governance model, VISA has become the largest financial institution in the world.

The history of the healthcare industry in the United States is one of shifting balances with one component or another gaining the upper hand, but these shifts have often not been in the best interest of the individual and the community. The healthcare domain—including, among others, providers, payers, regulators, vendors, and most importantly, consumers—could benefit greatly if these stakeholders could establish a method for collaborating as equal participants. The associated advances in health, medical, and information knowledge and technologies would soar as a byproduct of such a collaborative governance mechanism. Simultaneously, the competition among participants would steadily improve the health and care of individuals and communities in a manner that would drive up quality and safety while driving down cost.

We stand at an exciting moment in the history of health and care where a relatively modest advancement in technologies and in governance can have profound, lasting, positive effects far into the future. The creation in May 2004 of the post of National Health Information Technology Coordinator, and the appointment of David J. Brailer, MD, PhD, holds tremendous promise. We cannot let this moment pass, or let a single sector of the healthcare domain take it for its own. The challenge we face is clear and compelling: To seize the moment and to use it to benefit us all.

References

Balas EA, Boren SA. 2000. Managing clinical knowledge for health care improvement. In: Yearbook of medical informatics 2000: patient-centered systems. Stuttgart: Schattauer. p 65–70.

Bernstein LM, Siegel ER, Goldstein CM. 1980. The hepatitis knowledge base: a prototype information transfer system. Ann Intern Med 93(1 Pt 2):169–181.

Brailer DJ. 2001. Connection tops collection. Peer-to-peer technology lets caregivers access necessary data, upon request, without using a repository. Health Manag Technol 22(8):28–29.

Brown SH, Lincoln MJ, Groen P, Kolodner RM. 2003. VistA: the U.S. Department of Veterans Affairs national scale hospital information system. Int J Med Inf 69(2–3):135–156.

Chassin MR, Galvin RW, and the National Roundtable on Health Care Quality. 1998. The urgent need to improve health care quality. JAMA 280(11):1000–1005.

Committee on Quality Health Care in America, Institute of Medicine. 2001. Crossing the quality chasm: a new health system for the 21st century. Washington, DC: National Academy Press.

Fox S, Fallows D. 2003. Internet health resources. Washington, DC: Pew Internet and American Life Project. Available at www.pewinternet.org/PPF/r/a5/report_display.asp. Accessed 11/11/2004.

Gardner RM, Pryor TA, Warner HR. 1999. The HELP hospital information system: update 1998. Int J Med Inf 54(3):169–182.

Huber M, Orosz E. 2003. Health expenditure trends in OECD countries, 1990–2001. Health Care Financ Rev 25(1):1–22.

Kohn LT, Corrigan JM, Donaldson MS. 1999. To err is human: building a safer health system. Washington, DC: National Academy Press.

McDonald CJ. 1976. Protocol-based computer reminders, the quality of care and the non-perfectability of man. N Engl J Med 295(24):1351–1355.

Overhage JM, Dexter PR, Perkins SM, Cordell WH, McGoff J, McGrath R, McDonald CJ. 2002. A randomized, controlled trial of clinical information shared from another institution. Ann Emerg Med 39(1):14–23.

Pickering GW. 1956. The purpose of medical education. Br Med J 21(4985):113–116.

Public Law 104–191. H.R. 3103 21 Aug 1996. Stat. 110.1936, Title XI, section 263, 5(B), p 98.

Shiffman RN, Shekelle P, Overhage JM, Slutsky J, Grimshaw J, Deshpande AM. 2003. Standardized reporting of clinical practice guidelines: a proposal from the Conference on Guideline Standardization. Ann Intern Med 139(6):493–498.

Sowell SL. 1978. LATCH at the Washington Hospital Center, 1967–1975. Bull Med Libr Assoc 66(2):218–222.

Victora CG, Habicht JP, Bryce J. 2004. Evidence-based public health: moving beyond randomized trials. Am J Public Health 94(3):400–405.

Weiner M, Callahan CM, Tierney WM, Overhage JM, Mamlin B, Dexter PR, McDonald CJ. 2003. Using information technology to improve the health care of older adults. Ann Intern Med 39(5 Pt 2):430–436.

3
Health*e*People: Person-Centered, Outcomes-Driven, Virtual Health Systems

GARY A. CHRISTOPHERSON

Health*e*People is our vision of better health for all—and a collaborative strategy to transform to person-centered, outcomes-driven health systems. This strategy is built to realize three goals. Our first goal is to improve and achieve a high state of health. This involves more than medical interventions or traditional healthcare services; it requires a full range of resources from across the community and beyond. Second, its focus is on people—consumers, patients, enrollees, and members. They are the center of the health universe and must be treated as such, forming strong partnerships between individual patients and their healthcare providers. Third, creating this new healthcare universe requires what we call the enabling "*e*", the electronic capabilities provided by

- adopting national health information standards;
- making available personal health record (PHR) systems;
- supporting health information exchange (IE) when authorized and appropriate;
- greatly increasing the affordability, availability, and interoperability of high-performance, standards-based electronic health record (EHR) systems.

We are already implementing the Health*e*People strategy to improve the health of 26 million United States veterans served by the Veterans Health Administration (VA). Our successes there have led us to a vision that is much grander in scale—a vision of a person-centered virtual health system that better serves the health needs of Americans.

Succeeding with Health*e*People across potentially 100% of clinics, hospitals, nursing homes, community-based care centers, and integrated health systems will transform health care in the United States. In essence, it will electrify one seventh of the United States economy—about $1.8 trillion in 2004. This transformation will change the healthcare landscape as surely as the Rural Electrification Act of 1936 changed the national economy when it brought electrical power to farms and small towns across the country, improving the quality of life and increasing the productivity of rural America.

The enabling "*e*" and the electronic capabilities it provides are critical to the creation of virtual systems and their components—standards, EHRs, PHRs, and IE. Such virtual health systems are valuable beyond just national use. They are valuable for communities. They are valuable for linking together primary care physicians, subspecialty physicians, and hospitals. And they are valuable for individuals committed to self care.

While some may question the feasibility of achieving a virtual health system nationwide, we believe that the United States has reached the "tipping point" in the creation of this system. For this reason, we recommend strategies for achieving a paperless, person-centered, outcomes-driven, virtual health system by the year 2010.

1. Transforming to Person-Centered Health Systems

A virtual health system offers the best means to optimize health care and maximize people's health and ability. For 26 million veterans and their providers in the VA, much of this future is close at hand. Going beyond the VA and reaching essentially all persons and their providers will likely require much of the rest of this decade.

It is well worth the effort. Person-centered health systems are different. They address health differently, they organize differently, they operate differently, they use information differently, they use their scarce resources differently, and they function best when enabled by high-performance health information systems. To illustrate, we offer several vignettes within and across care settings.

1.1. Coordinating Care

As part of the clinical team, a care coordinator is responsible for a large number of patients, ranging from the well to the severely chronically ill. He uses the "electronic dashboard" on his computer screen to access the records of the patients he serves and to display the full array of health services available to patients registered at the clinic. On a day-to-day basis, he uses the service array to optimize scarce resources in producing target health outcomes. Via his electronic dashboard, he orchestrates a virtual health service delivery system that blends clinic-based and community-based services to improve the health of the patients he serves.

1.2. Managing Appointments

A patient makes and checks appointments any place and any time using the Internet and/or telephone. Using real-time scheduling, his primary care team matches their appointment schedule and his needed and/or desired visit. The scheduling system allows advanced access appointment making and provides decision support that optimizes appointments for patient and staff alike. To conserve patient time and scarce clinic resources, the system times the appointment to meet multiple healthcare needs during a single visit.

1.3. Optimizing Clinic Visits

Before his scheduled clinic visit, a patient updates his health and demographic information from home or workplace using phone or computer. When he enters the clinic building, he is electronically recognized and the clinic is notified of his arrival. His electronic record is uploaded, staff move into position, and ancillary services are prepared. He goes directly to an available exam room or ancillary service to start care. Subsequent parts of the visit are optimized based on his needs, his progression through the visit, and the availability of resources. All information, including specialty consultations necessary for diagnosis and treatment (provided via telehealth if needed), is obtained during the visit. Treatment is initiated prior to departure and prescriptions are waiting at the end of his visit or are already scheduled for quick delivery to his home or workplace. He electronically indicates satisfaction with his visit before his departure; if there is a problem, service recovery occurs before he leaves. Following the visit, the patient reports on his progress with the therapeutic interventions timed to clinician-initiated guidelines. Except when a clinic visit is necessary, he receives ambulatory care and eHealth services (telephone- or internet-based) in his home or workplace.

1.4. Optimizing Clinical Care

Entering one of the exam rooms to which she has access, a clinic physician carries a portable, wireless electronic device that moves with her throughout the clinic day after a single sign-on. All information on the patient from any authorized source is available real-time in computable form using standardized data. During the exam, all vital signs are automatically entered into the patient's health record by the respective medical device. A tablet computer is used for data entry and patient education. If a specialty consultation is needed, the physician can access a sub-specialist locally or in other parts of the nation. She orders ancillary services electronically, and they respond directly, minimizing patient time and inconvenience and optimizing clinic resources. In the future, the physician will use speech recognition, a wearable computer, and a head-mounted monitor to record and display information and allow hands-free handling of data input/output.

1.5. Reducing Health Risks

A health plan member uses her personal health record to complete a health risk assessment online or at her closest health facility. She then shares the information with her primary care team, works with them to set up a risk factor management strategy, feeds her risk reduction progress to her primary care provider, and receives reinforcement via electronic messaging. When behavior change is needed, she uses her health plan's electronic risk factor reduction program and/or enrolls in phone or online peer-to-peer support groups assisted by her plan's health staff. This information is recorded in her PHR and in her health plan's EHR.

1.6. Sharing Information

A health plan member has a primary care physician, receives chronic disease care from a sub-specialist, uses a teaching hospital for any needed inpatient care, worries about needing emergency care while on a hiking vacation, and accesses health information and services via the Internet. Via a nationwide health information exchange system and in real time, she uses the Internet to make appointments and get trusted information, to share her health record with her primary and subspecialty care physicians and with her hospital when hospitalized, to retrieve her health record for use by the emergency physician treating her hiking injury. Healthcare providers all have high functioning electronic health records that support care in those care sites and can send, receive, and use information shared with her and with other providers. Any information sharing is subject to privacy requirements, standards, encryption, authorization, and authentication.

1.7. Supporting a Person and Involving Family and Friends

A chronically ill veteran gives his family and friends access to his PHR, so they can help him make appointments, refill pharmacy prescriptions, and get trustworthy information. In short, they use his PHR as a family support tool, becoming informal members of his primary healthcare team, effectively extending the team's resources. On occasion, his family and friends engage in internet dialogues with his health advisors, or form peer-to-peer and family support groups. They rely on the PHR as a source for information on the facilities he uses and on his benefits, including registration and application requirements. All these efforts contribute to better person-centered care.

As these vignettes illustrate, virtual health systems, building on existing provider health systems, empower individuals to participate in improving their health and to partner with all their healthcare providers.

2. Optimizing Health Systems and Maximizing Health and Ability

Maximizing the health and ability of people—the insured, underinsured, and uninsured as well as America's veterans—requires that our health systems operate as close to the optimum as possible. At the service, facility, community, and regional levels, our systems must move beyond episodic care. They must coordinate the whole care of the person and the care of populations, whether they are defined by disease, functional status, risk status, or health plan enrollment. Care needs to be coordinated and delivered not just to the acutely or chronically ill, but also to those who are well. When there are care episodes, all evidence-based care needs to be brought to bear and delivered in an optimal manner. Few, if any, health systems today operate even close to optimally.

Health systems need to work within their walls and in collaboration with other health systems and academic institutions to determine best practices based on outcomes and to apply them rigorously. But this will not be enough. Current best practices may not be the best that can be done; we may need to design more "ideal" systems, systems that operate optimally to maximize health and ability at all levels—episode, person, and population. Further, health and information technology must be applied effectively to support these best practices and ideal systems.

Coordination of care using best practices and ideal health systems enabled by high-performance health and information technology will move us toward more optimized health systems producing substantially better health outcomes, as shown in Figure 3.1.

Even this will not be enough. Maximizing health requires going beyond the limitations of what any healthcare system can do by itself. The key is the person. For this effort to succeed, the person is and must be treated as the center of the health universe. To the extent possible, that person should engage in healthy behaviors and conduct self care using reliable information and proven health supplies, medications, and other health aids. In addition, the person should exercise choice in selecting health providers and partner with them as an active participant in the healthcare process.

Optimal care for the person and for populations and communities demands the use of outcomes-based measures for prevention and wellness, and the adoption and ongoing redefinition of best practices. Maximizing health and ability requires more than health information systems, and valuable work is being done to address these medical challenges.

We believe the use of affordable, high-quality, standards-based health information systems can help create virtual health systems, enabling substantial health improvements here in the United States and in other countries around the world. This is the heart of the HealthePeople concept and our focus in this book.

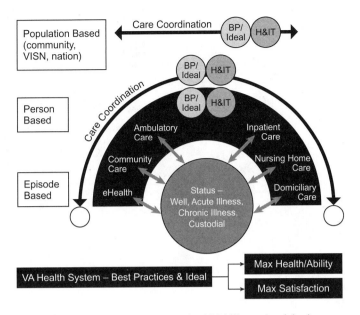

FIGURE 3.1. Maximize veterans' health/ability and satisfaction.

3. Creating a Virtual Health System

The Health*e*People concept places the person firmly at the center of the virtual health system. Supporting that person and serving as the foundation for the system are electronic health record systems. Electronic health records are essential. Without them, personal health record systems contain little of value, information exchange has little of value to share, and standards have limited applicability. Still, EHRs alone are not sufficient to transform health care. It is PHRs that bring the person into a more active role in improving health, and it is information exchange that enables information to flow where it is needed—to the person for personal use, to the emergency room outside the person's provider system, to a person's primary healthcare provider engaged in an outside subspecialty consultation, or to a new provider when a person moves, either short or long term.

For information to be clinically meaningful, there must also be standards to ensure that terminology is the same across providers. Standards are essential to moving health information, as appropriate and authorized, by the person, primary provider, and other providers. Standards also allow the sharing of de-identified information with public health systems, including the Centers for Disease Control and state and local health departments, for disease surveillance.

As shown in Figure 3.2, four components are key to the creation of a virtual health system: electronic health records, personal health records, information exchange, and standards. The Health*e*People strategy builds upon all four and offers models for what these individual components should be and how they should operate.

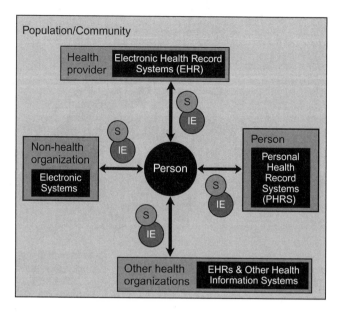

FIGURE 3.2. Virtual health system: EHRs, PHRs, EHR/PHR information exchange (IE), and standards (S).

3.1. *Electronic Health Record Systems*

Electronis health records systems are the foundation for the virtual health system. The other components cannot function effectively without them. Thus, we must implement EHRs in this country's clinics, hospitals, community-based care, and integrated health systems. Our goal is to come as close to 100% as possible by the year 2010. We know this is very, very ambitious. We also know it is possible.

It is possible because we already have functional models defining and setting the standards for an EHR. Such models are being developed by the health community in initiatives involving both private and public organizations. One major effort is being coordinated by the Institute of Medicine (IOM) and the health standards group Health Level Seven (HL7). Participants from the public sector include the VA, the Centers for Medicare and Medicaid Services (CMS), the Agency for Health Research and Quality (AHRQ), and the Assistant Secretary for Planning and Evaluation in the Department of Health and Human Services (HHS). Private sector representatives come from the Health Information Management and Systems Society (HIMSS) and the Robert Wood Johnson Foundation.

Within our vision of HealthePeople, high-performance EHRs collectively support the full range of functions and settings for health care, including public health. The range of functions includes health data storage, clinical tools (clinical interface, clinical reminders, clinical guidelines, access to current medical/health information), and analytical tools (management, research). The range of settings reaches across the full spectrum of care: integrated health systems, community-based care (home and workplace), ambulatory care, inpatient care, nursing home care, primary and specialty care, mental health care, emergency care, laboratory, radiology, pharmacy, and rehabilitation.

Such EHRs exist today at leading institutions in the private sector. In the public sector, the VA systems have a high level of functionality and will offer progressively higher levels over the next several years.

Although the VA EHR is not functionally different from any other high-performance EHR, it stands as a proof of concept. It demonstrates what EHRs can do and how they can work in the varied settings that make up the VA, America's largest integrated health system, ranging from small clinics and nursing homes to large research hospitals. Figure 3.3 depicts a potential model, high-performance health information system, based on the VA HealtheVet/HealthePeople-VistA.

A few private sector software vendors have high-performance EHRs. More could offer such a system as a single suite of applications, either from a single vendor or a number of different vendors. As part of the HealthePeople vision, we strongly encourage vendors to make such highly functional systems available in all these different settings.

3.2. Personal Health Record Systems

Building on the EHR, PHR systems allow individuals to manage their own health care. Within the HealthePeople vision, PHRs enable persons to access their own health records and to link those records, if they choose, with records from multiple healthcare providers. Individuals are able to record and share their personal health information, such as weight, blood pressure, glucose levels, pain, and tobacco and alcohol use. The PHR gives people access to trusted information and helps them link up with support groups and other resources to help maintain and improve their health. Personal health

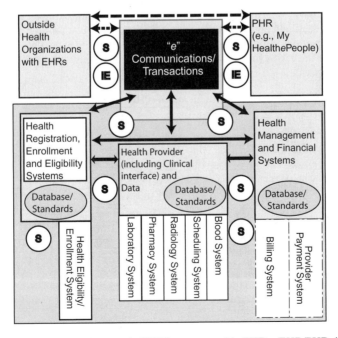

FIGURE 3.3. Electronic health record (EHR) systems with PHRs, EHR/PHR information exchange, and standards.

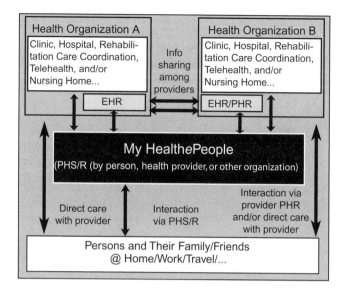

FIGURE 3.4. My Health*e*People: person-centered view.

records also assist individuals with health-related tasks such as making appointments, filling prescriptions, and making co-payments. These capabilities are provided via secure use of the Internet and other appropriate technologies.

This concept works, and there are models for a PHR developed and tested in the VA. The first working model, My Health*e*Vet, had many of the functions a strong PHR should have; this PHR was used by tens of thousands of veterans. The next version, My Health*e*People, shown in Figure 3.4, offers a model of how a PHR system could function and interoperate with EHRs using information exchange and standards. The VA is continuing to build upon their experience to refine the functions that PHRs provide to individuals; these services are listed in Table 3.1.

TABLE 3.1. Personal health record (PHR) capabilities.

Health record
   Access to health records
   Share health records
   Self-entered health record
Services
   Check/fill prescriptions
   Check/confirm/make appointments
   Check/pay co-payments
   Participate in support groups
   Health decision support
   Health self-assessment
   Risk reduction programs
   Message with health provider
   Diagnostic/therapeutic tools
   Reminders
   "Check in"
   Safety services/tools
   Links to other health sites
Information
   Trusted information

Despite these promising advances, PHRs remain relatively immature at this time. There must be a substantial amount of public–private sector collaboration and development to make a good PHR system available to everyone who wants one.

3.3. Health Information Exchange

Health information exchange (IE) is the capability and the associated system or systems to securely and effectively exchange information among the person, the primary health provider, other health providers, and other health organizations (public health, payers, quality improvement) when appropriate and authorized. In the health sector today, exchanges tend to be limited and bilateral in nature, for example, between two health providers, between a person and his/her primary health provider, between a health provider and a payer, between a health provider and a public health agency, and so on. These differ markedly from multilateral exchanges, as Figures 3.5 illustrates.

There are efforts trying multilateral approaches at the community level and a couple of efforts are experimenting on a larger scale. Achieving the health information

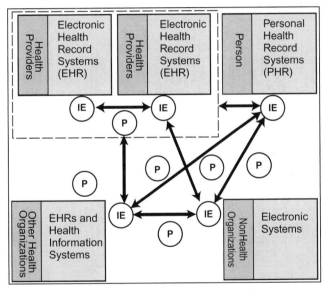

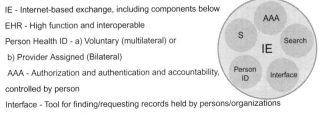

P - Person

IE - Internet-based exchange, including components below

EHR - High function and interoperable

Person Health ID - a) Voluntary (multilateral) or

 b) Provider Assigned (Bilateral)

AAA - Authorization and authentication and accountability, controlled by person

Interface - Tool for finding/requesting records held by persons/organizations

S - Standards, e.g., HL7

FIGURE 3.5. EHR/PHR information exchange (IE).

exchange capability essential to greatly improve health requires a quantum leap. Efforts to implement multilateral approaches at community and regional level are helpful, but there must be a much greater speed of development and rate of adoption.

A complementary approach is enable EHR and PHR health information exchange similar to the Internet or the banking system, each of which offer working models that incorporate a wide range of users and functions. Such a system might:

- provide multilateral capability across persons, providers, and other health organizations;
- utilize HL7 messaging as the standard for moving messages among the users;
- employ authorization and authentication systems to ensure that only authorized persons/providers exchange authorized information;
- provide EHRs on both ends of an exchange that have the functionality to share (send and receive/use) information;
- use encryption to secure the exchange system if we are to obtain and sustain the trust of users;
- provide an identifier (possibly a voluntary ID similar to what we do with phone numbers and e-mail addresses) so that we can ensure that we have the right person's health information to be shared;
- leverage the infrastructure provided by the Internet and its ability to move information securely and effectively.

3.4. Standards

After decades of work, standards are being adopted by the federal government and by many other public and private sector organizations. Table 3.2 provides a current list of standards that have been approved by the federal initiative known as Consolidated Health Informatics (CHI).

While there are many areas for standards, we focus on five areas: health data, health information exchange, security, EHRs, and PHRs.

Health data standards, in terms of a common language and common terminology, are critical across health providers and within large health systems. They include

TABLE 3.2. Consolidated Health Informatics (CHI) standards.

Twenty standards adopted by CHI through 2004
- Health Level 7® (HL7®) messaging
- National Council on Prescription Drug Programs (NCDCP)
- The Institute of Electrical and Electronics Engineers 1073 (IEEE1073)
- Digital Imaging Communications in Medicine® (DICOM®)
- Laboratory Logical Observation Identifier name Codes® (LOINC®)
- Health Level 7® (HL7®) vocabulary standards for demographic information, units of measure, immunizations, and clinical encounters, and HL7®'s Clinical Document Architecture standard for text based reports. (Five standards)
- The College of American Pathologists Systematized Nomenclature of Medicine Clinical Terms® (SNOMED CT®). (Five standards)
- Laboratory Logical Observation Identifier Name Codes® (LOINC®) to standardize laboratory test orders and drug label section headers.
- The Health Insurance Portability and Accountability Act (HIPAA) transactions and code sets
- Federal medication terminologies, including the Food and Drug Administration's, the National Library of Medicine's RxNORM, and the Veterans Administration's National Drug File Reference Terminology (NDF-RT)
- The Human Gene Nomenclature (HUGN)
- The Environmental Protection Agency's Substance Registry System for non-medicinal chemicals of importance to health care

LOINC for laboratory, SNOMED for a broad range of clinical terminology, and NCPDP Script for drugs. In the future, we will move beyond terminology to have robust reference models in key areas such as drugs. Data standards support a wide range of decision support needs such as drug–drug and drug–allergy interactions, clinical reminders, and visual displays of laboratory results and vital signs. Such standards help ensure that information from multiple sources is clinically meaningful and comparable.

With respect to health communications, standards help ensure that information can be moved between health providers (e.g., HL7) and between medical equipment and EHRs (e.g., DICOM for imaging and IEEE 1073 for medical devices). As a potential solution for health information exchange is developed, additional standards will likely be needed.

Functional models and standards for EHRs are needed to guide vendors, providers, and payers to what functionality is needed, for what setting, and when. The key is to determine what functions (e.g., ordering, a longitudinal record, a clinical interface, decision support, interoperability with other EHRs) are needed for different care settings (clinics, hospitals, nursing homes, care in the community, public health, and integrated health systems) and when (what should be core to a good EHR in the near term; what should be the future progression of this core in the longer term; what should be the desired functions in an "ideal" EHR for the long term). These standards focus on what functions a good EHR should have and not on how those functions are delivered by a particular vendor.

Much of the work now being done on EHRs should help guide the development of standards and models for PHRs, even though the two types of records are substantially different. Standards for both records are critical to the high levels of functionality and interoperability a virtual health system requires.

4. The Challenge

Achieving positive, large-scale change is not simple or easy, but it can and must be done. Success requires recognizing complexities of the environment in which change must occur and of the key players who can bring about quantum-level change.

Until about 2001, relatively little had been achieved nationally or internationally to accomplish the changes demanded by modern health practice, healthcare providers on the front line, and individuals wanting and needing to improve their health. That is not to say that a lot of good work had not been done. The contrary is the case: Much of what is being achieved today and will be accomplished in the days ahead is heavily dependent on the pioneering work of the past two decades.

In the United States and around the world, there are hundreds, perhaps thousands, of health information systems and health information standards. The lack of standardization for health data and for communicating health records makes it extremely difficult to share health information. As Figure 3.6 illustrates, the result is a very complex environment, where healthcare organizations often recreate and reinvent health information systems at great expense. This situation persists despite the fact that the delivery of health care is very similar, regardless of the particular settings, across healthcare organizations, and that data and communications needs are also very similar.

The demands on healthcare providers to have current and complete information in real time are intensifying. Healthcare providers must deal with an ever-growing, ever-changing body of medical knowledge. Patient demands and knowledge are increasing

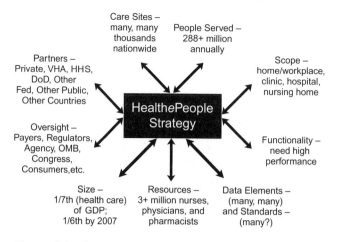

FIGURE 3.6. Dimensions of complexity for HealthePeople strategy.

as availability and sources (e.g., the Internet) of information increase. People move from place to place and have emergency care needs as they travel. Care is being provided in a wide range of settings—hospitals, clinics, nursing homes, and in the community (e.g., home, workplace). And all this is occurring amid rising expectations for healthcare satisfaction, efficiency, quality, and outcomes.

The Institute of Medicine has called for paperless health information systems by the year 2010 [Institute of Medicine (IOM) 2002]. Many organizations, including the VA, are working to reach that goal, as shown in Figure 3.7. To achieve the widespread adoption of the paperless, high-performance electronic health records and personal health records, we must have all the necessary components in place. Health data and communications standards must be adopted. Personal health record systems, electronic health record systems, and health information exchange must be available, affordable, standards-based, and high quality.

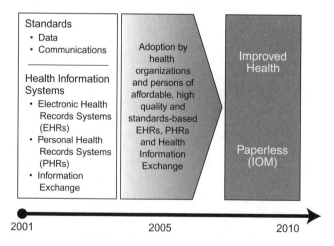

FIGURE 3.7. Improve health and become paperless system.

Until recently, the efforts of public and private sector healthcare organizations were disparate in nature, and the lack of standards made systems expensive to create and recreate. This situation is changing. New opportunities are emerging and being aggressively pursued. Today, key organizations in both sectors are developing or adopting the next generation of health information systems that are very similar. Both sectors have common needs and face common challenges; both have limited resources with which to execute their individual strategies.

4.1. Data Standardization: A Case in Point

In the private sector, healthcare organizations like Kaiser Permanente are working to migrate from multiple versions of clinical and demographic data to one national standard. In the public sector, the Department of Defense (DoD) is migrating its 104 variations of clinical data to one standard to support its Composite Health Care System (CHCS II). The Indian Health Service (IHS) has to migrate over 200 variations of clinical and demographic data to one standard. To support its Health*e*Vet strategy and its health data repository, the VA is migrating between 150 and 170 variations of clinical and demographic data to one standard. Other health organizations are making similar moves. Across the healthcare sector, these efforts pose tremendous challenges and consume scarce resources. Clearly, it would be preferable to move to one national or international set of data and communications standards and to deploy high-performance health information systems.

5. The Tipping Point

Our country is at a tipping point, an opportune moment in history. Together, private and public sector health organizations can help change how health information and related systems support health delivery. Such change can transform health care in both the private and public sectors.

An immediate opportunity arises from the needs of payers to ensure that they are good stewards on behalf of the ultimate payers—taxpayers, employers/employees, and individuals. The largest of the major payers, the Centers for Medicare and Medicaid Services (CMS), has identified a great need for more information on health providers for their beneficiaries and on the quality and outcomes CMS is receiving for payments made. In partnership with VA and AHRQ, CMS is strongly encouraging the widespread adoption of health information standards, personal health records, information exchange, and electronic health records—the four components that make up Health*e*People.

5.1. Collaborative Efforts

Recognizing that they share common goals, many health organizations are supporting collaborations with other entities in the public and private sectors, including foundations, professional organizations, commercial technology companies, and state and local agencies. For example, there are the eHealth Initiative (eHI) and the Electronic Health Record Collaborative. In addition, there are the following:

Connecting for Health. Convened by the Markle Foundation, a New York–based philanthropy, Connecting for Health brought together over 100 public and private organizations representing every part of the healthcare system to advance standards, privacy and security practices, and personal health records.

Public–Private Electronic Health Record Initiative. Federal agencies, including the VA, CMS, and AHRQ, have joined with the American Academy of Family Physicians to campaign for the adoption of electronic health records, personal health records, and health information standards. The availability of affordable, standards-based, high-quality EHRs in the private sector, including VA's HealthePeople-VistA, will substantially increase their use in clinics, hospitals, nursing homes, community-based care, and integrated health systems. The widespread adoption of standards will enable the sharing health information, when authorized and appropriate. The availability of PHRs gives people and their health providers more capabilities to provide health support any place and any time.

Consolidated Health Informatics (CHI). This collaborative is a joint effort of federal agencies, including VA, DoD, and HHS (including CMS and FDA). Through its partnership with the National Committee for Vital and Health Statistics and its members, CHI has links to standards development organizations and health providers like Kaiser-Permanente. The initiative builds on the decisions of the VA and DoD, first, to move a single standard individually and, second, to go to a single standard for both. Thus, CHI is defining a common set of data and communications standards to be used across all federal health agencies, as shown in Table 3.2. The first five standards were jointly adopted in 2002 and an additional fifteen standards were jointly adopted in 2004. These may prove to be the tipping point in the adoption of health data and communications standards across public and private health organizations nationally and internationally.

6. HealthePeople

HealthePeople is a collaborative strategy for helping accomplish this critical change. As its name declares, HealthePeople focuses on health, not just medicine. It focuses on people, including beneficiaries, members, and patients. And it relies heavily on electronic means—the "*e*"—as a key enabler. Public and private sector organizations have been participating with this effort since 2001 and together are helping adopt health information standards and develop and deploy affordable, high-performance health information systems.

Among HealthePeople's goals are to do the following:

- adopt national and international health information standards for health information systems;
- make public and private sector high-performance health information systems, including EHRs, more affordable, available, standards-based, and interoperable—as appropriate, provide health information system software (e.g., HealthePeople-VistA) to public organizations and to private sector organizations that serve the poor and near poor at as close to no cost as is possible;
- make PHRs available to people and their healthcare providers that enable people to access and share their health records, access trusted health information and access key supportive services, including prescription drugs and appointments;
- help develop a national solution to enable the appropriate and authorized health information exchange.

Part of the HealthePeople strategy is to advance on multiple fronts and collaborate with different federal partners. In one such effort, the VA is working jointly with the Department of Defense to:

- improve sharing of health information;
- adopt common standards for architecture, data, communications, security, technology, and software;
- seek joint procurements and/or build applications, where appropriate;
- seek opportunities for sharing existing systems and technology;
- explore convergence of VA and DoD health information applications consistent with mission requirements;
- develop interoperable health records and data repositories.

In a second effort, the VA is building on its long-term partnership with the IHS0. Converging on the same EHR (while still addressing unique IHS needs) and adopting common standards for data and communications will enable IHS to use current and future versions of the VA's HealthePeople-VistA.

7. HealthePeople by 2010

7.1. The Strategy

In 2001, those of us working on HealthePeople and like efforts arrived at consensus as to the conditions necessary to a paperless, virtual health system, but we were still unclear what steps we needed to take to make it happen. Thanks to initiatives like those discussed in this chapter, an overall approach has emerged. From where we now stand, there is a fairly clear though challenging path to achieving this goal. HealthePeople and related efforts are bringing about needed changes. The progress being made now and the progress projected for the next five years make it possible to arrive at this goal by 2010, as laid out in Figure 3.8. But we cannot and do not underestimate the work that lies ahead. Electrifying one seventh of the national economy is a huge but doable undertaking.

The overall strategy requires that data and communications standards and high-performance health information systems be in place. In 2003, the HealthePeople initiative focused on joint standards efforts, targeting the adoption of key standards by the federal sector no later than the end of 2004 and nationally shortly thereafter. The focus now is to make high-performance systems, like VA's current VistA and future HealthePeople-VistA system, fully operational by 2005. Along with several existing private sector EHRs, these VA systems demonstrate feasibility, deliver value, and offer proof of concept. According to the IOM, "VHA's integrated health information system, including its framework for using performance measures to improve quality, is considered one of the best in the nation" (IOM 2002).

To meet the ever-increasing demands of clinicians, payers, and regulators, even high-performance systems need more enhancements. The overall strategy requires quickly moving PHRs from their current immature state, making several viable and available by the end of 2005. To make these components work together and move information, the approach also requires the creation of a health information exchange at the national level by the end of 2005.

Meeting these targets will rely upon much of the work already done or underway in the public and private sectors. By making affordable standards-based, high-

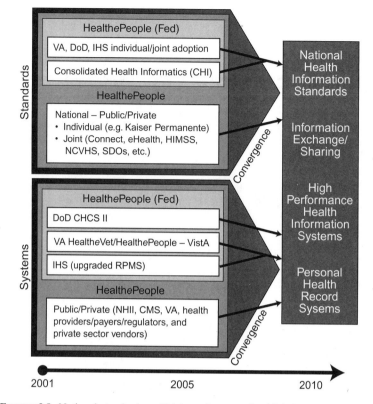

FIGURE 3.8. National standards and high-performance health information systems.

performance EHRs and PHRs available, efforts like Connecting for Health and HealthePeople are helping "early adopting" health organizations put highly effective health information systems into place, here in the United States and beyond. Other collaborative efforts are advancing standards for communication of health records and for health data within health records. Once fully implemented, such standards will enable people and their healthcare providers and healthcare payers and regulators to secure and, when appropriate, share data.

7.2. Actions to Take

Achieving a virtual health system in the United States by the year 2010 requires that the components essential to HealthePeople are in place. We must support efforts underway in the private sector and continuing initiatives ongoing in the VA, and we must do more. We must act now.

These are the actions we must take in critical areas:

7.2.1. Electronic Patient Records

• Strongly encourage private sector vendors to make affordable, high-quality, standards-based EHRs available.

- Strongly encourage provider-based efforts like American Academy of Family Physicians (AAFP).
- Provide financial incentives to healthcare providers through differential payments and/or grants.
- Continue to improve and make available HealthePeople-VistA.

7.2.2. Personal Health Records

- Strongly encourage the public and private sectors to work together to develop PHRs and make them available to individuals.
- Encourage primary healthcare providers to offer PHRs that individuals can operate on their home computers.
- Support the development of PHRs by independent "vaulting" services or as a kind of "personal banking."
- Foster a public/private initiative to make PHRs available to Americans with limited or no ability to pay.

7.2.3. Health Information Exchange

- Strongly encourage the public and private sectors to work together to develop and make available a national "exchange" solution.
- Urge the development of a multilateral national exchange system to link the individual at the center of care with multiple providers and health organizations.
- Encourage health providers to establish bilateral systems with colleagues with whom they have close, day-to-day working relationships.
- Strongly encourage public/private adoption of an "identifier," most likely voluntary, to be used as telephone numbers or e-mail addresses are now.
- Build upon the experience of the banking community and the growing adoption of Health Level Seven (HL7) messaging.

7.2.4. Standards

- Strongly encourage public/private development and adoption of national standards.
- Assign the federal Consolidated Health Informatics (CHI) initiative a leadership role nationally and internationally.

7.2.5. Security

- Utilize established authorization and authentication systems to ensure only appropriately designated individuals exchange information.
- Take advantage of the infrastructure provided by the Internet and the ability it gives us to securely move information across it.

8. Moving Toward 2010

Together, these actions will help us move toward virtual systems that provide

- more affordable, more available, higher performance electronic heath record systems and greater interoperability among such systems;
- more available personal health record systems;
- more adoption of national and international health information standards;

- easier, more secure health information exchange among people, healthcare providers, payers, and regulators when appropriate and authorized.

Beyond these actions, Healt*he*People calls upon us to change how we deliver health care, to go beyond episodic care to care for the whole person and, ultimately, for entire populations. It requires that we develop and incorporate best practices into ideal health systems, and make the best possible use of technology.

If we do all these things, and do them well, we will create a virtual health system that contributes substantially to improving the health of people it serves, beginning with 26 million United States veterans, and from there reaching out across the United States and around the world.

Reference

Institute of Medicine (IOM). 2002. Leadership by example: coordinating government roles in improving healthcare quality. Washington, DC: National Academy Press.

4
The Value of Electronic Health Records

BLACKFORD MIDDLETON

The electronic health record (EHR) has finally come of age (Kohn 2000; Teich 2000; Bates and Gawande 2003). Modern clinical practice requires a clinician to be mindful of best practices, and wary of excess utilization and cost. Yet abundant data show that gaps exist between best evidence and practice, wide variations persist in clinical practice patterns, and escalation of healthcare costs continues largely unabated (Haynes 1995; McGlynn et al. 2003). Many studies have shown the impact of electronic health records and clinical decision support tools in leading academic medical centers (Hunt 1998; Teich 1999), but similar effects in other settings are harder to demonstrate.

Physicians are increasingly willing to consider information technology (IT) to support clinical practice, insisting that it fit into their workflow (Teich 1995) or at least be time and revenue neutral or positive. Recently, it appears that financial incentives for physicians attaining quality benchmarks in their patient care, and the possibility of other programs aimed at providing rewards for EHR use or even low interest loans for acquiring EHRs, will reduce the financial hurdles physicians face in adopting IT in practice. This chapter describes what an electronic health record is and should do, examines the evidence suggesting how this technology may impact the cost and quality of care, and discusses of potential futures for the use of the EHR.

1. Defining the Electronic Health Record

As a base for understanding the value of the EHR, a functional definition of the EHR is provided, and common modes of use in practice are examined. The Institute of Medicine recently convened an expert panel to analyze patient safety data standards. As a byproduct of their work, this group produced a special report for the Secretary of the Department of Health and Human Services outlining essential functional standards for the EHR (Tang and the Committee on Data Standards for Patient Safety 2003). The core functionalities recommended for an EHR by this group are listed in Table 4.1. For each of the areas identified, a brief descriptive overview is given.

1.1. Results Management

In general, *results management* refers to the presentation of a laboratory and other data gathered from ancillary services in the clinical environment. In the hospital setting, results are returned from a wide variety of ancillary departments performing labora-

39

TABLE 4.1. Core Functionalities for an Electronic Health Record (EHR) system

Core EHR System Functionalities
Results Management
Health Information and Data
Order Entry/Management
Decision Support
Electronic Communication and Connectivity
Patient Support
Administrative Processes
Reporting & Population Health Management

tory tests, radiological investigations, and other investigations or procedures. In the ambulatory care setting, similar data are returned from internal or external laboratories and ancillary service providers. In either case, results are typically sent to an EHR database through an interface engine.

1.2. Health Information and Data

Results retrieved from external sources are appended to the EHR, which contains patient demographic information. Typically, an EHR will have information about the patient's current medical problems and conditions, current medications, current allergies, and advance directives, as well as electronic documentation from clinical encounters or patient care contacts. The clinical narrative should also be captured and made available within the EHR. This includes all clinicians' notes (physician, nurse, ancillary care providers) which can be captured by a wide variety of means ranging from free text dictation and text templates to fully structured documentation.

1.3. Order Entry/Management

An EHR transitions from becoming a passive storage center for a patient's health information and data to a more active care management tool when the provider begins to use it for order entry. Typically, the first orders written in EHRs in the ambulatory care setting are prescriptions. In the inpatient setting, provider order entry systems allow for writing not only medication orders, but potentially all other therapeutic and diagnostic orders as well. If the order entry capability of the EHR is interfaced to or includes an order communication capability, the system may contain some knowledge of order status so that a provider can determine whether an order has been fulfilled and results returned.

1.4. Decision Support

With use of EHRs for more than data storage alone, the opportunity arises for providing clinical decision support to the healthcare provider. In the simple context of writing an outpatient electronic prescription, providers may receive alerts about potential drug–drug interactions, drug and laboratory interactions, as well as indications of potential interactions between medications and selected laboratory tests, and a patient's symptom profile.

1.5. Electronic Communication and Connectivity

To obtain results from external systems and ancillary departments, EHRs must have connectivity with an interface engine that manages electronic communications and data messaging. At the simplest level, the interface engine routes transactions from one system to another. In this process, data may be transformed from the format of the sending system to the format of the receiving system. This translation allows the data to be integrated into the appropriate data structures of the receiving EHR.

Beyond connectivity for health information exchange, however, certain electronic health records provide for electronic communication among members of the healthcare delivery team, and some facilitate direct communication with the patient or the patient's personal health record (PHR). Typically, these capabilities provide for secure clinical communication and do not interact with the provider's electronic mail system.

1.6. Patient Support

Most EHR systems have facilities for providing care information on health conditions, medications, tests, and procedures for the patient. This patient care information facilitates doctor–patient communication and supports patient education.

1.7. Administrative Processes

In the ambulatory setting, many EHR systems are distinct from the practice management system. In such an environment, the same interface engine described above may facilitate the exchange of clinical information to the practice management system for the purpose of creating the patient's bill. In the hospital environment, clinical information management systems are usually distinct from financial information management systems, with interfaces for the exchange of clinical and financial information as appropriate for patient accounting.

1.8. Reporting and Population Health Management

Newer EHR systems allow for reporting on the patient care database. Such reports may examine how well a population of diabetics are being managed, or what fraction of women of appropriate screening age have had mammography, for example. Certain EHR systems allow the provider to provide a service for an entire cohort, for example, writing a patient letter about a drug recall.

2. Assessing the Value of Electronic Health Records

The EHR has value in three dimensions: clinical, financial, and organizational.

2.1. Clinical Value

To assess the clinical value of EHRs, three areas are examined: information access; clinical decision support, including alerts and reminders, test ordering, and medications; and workflow support, including clinical communication, test notification, and referral support.

2.1.1. Information Access

Simply having clinical data available in the EHR without any other form of clinical decision support undoubtedly improves clinical decision making, utilization, and, probably, patient outcomes. The paper-based record has limited information management and retrieval capabilities. Physicians may not be able to find relevant information in the paper chart when it is available, and often the chart itself may not be available (Finnegan 1980; Hughes 1995; Kuilboer et al. 1997; Gibby and Schwab 1998). Simply having the information online and available in an EHR may impact utilization. Studies in the outpatient setting find that displaying test results (Wilson et al. 1982; Tierney et al. 1987) or predicting test results (Tierney et al. 1988) can reduce test utilization. The EHR may also be made available in settings beyond the care environment. Even having access via wireless methods to only certain components of the medical record, such as laboratory results, can influence utilization and management (Shabot et al. 2000). Thus, a key determinant of value of the EHR is the extent to which it collates, organizes, and makes available all relevant patient care information for the provider.

2.1.2. Clinical Decision Support

The most profound impact of the EHR, however, comes when it provides clinical decision support to the clinician at the point of care at the time of clinical decision making. This may occur in a variety of different ways in an EHR, as the following discussion of the impact of alerts and reminders, decision support for test ordering, and decision support for medications explains.

2.1.2.1. Alerts and Reminders

Review of the effectiveness and impact of various alerts and reminders shows the most predictable impact is achieved when the decision support is delivered through computer-based, patient-specific reminders that integrate into the clinician's workflow (Zielstorff 1998). Preventive care is an area where adherence to guidelines has been well studied (Bates 1998). Despite the abundance of preventive care guidelines, large gaps persist between appropriate levels of preventive care and what is actually done in practice. A recent review (Shea 1996) of the effectiveness of computer-based reminder systems in the use of preventive care measures in ambulatory settings demonstrated that computer reminders can be effective. According to Shea's meta-analysis, computerized reminders would increase compliance among practitioners to 64% from an estimated 50% baseline rate. Thus, although the reminders do enhance guideline compliance, these systems still often fail to achieve desired rates of compliance.

New evidence suggests alerts and reminders can impact disease-state specific care guidelines as well. Studies have demonstrated benefits in reminding care providers about drug selection and dosing (Pestotnik 1996; Bates et al. 1998; Raschke 1998; Persson 2000), care plan creation for chronic conditions such as diabetes (Lobach 1997), and in-hospital error prevention (Overhage 1997). Several studies have demonstrated that information technology can improve care (Hunt 1998), although much work remains to be done.

2.1.2.2. Test Ordering

Some quip that the pen is the most expensive instrument in the hospital, as it is the means by which physicians write orders for all tests and procedures. Using the EHR with clinical decision support for test ordering can impact utilization of expensive tests and procedures. Substantial recent research has focused on variation in rates of medical and surgical procedures, and large variations in virtually all areas have been demonstrated (Eisenberg 1986). Such variation has been found in ancillary test use as well as for more expensive procedures (Schroeder 1973; Epstein and McNeil 1987). Studies of test ordering have found that as much as 50% of diagnostic tests in teaching hospitals may be unnecessary, and many outpatient tests are also low yield (Schroeder 1973; Dixon and Laszlo 1974; Williams and Eisenberg 1986; Schoenenberger 1995; Eisenberg et al. 1977; Canas 1999). However, the few studies evaluating high utilization more closely have not found it to be correlated with high levels of inappropriateness. In fact, high levels of inappropriateness have been noted at all levels of utilization (Chassin 1987; Tierney 1988; Welch 1993). This suggests that decreasing inappropriateness requires more than identifying high levels of utilization; the next critical step is to develop decision support interventions that occur at the level of the individual decision and are targeted at decisions which are likely to be inappropriate.

Many such interventions have been attempted to decrease inappropriate utilization of tests (Schroeder 1973; Dixon and Laszlo 1974; Martin 1980; Marton 1985; Williams and Eisenberg 1986; Spiegel 1989; Eisenberg et al. 1977). The major types of intervention studied have been feedback, education (including providing information about clinical decision making and cost issues), rationing, and financial incentives (Grossman 1983). Each of these strategies in the most successful studies has produced transient reductions of about 25% for targeted tests. Despite a growing information base about what represents unnecessary utilization, physician behavior with respect to test ordering has been remarkably resistant to change over the long term (Sox 1986; Tierney et al. 1990; Wennberg 1998). In the past, there were few direct incentives for physicians to modify behavior, but this is changing rapidly as a high percentage of patient care is now reimbursed under capitation or, more often recently, directly rewarded when high quality benchmarks are achieved.

Using the EHR with clinical decision support in the clinical workflow may be the best means of effecting physician behavior change with respect to inappropriate utilization. Certain EHR decision support interventions have resulted in decreased test ordering in the outpatient setting. The Regenstrief group has demonstrated that providing information at the time of test ordering regarding charges for tests (Tierney et al. 1990), the time and result when they were most recently performed (McDonald 1992), and the probability of obtaining an abnormal result (Tierney 1988) all decreased the number of tests that were performed by 9% to 14%. Decision support can help physicians by making them more aware of information such as costs of tests and previous results, giving them guidelines at the time they are ordering, and suggesting additional testing when appropriate (e.g., hemoglobin A1c in diabetes or viral loads for HIV).

2.1.2.3. Medications

Like diagnostic and therapeutic test ordering, pharmacy is a high-volume and high-expense component of health care where there is considerable variability in practice patterns (Schroeder 1973). One study (Gonzales 1997) demonstrated widespread inappropriate antibiotic use for colds, upper respiratory tract infections, and bronchitis nationwide. Other examples exist in the post–myocardial infarction (MI) population. National guidelines support the use of aspirin and beta-blockers, yet several studies have shown that there is substantial non-adherence to these recommendations (Krumholz 1996, 1998; Marciniak 1998). Only 76% of eligible elderly patients in the studies cited received aspirin; in one study, only 50% of eligible patients received beta-blockers. National guidelines have been developed regarding when to treat and which drugs are most cost effective. However, the impact of these guidelines on physician behavior is limited. While it may be difficult to provide computerized clinical decision support on medication utilization appropriateness given the idiosyncracies of care, it is clear that decision support can impact adverse outcomes.

Adverse drug events (ADEs) and medication errors are common in the inpatient setting (Kellaway and McCrae 1973; Hutchinson et al. 1986) and are increasingly being recognized in the outpatient environment as well. In one study of primary care patients at 11 ambulatory care clinics, 18% of the patients reported problems or symptoms related to their medications on a patient survey (Gandhi et al. 2000a). In the same study, patients whose ADEs were detected by chart review were found to have a previously documented allergy to the medication in 11% of the cases, and 4.5% required hospitalization. These data suggest that drug complications in the ambulatory setting are common and can be serious and preventable. A prospective study of four outpatient clinics using prescription review and patient survey identified adverse drug events in 25% of patients and medication errors in 9% of prescriptions (Gandhi et al. 2001). Of these, almost half had potential to harm patients. Of 182 ADEs, 25 (14%) were serious, 21 (12%) were preventable, 50 (27%) were ameliorable, and 11 (6%) were both serious and preventable or ameliorable.

While many strategies for preventing medication errors and ADEs have been proposed (Bates et al. 1996), the evidence supporting their efficacy is, with some exceptions, limited. Bates and colleagues showed that implementation of a physician order entry system resulted in a 55% decrease in the serious medication error rate (Bates et al. 1998) and others found that delivery of computerized decision support for antibiotics reduced costs and improved outcomes (Evans 1998). Computerization of prescribing with accompanying decision support seems likely to be important in all settings, although its yield and the most important types of decision support are likely to vary by setting. Another study assessed the impact of basic computerized prescribing on medication errors, potential ADEs, and ADEs in the outpatient setting (Gandhi et al. 2001). Basic computerized prescribing at two study sites included printed prescriptions and required fields, but the programs contained few defaults or checks for allergies and drug interactions. Prescriptions from these computerized sites contained significantly fewer medication errors (7% vs. 15%, $p < 0.0001$) and rule violations (32% vs. 40%, $p < 0.0001$). The majority of medication errors could have been prevented with requiring complete prescriptions (44 of 92, 48%), frequency checking (20 of 92, 22%), and dose checking (13 of 92, 14%). Requiring complete prescriptions and dose checking were much more important for handwritten sites. More advanced decision support would also have prevented one third of preventable ADEs. Other advantages of computerized prescribing systems include the ability to reduce transcription and verbal orders by automatically sending prescriptions to pharmacies and to improve the upkeep of accurate medication lists in the medical record.

2.1.3. Workflow

Electronic health records may impact clinical workflow in a variety of ways. For simplicity, *workflow* in this context is defined as the actions taken by an individual to perform tasks related to patient care and communication. Many EHR features are designed to improve an individual's workflow, completing tasks such as writing a prescription, ordering tests, or documenting a visit. Certain EHRs may also support the workflow of care teams, largely through improved clinical communication, notification of test results, and referral processes.

2.1.3.1. Clinical Communication

Little solid evidence is available to address how well EHRs may support clinical communication among a care team in the provision of care during a unique patient encounter, or over time, in care delivery. Simple embedded e-mail systems in the EHR allow providers to message each other conveniently; for example, the physician may message the nurse that a test is due for a particular patient or a nurse may message the physician regarding a patient's prescription refill request. These messages may form a task list for either physician or ancillary staff. Like e-mail in any setting, this asynchronous messaging capability supports communication and task management. In addition, users of an EHR may also write a message to themselves or others and postdate it so that it is not delivered until a future date. This forms a tickler or reminder system that may be used to queue future tasks or prompt the provider to review a chart at a future date.

2.1.3.2. Test Notification

An equally or more important communication capability of more advanced EHR systems is the ability to notify ordering or covering clinicians of abnormal test results. Critical laboratory results occur frequently in inpatients and delays in physician response are common (Bates et al. 1996; Wyrwich 1999). One study showed that using an inpatient computerized alerting system to notify physicians of critical laboratory results reduced the time until an appropriate treatment was ordered by 38% (Kuperman et al. 1999). Similar benefits would be expected in the outpatient setting, especially because delays in obtaining test results are likely to be more common due to testing being performed offsite. Some ambulatory EHR systems message the ordering physician if a panic laboratory result is obtained.

2.1.3.3. Referral Support

Select EHR systems may also support the clinical referral process. The referral process is the critical communication link between primary care and subspecialty care for outpatients. Ideally, a referral communication should include a specific goal or question, pertinent clinical information, and the referring physician's initial assessment. Feedback from the specialist should occur soon after the consultation visit so that continuity of care is not disrupted. However, evidence from physician surveys indicates that neither the initial communication nor feedback from the specialist occurs reliably. This breakdown in physician-to-physician communication has led to delayed diagnoses, poly-pharmacy, increased litigation risk, and unnecessary testing (Epstein 1995). Referral letters are the standard communication medium of consultations, and have been the focus of prior research. Ninety percent of generalists and consultants agree that referral requests should include a statement of the medical problem, current medications, and specific clinical question. However, while 98% of referrals contain patient background information, only 76% state an explicit purpose for the referral (McPhee et al. 1984). This discrepancy may explain why, in 14% of inpatient consultations, the referring physician and consultant disagree on the reason for the consultation (Lee et al. 1983). In the inpatient setting, the availability of all care notes online, whether from the primary care provider team in the academic setting or the attending physician in the community setting, in addition to consultant's notes, facilitates referral and consultation communication.

In the outpatient setting, however, the interaction between referrer and specialist is presently inadequate and frequently a source of dissatisfaction. Sixty-three percent of primary care physicians in one system were dissatisfied with the referral process (Gandhi et al. 2000b). Reasons most often cited were late consultation reports, redundancy in the referral process, and the time required to create an adequate referral note. Forty percent of primary care physicians had not received feedback from the consulting specialist two weeks after the initial evaluation (Gandhi et al. 2000). The problem of late or missing feedback has not automatically resolved with the advent of new communication technologies. In 1980, physicians received follow-up information from consultants in 62% of cases while 18 years later the follow-up rate is reported at 55% (Cummins et al. 1980; Bourguet et al. 1998). Specialists are likewise dissatisfied with the referral process. In one study, 48% stated the information from the referring physician was untimely, while 43% felt the content of the referral request was inadequate (Gandhi et al. 2000b). Their primary concern was the failure of referring physicians to include a specific question and pertinent past medical history in the request. This missing information may be a substantial drain on physician time and office resources. Supplying the necessary information from the paper chart is difficult.

Little research has been done to study systematic changes to the referral process that could improve these deficits in communication. Computerizing the referral process and substituting electronic messaging for paper-based communications could help solve the problem of insufficient information exchange. Implementing referrals within a networked environment could facilitate communication between primary care physicians and specialists by making it easier to send a complete referral letter and more quickly receive feedback (Sittig et al. 1999). Computerized referral templates could require necessary data elements, and, unlike paper-based forms, can enforce those requirements. Coded information already stored within the electronic medical record could be automatically included in the communications, eliminating time-consuming data re-entry. Referral messages also could be routed to multiple recipients, ensuring that the clinical process and managed care approval process proceed in tandem without physician intervention. Finally, the status of referrals on multiple patients could be tracked in a central location, so that primary care providers can more quickly know when a specialist's evaluation is complete.

2.2. Financial Value

While most of the value of EHRs may be appreciated first in the clinical domain, important dimensions of value arise in the financial domain.

2.2.1. Improved Utilization

One of the most dramatic ways in which EHRs can produce venture value is through improved utilization of expensive laboratory tests, medications, and radiology procedures.

2.2.1.1. Medications

Electronic health records, with medication decision support offered at the time of writing electronic prescriptions in the ambulatory setting or provided during writing medication orders in the inpatient setting, can profoundly impact utilization. Appropriate clinical decision support at the time of medication ordering can help eliminate overuse, underuse, and misuse of medications. For example, as noted above, the system can censure a complete prescription, with all necessary information entered and checked, check for duplicate medications, drug interactions, or other forms of clinical decision support. In addition, suggestions for brand-to-generic substitution and for alternative cost-effective therapies can also reduce expenses associated with medications. Complying with a patient's health plan formulary can provide savings to the provider if she shares in the medication risk. Even if she does not, formulary compliance produces savings for the health plan, the employer-purchaser of healthcare services, and, ultimately, the patient.

The Center for Information Technology Leadership (CITL) modeled these effects in the ambulatory care setting (Johnston et al. 2003). In the analysis, CITL modeled EHRs with basic, intermediate, and advanced clinical decision support in ambulatory computerized provider order entry. Center for Information Technology Leadership estimates of medication savings per provider year from EHRs with clinical decision support predict that basic systems could save providers $2000 annually at an assumed 11.6% capitation rate, or as much as $17,000 annually per provider with advanced decision support capabilities. At the national level, these systems would produce savings of $3.3 billion for basic systems, $18 billion for intermediate systems, and $27 billion for advanced systems.

2.2.1.2. Laboratory

Similarly, decision support systems in laboratory order entry can help users reduce duplicate test ordering, or improve utilization through other effects. Systems that display test costs, prior results, or the probability of future abnormal test results to physicians during order entry can each save from 5% to 15% in laboratory expenditure (Tierney et al. 1988, 1990; American Billing Systems 2003). Center for Information Technology Leadership analysis predicts that order entry systems in electronic health records may reduce redundant laboratory expenditures anywhere from 0.4% for basic systems all the way up to 19.4% for advanced decision support systems. If such systems were adopted nationally, CITL estimates reduced laboratory expenditures of $14,000 per provider per year with intermediate class decision support, and as much as $32,000 per provider per year with advanced decision support system. Note these are total savings that are shared between the provider and payer. If such systems were adopted nationally, this would result in savings of as much as $5.8 billion per year.

2.2.1.3. Radiology

Similarly, order entry systems with decision support may improve expensive radiology test ordering. These systems may recommend appropriate radiological examinations, reduce inappropriate as ordering, improve radiology utilization with appropriate indications or consequent and corollary orders, and provide reminders about recent or redundant tests. According to CITL estimates of the impact of radiology decision support, such systems could avoid anywhere from 0.8% to 20% of redundant laboratory investigations with sophisticated decision support. Center for Inforamtion technology Leadership estimates that EHRs with intermediate and advanced radiology decision support would lead to savings from avoided radiology test redundancy on the order of $32,000 per provider per year up to $71,000 per provider per year. At the national level, if such systems were adopted nationwide in the ambulatory setting alone this could result in savings of as much as $12.9 billion per year.

2.2.2. Coding and Charge Capture

Electronic health record systems may also improve coding and charge capture in clinical practice. The literature suggests that more than 30% of a provider organization's claims may be rejected initially, with the eventual losses ranging from 5% to 10% of total revenues (American Billing Systems 2003; Independent Billing Services 2002). Order entry with decision support at the time of clinical documentation may assist the user in applying the appropriate billing code for a clinical encounter. In addition, some EHR systems facilitate charge capture for all procedures rendered in the clinical environment. Also, EHR health record systems may improve the quality of support data provided with financial claims. In this way rejected claim rates may be reduced. Center for Information Technology Leadership estimates that the EHR with decision support could reduce rejected claims by as much as 40% by highlighting missing diagnoses codes and suggesting appropriate cuts from the patient's record when necessary. In the aggregate, this would eliminate approximately $10 worth of rejected claims per visit.

2.3. Organizational Value

Perhaps the least well understood, and least studied, aspect EHR value is the dimension of organizational value. The following discussion examines organizational value from three perspectives: philosophical perspectives on value, quality and patient safety value, and organizational efficiency and culture.

2.3.1. Philosophical Perspectives on Value

Two principal philosophical perspectives on the value of IT in health care exist. The first views IT as a necessary component of the healthcare delivery system infrastructure. In this view, IT investments are made to support the business of healthcare delivery as a whole; typically, individual return-on-investment calculations for select projects and products are not done. The second competing perspective views IT investments as optional, or discretionary, in that they are associated with alternative business initiatives or care programs; thus, each requires a business case justification or return-on-investment analysis. The most coherent viewpoint lies somewhere in between, where mission critical services or initiatives are viewed as necessary components of the information systems infrastructure for the healthcare enterprise. Less central components, which are not part of the information systems infrastructure, are viewed with an eye toward meeting unique strategic objectives and thus are more amenable to a business case analysis.

2.3.2. Quality and Patient Safety Value

The dimension of organizational value that is easiest to understand is in the area of quality and patient safety. The evidence summarized above clearly demonstrates that IT can impact the quality of health care delivered and improve patient safety in both the hospital and the outpatient care environment. In addition, purchasers of healthcare services such as the federal government, self-insured employer purchasers, and other employer coalitions increasingly recognize the impact of IT on quality and patient safety and make its use a requirement in the delivery of healthcare services they purchase.

2.3.3. Organizational Efficiency and Culture

Less well understood is the impact of the EHRs, or IT in general, on organizational efficiency and the culture in health care. The experiences of other industries suggest that IT technology can lead to improved service delivery and organizational efficiency, although debate continues on its net impact on productivity. Further work needs to be done to assess the impact of IT on organizational efficiency in the healthcare environment, whether in the context of a solo provider in ambulatory care or a multi-institutional integrated delivery network. What is becoming clear, however, at least anecdotally, is that the use of IT in healthcare delivery is increasingly expected by both providers and patients as the norm. New trainees in health care and younger clinicians have grown up with IT as part of their daily experience in schooling and in society. Moreover, patients are experiencing the application of IT in all other service industries and bring an expectation for IT-enabled services and convenience to health care.

3. Enhancing the Value of Electronic Health Records

Beyond the clinical, financial, and organizational value of the EHR discussed above, three additional areas will undoubtedly contribute to the value of the EHR in the future, namely, the use of EHR systems for improved patient-centered care and communication, and improved healthcare services delivery through regional connectivity.

3.1. Patient-Centered Care and Communication

The EHR will become the foundation for doctor–patient communication, shared clinical information management, knowledge access, and decision support. Healthcare consumers are flocking to the Internet in advance of clinicians to find second opinions (Patrick 1999), and general health resources (Wyatt 2000; Pagon et al. 2001). Patient involvement in their plan of care, including preventive health screening and follow up of abnormal test results, is critical to improving compliance with guidelines (Roth et al. 1996; van Dulmen et al. 1997). With the widespread adoption of electronic mail and use of the Internet, e-mail communications between providers and patients may potentially improve information exchange (Ball and Lillis 2001) and ultimately impact healthcare outcomes.

In addition, as patients have become better informed about health care, they have developed higher expectations for follow up (Schofield et al. 1994; Meza and Webster 2000). Evidence from malpractice litigation suggests that incomplete follow up of test results is an important issue (Risk Management Foundation 2000): more than one fourth of diagnosis-related malpractice cases can be attributed to failure in the follow-up system. In response to these concerns, the National Committee for Quality Assurance (NCQA) has proposed missed follow up of abnormal test results as one of its outcome measures to be included in the new Health Plan Employer Data and Information Set (HEDIS) criteria.

There is a relatively large body of literature on efforts to increase patient adherence with recommendations for further evaluation of abnormal pap smears or breast cancer screening. However, very little literature on the follow up of test results exists. One study (Burstin et al. 1999) examined the documentation of transmitting results to patients and documentation of follow-up plans for abnormal mammograms, pap smears, and cholesterol tests. Significant deficiencies were found: on average 47% of records had no documentation of results transmitted to patients (mammogram 44%, pap smears 50%, cholesterol 45%) and 20% of records had no documentation of follow up of abnormal results (mammogram 16%, pap smears 7%, cholesterol 35%).

This study also used the Picker ambulatory survey to assess patient satisfaction reports with testing, including understanding why they need tests and how they can get the results and a comprehensible explanation of their meaning. Patient satisfaction with testing appeared to be associated with documentation of the communication. Among patients to whom results were transmitted, 86% reported satisfaction with the testing scale, compared to 72% of those without such documentation ($p < 0.05$). Those with a documented follow-up plan in the record were more likely to be satisfied with testing (85%), compared to 75% for patients without a follow-up plan in the record ($p < 0.05$). This study emphasizes the deficiencies that exist in documentation and communication of test results and in the follow up of abnormal results. Electronic health record systems, coupled with Internet-based patient portals providing access to their online EHRs and communication with their providers, will be an important part of patient care follow up.

3.2. Regional Connectivity

Recent work in regional healthcare information exchange and interoperability suggests that significant value will be obtained when individual EHR systems, in hospital environments or in ambulatory care settings, can communicate in a secure and confidential way with one another. The above review of the value of EHRs in clinic and hospital settings assesses the value of these products in a myopic way: that is, the value that is obtained within a clinic, hospital, or integrated delivery network. It is analogous to considering the value of automating individual banks without linking them together through the financial networks. Pundits suggest the value of a network increases with the square of the number of nodes on it. Hence, it is reasonable to expect that significant value will accrue when EHR systems are linked one to the other across local care regions and, potentially, across the country.

Recently, the CITL analyzed the value of healthcare information exchange and interoperability (Pan et al., 2004). The analysis included all the healthcare transactions occurring in a clinical encounter between provider and payer, pharmacy, laboratory, radiology center, other providers, and public health reporting. It did not include other transactions, such as those that might occur between payer and pharmacy or pharmacy benefits manager. Thus, this analysis focused only on those first-order transactions arising directly from the provider to other stakeholders in the healthcare system. Despite this narrow focus, the savings potential from interoperability in electronic information systems is profound. This work suggests that labor savings and avoided costs (related to duplicate medication and diagnostic and therapeutic test ordering) could total approximately $78 billion per year for the U.S. healthcare delivery system after a 10-year implementation period of fully standardized, interoperable systems. The savings potential for providers is approximately $34 billion.

We believe these potential savings will be in addition to the savings arising from EHR effects within the individual care setting. While savings from reduced redundant diagnostic tests and medications should be readily obtainable, it is clear that reducing labor costs with improved efficiency of information exchange may be difficult. However, personnel who previously managed paper and fax information exchange could be directed toward improving the care experience or possibly into revenue generating activities.

4. Conclusion

This chapter has reviewed the basic functionality of EHRs in healthcare delivery. The core features provide value in a variety of ways. They may impact the quality of patient care services rendered and the incidence of an adverse events relating to patient safety. These clinical effects are complemented by evidence suggesting EHRs provide value in both the financial and organizational dimension. Financial value of EHRs is largely determined by improvement in utilization of medications and of expensive diagnostic and therapeutic tests and procedures. Other dimensions of financial value include improved financial management of healthcare claims related to better charge capture, and decision support for administrative issues in the HER, such as appropriate coding. Lastly, electronic health records are the foundation for a national healthcare information infrastructure which will undoubtedly have beneficial clinical and financial effects.

Acknowledgments. The author gratefully appreciates the input to this chapter from Drs. David Bates and Tejal Gandhi.

References

American Billing Systems. 2002. Electronic claims filing. American Billing Systems. Available from: http://www.americanbilling.com/ecf.htm. Accessed 2003 15 Jan.

Ball MJ, Lillis J. 2001. E-health: transforming the physician/patient relationship. Int J Med Inf 61(1):1–10.

Bates DW. 1998. Effect of computerized physician order entry and a team intervention on prevention of serious medication errors. JAMA 280(15):1311–1316.

Bates DW, Gawande AA. 2003. Improving safety with information technology. N Engl J Med 348(25):2526–2534.

Bates DW, Burrows AM, Grossman DG, Schneider PJ, Strom BL. 1996. Top-priority actions for preventing adverse drug events in hospitals: recommendations of an expert panel. Am J Health Syst Pharm 53:747–751.

Bates DW, Leape LL, Cullen DJ, Laird N, Petersen LA, Teich JM, et al. 1998. Effect of computerized physician order entry and a team intervention on prevention of serious medication errors. JAMA 280(15):1311–1316.

Bourguet C, Gilchrist V, McCord G. 1998. The consultation and referral process. A report from NEON. Northeastern Ohio Network Research Group. J Fam Pract 46(1):47–53.

Burstin HR, Cook EF, Puopolo AL, Brennan TA. Follow-up of test results in primary care: an opportunity to reduce errors. Submitted for publication 1999.

Canas F. 1999. Evaluating the appropriateness of digoxin level monitoring. Arch Intern Med 159:363–368.

Chassin MR. 1987. Does inappropriate use explain geographic variations in the use of health care services? A study of three procedures. JAMA 258:2533–2537.

Cummins RO, Smith RW, Inui TS. 1980. Communication failure in primary care: failure of consultants to provide follow-up information. JAMA 243(16):1650–1652.

Dixon RH, Laszlo J. 1974. Utilization of clinical chemistry services by medical house staff: an analysis. Arch Intern Med 134:1064–1067.

Eisenberg JM, Williams SV, Garner L, Viale R, Smits H. 1977. Computer-based audit to detect and correct overutilization of laboratory tests. Med Care 15(11):915–921.

Eisenberg JM. 1986. Doctors' decisions and the cost of medical care. Ann Arbor, MI: Health Administration Press.

Epstein RM. 1995. Communication between primary care physicians and consultants. Arch Fam Med 4(5):403–409.

Epstein AM, McNeil BJ. 1987. Variations in ambulatory test use: what do they mean? Med Clin North Am 71:705–717.

Evans RS, Pestotnik SL, Classen DC, Clemmer TP, Weaver LK, Orme JF Jr., Lloyd JF, Bouke JP. 1998. A computer-assisted management program for antibiotics and other antiinfective agents. N Engl J Med 338(4):232–238.

Finnegan R. 1980. Dual challenge: medical record continuity and availability. J Am Med Rec Assoc 51(5):28–36.

Gandhi TK, Burstin HR, Cook EF, Puopolo AL, Haas JS, Brennan TA, Bates DW. 2000a. Drug complications in outpatients. J Gen Intern Med 15(3):149–154.

Gandhi TK, Sittig DF, Franklin M, Sussman AJ, Fairchild DG, Bates DW. 2000b. Communication breakdown in the outpatient referral process. J Gen Int Med 15(9):626–631.

Gandhi TK, Weingart SN, Seger A, Seger DS, Borus JS, Burdick E. Impact of basic computerized prescribing on outpatient medication errors and adverse drug events. J Gen Intern Med 16(Suppl 1):195.

Gibby GL, Schwab WK. 1998. Availability of records in an outpatient preanesthetic evaluation clinic. J Clin Monit Comput 14(6):385–391.

Gonzales R. 1997. Antibiotic prescribing for adults with colds, upper respiratory tract infections, and bronchitis by ambulatory care physicians. JAMA 278:901–904.

Grossman RM. 1983. A review of physician cost-containment strategies for laboratory testing. Med Care 21:783–802.

Haynes RB. 1995. Bridges between health care research evidence and clinical practice. J Am Med Inform Assoc 2:342–350.

Hughes G. 1995. A case study in chart availability: University of Texas Medical Branch Hospitals and Clinics. J AHIMA 66(10):70–71.

Hunt DL. 1998. Effects of computer-based clinical decision support systems on physician performance and patient outcomes: a systematic review. JAMA 280:1339–1346.

Hutchinson TA, Flegel KM, Kramer MS, Leduc DG, Kong HH. 1986. Frequency, severity and risk factors for adverse drug reactions in adult out-patients: a prospective study. J Chronic Dis 39:533–542.

Independent Billing Services. 2002. The need for medical billing. Independent Billing Services. Available from: http://www.independentbilling.com. Accessed 2003 Jan 15.

Johnston J, Pan E, Walker JD, Bates DW, Middleton B. 2003. The value of computerized provider order entry in ambulatory settings. Boston, MA: Center for Information Technology Leadership.

Kellaway GS, McCrae E. 1973. Intensive monitoring for adverse drug effects in patients discharged from acute medical wards. N Z Med J 78:525–528.

Kohn LT, Corrigan J, Donaldson MS, editors. 2000. To err is human: building a safer health system. Washington, DC: National Academy Press.

Krumholz HM. 1996. Aspirin for secondary prevention after acute myocardial infarction in the elderly: prescribed use and outcomes. Ann Intern Med 124:292–298.

Krumholz HM. 1998. National use and effectiveness of beta-blockers for the treatment of elderly patients after acute myocardial infarction: National Cooperative Cardiovascular Project. JAMA 280:623–629.

Kuilboer MM, van der Lei J, Bohnen AM, van Bemmel JH. 1997. The availability of unavailable information. Proc AMIA Symp 749–753.

Kuperman GJ, Teich JM, Tanasijevic MJ, Ma'luf N, Rittenberg E, Fiskio J, Winkelman J, Bates DW. 1999. Improving response to critical laboratory results with automation: results of a randomized controlled trial. J Am Med Inform Assoc 6:512–522.

Lee T, Pappius EM, Goldman L. 1983. Impact of inter-physician communication on the effectiveness of medical consultations. Am J Med 74(1):106–112.

Lobach DF. 1997. Computerized decision support based on a clinical practice guideline improves compliance with care standards. Am J Med 102:89–98.

Marciniak TA. 1998. Improving the quality of care for Medicare patients with acute myocardial infarction: results from the Cooperative Cardiovascular Project. JAMA 279: 1351–1357.

Martin AR. 1980. A trial of two strategies to modify the test-ordering behavior of medical residents. N Engl J Med 303:1330–1336.

Marton KI. 1985. Modifying test-ordering behavior in the outpatient medical clinic: a controlled trial of two educational interventions. Arch Intern Med 145:816–821.

McDonald CJ. 1992. Effects of computer reminders for influenza vaccination on morbidity during influenza epidemics. MD Comput 9:304–312.

McGlynn EA, Asch SM, Adams J, Keesey J, Hicks J, DeCristofaro A, Kerr EA. 2003. The quality of health care delivered to adults in the United States. N Engl J Med 348(26):2635–2645.

McPhee SJ, Lo B, Saika GY, Meltzer R. 1984. How good is communication between primary care physicians and subspecialty consultants? Arch Intern Med 144(6):1265–1268.

Meza JP, Webster DS. 2000. Patient preferences for laboratory test results notification. [see comments]. Am J Manage Care 6(12):1297–1300.

Overhage JM. 1997. A randomized trial of corollary orders to prevent errors of omission. J Am Med Inform Assoc 4:364–375.

Pagon RA, Pinsky L, Beahler CC. 2001. Online medical genetics resources: a US perspective. BMJ 322(7293):1035–1037.

Pan E, Johnston D, Walker JD, Adler-Milstein J, Bates DW, Middleton B. 2004. The value of health-care information exchange and interoperability. Boston, MA: Center for Information Technology Leadership.

Patrick K. 1999. How patients use the web for second opinions. West J Med 170(6):332–333.

Persson M. 2000. Evaluation of a computer-based decision support system for treatment of hypertension with drugs: retrospective, nonintervention testing of cost and guideline adherence. J Intern Med 247(1):87–93.

Pestotnik SL. 1996. Implementing antibiotic practice guidelines through computer-assisted decision support: clinical and financial outcomes. Ann Intern Med 124:884–890.

Raschke RA. 1998. A computer alert system to prevent injury from adverse drug events: development and evaluation in a community teaching hospital. JAMA 280:1317–1320.

Risk Management Foundation. 2000. Reducing office practice risks. Forum 20(2).

Roth CS, Schlossberg L, Woods S. 1996. Physician-patient communication in ambulatory settings. Acad Med 71(5):558–559.

Schoenenberger RA. 1995. Appropriateness of antiepileptic drug level monitoring. JAMA 274:1622–1626.

Schofield MJ, Sanson-Fisher R, Halpin S, Redman S. 1994. Notification and follow-up of Pap test results: current practice and women's preferences. Prev Med 23(3):276–283.

Schroeder SA. 1973. Use of laboratory tests and pharmaceuticals: variation among physicians and effect of cost audit on subsequent use. JAMA 225:969–973.

Shabot MM, LoBue M, Chen J. 2000. Wireless clinical alerts for physiologic, laboratory and medication data. Proc AMIA Symp 2000;789–793.

Shea S. 1996. A meta-analysis of 16 randomized controlled trials to evaluate computer-based clinical reminder systems for preventive care in the ambulatory setting. J Am Med Inform Assoc 3:399–409.

Sittig DF, Gandhi TK, Franklin M, Turetsky M, Sussman AJ, Fairchild DG, Bates DW, Komaroff AL, Teich JM. 1999. A computer-based outpatient clinical referral system. Int J Med Inf 55(2):149–158.

Sox HC. 1986. Probability theory in the use of diagnostic tests: an introduction to critical study of the literature. Ann Intern Med 104:60–66.

Spiegel JS. 1989. Changing physician test ordering in a university hospital. An intervention of physician participation, explicit criteria, and feedback. Arch Intern Med 149:549–553.

Tang PC, Committee on Data Standards for Patient Safety. 2003. Letter report: key capabilities of an electronic health record system. Institute of Medicine. Washington, DC.

Teich JM. 1995. Enhancement of clinician workflow with computer order entry. Proc Annu Symp Comput Appl Med Care 1995;459–463.

Teich JM. 1999. The Brigham integrated computing system (BICS): advanced clinical systems in an academic hospital environment. Int J Med Inf 54:197–208.

Teich JM. 2000. Clinical decision support systems come of age. MD Comput 17(1):43–46.

Tierney WM, McDonald CJ, Martin DK, Hui SL, Rogers MP. 1987. Computerized display of past test results: effect on outpatient testing. Ann Intern Med 107:569–574.

Tierney WM, McDonald CJ, Hui SL, Martin DK. 1988. Computer predictions of abnormal test results: effects on outpatient testing. JAMA 259:1194–1198.

Tierney WM, Miller ME, McDonald CJ. 1990. The effect on test ordering of informing physicians of the charges for outpatient diagnostic tests. N Engl J Med 322:1499–1504.

van Dulmen AM, Verhaak PF, Bilo HJ. 1997. Shifts in doctor-patient communication during a series of outpatient consultations in non-insulin-dependent diabetes mellitus. Patient Educ Couns 30(3):227–237.

Welch WP. 1993. Geographic variation in expenditures for physicians' services in the United States. N Engl J Med 328:621–627.

Wennberg DE. 1998. Variation in the delivery of health care: the stakes are high. Ann Intern Med 128:866–868.

Wennberg JG. 1973. Small area variations in health care delivery. Science 182:1102–1108.

Williams SV, Eisenberg JM. 1986. A controlled trial to decrease the unnecessary use of diagnostic tests. J Gen Intern Med 1(1):8–13.

Wilson GA, McDonald CJ, McCabe GP Jr. 1982. The effect of immediate access to a computer-medical record on physician test ordering: a controlled clinical trial in the emergency room. Am J Public Health 72(7):698–702.

Wyatt JC. 2000. Information for patients. J R Soc Med 93(9):467–471.

Wyrwich KW. 1999. Linking clinical relevance and statistical significance in evaluating intra-individual changes in health-related quality of life. Med Care 37:469–478.

Zielstorff RD. 1998. Online practice guidelines: issues, obstacles, and future prospects. J Am Med Inform Assoc 5:227–236.

5
Personal Outcomes in Health Care

Thomas L. Garthwaite

The ultimate test of the quality of a health care system is whether it helps the people it intends to help. (Institute of Medicine 2001)

Over the past four years, I have retold stories of healthcare experiences of my family members and me. Each audience reacts similarly. Each listens intently, and many individuals smile or nod knowingly. At the end of the stories, I ask that anyone who has similar experiences regarding themselves or their family or friends to please raise their hands. Invariably, between one third and one half of the audience members do so.

1. My Stories ...

1.1. My Nephew

My nephew Chris came to visit his grandmother and volunteered to trim her hedges. He borrowed my heavy-duty hedge trimmer and did a fine job on the hedges and on his index finger. I was called, and we rushed to a nearby emergency room. The triage nurse glanced at his finger and told him to rewrap it and to sign in. We spent the next 25 minutes giving the usual demographic information and trying to convince the clerk that he was insured despite the fact that he was covered by three separate policies. We were seated and eventually called and placed in an examination room. The emergency room physician looked at the wound and informed us that all through-and-through lacerations of the nail bed mandated a plastic surgery consultation. The plastic surgeon was paged; we later learned that he received the page just as he was getting out of his car after returning home from the same hospital. He came back to the hospital and sutured the nail bed. We went home about six hours after we left.

1.2. My Mother

My mother, 82 years old at the time, called me on a Sunday morning to tell me that she had abdominal pain and to ask me to come over and check it out.

"Of course, I'll be right there," was my response.

After examining her abdomen, I asked, "What do you want to wear to the hospital?"

She retorted, "I'm not going to hospital. Just let me go. Just give me something for the pain."

I insisted, "Mom! No one is 'letting you go.' It's just your gallbladder. It's easy to fix!"

We drove to the emergency room. The ER intern felt her abdomen. "Gallbladder," he proclaimed.

The ER resident concurred, "Gallbladder."

The ER staff physician confirmed, "Gallbladder."

The surgery team was called. The intern on the surgery team proclaimed, "Gallbladder."

The surgery resident agreed, "Gallbladder."

Finally, the staff physician examined her abdomen and said, "I'm not so sure. The findings seem more diffuse."

Some 36 hours later, as her white count continued to rise and she continued to deteriorate, the last film of the endoscopic retrograde cholecystopancreatography (ERCP) study showed leakage of fluid from the gallbladder into the peritoneum. Sometime during the multiple abdominal exams or during the admission ultrasound study, her gallbladder ruptured, spilling several hundred small stones and infected bile into her abdominal cavity. After emergency surgery (a cholecystectomy with T-tube placement) and several additional complications, she recovered and is doing amazing well at age 92.

1.3. My Mother-in-Law

My mother-in-law called to say that she had been placed on estrogen therapy for menopausal symptoms. Shortly after she started the estrogen, she noted swelling in her armpit, the axilla in medical speak. She wondered what I thought might be happening. Based on my training in endocrinology, I said that I was concerned that the estrogen-sensitive tissue in that area was the breast and that I was worried that lymph nodes in her axilla were reacting to or contained breast cancer. I advised that she go to her doctors and be examined for breast cancer and have a biopsy of the swelling in her axilla taken.

She returned to her doctor who advised her that she had had a mammogram not that long ago and that rather than biopsy the swelling or repeat the mammogram, he would simply stop the estrogen. She went to another doctor who did not challenge the judgment of the first. The swelling diminished after the estrogen was stopped.

About a year later, a repeat mammogram was abnormal. At radical mastectomy, an estrogen-receptor–positive adenocarcinoma of the breast with evidence of spread to 10 of 13 axillary lymph nodes was removed.

1.4. My Wife

My wife had an upper respiratory infection that was very similar to the illness I was seeing in my co-workers and patients. When I came home from work, she would say she felt lousy and I would feel her forehead, listen to her lungs, and tell her that she had a virus and it was "going around." Several days later, I came home from work and went upstairs to see how she was doing. She did not look good—listless, short of breath, high fever. I took her to the emergency room.

The emergency room resident came in to see her. I could tell that the resident was a little skeptical that someone with the "flu" needed to come to the emergency room. After listening to the story and listening to her lungs, the resident suggested that we go home. "I guess we could get a CBC and a chest x-ray," she said in a tone that conveyed her opinion that they would be normal.

"I really think she needs a chest film," I said. The x-ray showed her lobar pneumonia and the CBC showed that her white blood cell count was markedly elevated, indicating a bacterial process. She responded very well to penicillin.

1.5. My Colleague

Alex was a member of my extended family—the Division of Endocrinology where I worked. He was a 42-year-old physician who had diabetes, asthma, and hypertension. He treated himself too much but also sought advice from specialists he knew regarding his illnesses. Neither Alex nor the doctors he consulted felt that they were in charge of his health care. Alex noted epigastric pain on a Monday. On the following Saturday, while he was shopping at a mall with his young son, Alex collapsed and died of an acute myocardial infarction. Underappreciated by Alex and his consultants was the fact Alex's father had died at age 42 of a myocardial infarction.

1.6. Myself

I have worn glasses since the ninth grade. In 1990, I noted that my glasses could no longer correct the vision in my right eye and that I was seeing halos around lights at night. My ophthalmologist noted a cataract in my right eye and since my best corrected vision was 20/50, we decided to have the cataract removed and a prosthetic lens inserted. In January 2001, the operation was performed and was a great success. My vision in my right eye had never been better or clearer. The yellow tint from the cataract was gone and colors were vibrant.

In May of 1991, while on business travel back to the Washington, D.C., area, I noted a blurry, dark area in the visual field of my right eye. I thought it was related to the implanted lens and thought I'd have it checked out as soon as I returned home. Two days later, the dark area expanded and a larger portion of my vision was compromised. Since I was still in Washington, D.C., where my cataract surgery was performed, I called the ophthalmologist who had performed the cataract surgery. He saw me that morning and determined that I had a retinal detachment. He said that I was at increased risk of a retinal detachment because I had myopia and cataract surgery. I was previously unaware of my risk for retinal detachment and of the signs and symptoms related to that condition. After two surgeries and special lenses, I am now able to see 20/50 in my right eye although my vision in that eye is significantly distorted.

2. The Test of Quality

The Institute of Medicine (IOM) suggests using measures "determined by the outcomes patients desire" to define the components that constitute quality: safety, effectiveness, patient-centeredness, timeliness, efficiency, and equity. Further, the IOM defines outcomes in a way that goes far beyond the success of specific procedures or "what is done to" patients to "what is accomplished for them" (p 46).

According to the IOM, desirable personal health outcomes include "improvement (and prevention of deterioration) of health status and health related quality of life, and management of physical and psychological symptoms." In expanding the definition, the IOM incorporates "interpersonal aspects of care" as health outcomes, citing "patients' concerns and expectations, their sense of dignity, their participation in decision making, and in some cases reduced burden on family and caregivers and spiritual well being" (p 46).

Using the IOM's measures, I have tried to learn what I can from the outcomes my family had. On the first set of measures, health status and management of symptoms, outcomes were varied. My nephew and wife ended up getting the care they needed, and neither was severely harmed. It took longer—and involved great risk—for my mother. Her survival was fortunate and more a testament to her toughness than to the ability of the system to properly diagnose and treat her. My mother-in-law's diagnosis of cancer was delayed, I have some permanent visual disability, and my friend Alex died too young.

When it comes to the interpersonal aspects of care, the outcomes certainly are not what my family and I would expect. Though it was essentially harmless, the wait in the emergency department was symptomatic of a system that fails on measures of timeliness and efficiency. Much more seriously, it shows a system that is not focused on the patient.

3. Curing Health Care

As a physician, I have tried to learn from my own family's stories. As I see it, there are three key lessons:

- Health care is focused on many things but frequently not on the person who is the patient.
- Most imperfections go unnoticed and/or no changes are made in the processes or systems that gave rise to the unintended outcomes. Thus, patients will continue to receive less than ideal care despite the opportunity to learn that presented itself.
- There is no way to infuse new information into the care system and to regularly apply it, regardless of whether that new information derives from new research or from knowledge gained by system failures.

A closer look at what went wrong in each case suggests that specific information systems that could help reduce variability, improve accuracy, and avoid previously made mistakes. Longitudinal, patient-owned health records would be of significant help in integrating what is known about the patient with what is known about medical science and the delivery of care.

Specifically, the care my family and I received could be improved by using information technology (IT) tools:

- Nephew: Simplify and automate registration, coverage determination, benefit coordination, and billing.
- Nephew, Mom, Wife: Develop and deploy smart systems to aid in triage.
- Mother-in-law, Wife: Develop and deploy smart systems to warn of dangers when certain conditions are met.
- Alex: Trigger reminders and alter probability algorithms based on the patient's family history (and work and exposure histories).
- Self: Educational modules and checklists for completion based on condition of the patient and the risk to the patient.

We face much more than an IT challenge. Each of these tools can function only as part of larger systems. Smart systems and decision support require access to patient data and medical knowledge, and the ability to link across time and across systems. In *The Quality Chasm*, the IOM concludes that "[t]he current care systems cannot do the job." Only a new health system can deliver high quality care—care that is *safe, effective, patient-centered, timely, efficient,* and *equitable* (IOM 2001).

Creation of a new system requires change on a massive scale, and it requires vision to guide that change. The HealthePeople concept offers this vision.

Reference

Institute of Medicine. 2001. Crossing the quality chasm: a new health system for the 21st century. Washington, DC: National Academy Press.

6
Human Factors: Changing Systems, Changing Behaviors

MARION J. BALL and JUDITH V. DOUGLAS

Transforming the healthcare system is not simply a technical undertaking. It requires much more than implementing new information systems or providing new computerized tools for clinicians. Simply stated, "Technology offers challenging capabilities, not solutions. New evidence and new tools demand new approaches and attention to human factors" (Ball and Douglas 2002).

1. The Role of Information Technology in Health Care

In its 1991 report advocating the computer-based patient record as "an essential technology for health care," the Institute of Medicine (IOM) acknowledged the problems caused by clinician resistance, suggesting mechanisms to encourage clinician input and recommending programs to educate students and practitioners in computer use (Institute of Medicine 1997).

In two more recent, high-profile studies on medical errors and quality of care, the IOM clearly assigned information technology (IT) to a supporting role. Its report calling for a safer health system (2000) described technology (not just IT) as "a 'member' of the work team." And this technology was "not restricted" to technology used by health care professionals, but included non-health professionals and "people at home" (p 62–63). The IOM made the supporting role of IT clearer still in its second report calling for a new health system. There, using information technology was given billing equal to that accorded to four other areas: building organizational supports, applying evidence to healthcare delivery, aligning payment policies with quality improvements, and preparing the workforce.

Both organizational and workforce issues involve "interrelationships between humans, the tools they use, and the environment in which they live and work," or what is defined as human factors (Institute of Medicine 2000, p 63). These factors received growing attention throughout the 1990s. By 1998, a prize-winning system implementer, Reed Gardner, formulated the 80/20 rule, stating that "the success of a project is perhaps 80% dependent on the development of the social and political interaction skills of the developer and 20% or less on the implementation of the hardware and software technology" (Gardner 1998). Nancy Lorenzi and Bob Riley offered a corollary of sorts, noting that "people who have low psychological ownership in a system and who vigorously resist its implementation can bring a 'technically best' system to its knees" (Lorenzi and Riley 2000).

1.1. Technology and the Challenge of Change

"A new technology does not add or subtract something. It changes everything." New technologies, like the printing press, "alter the structure of our interests: the things we think *about*. They alter the character of our symbols: the things we think *with*. And they alter the nature of community: the arena in which thoughts develop," according to communications theorist Neil Postman (Postman 1992, p 18, 20).

This is true even of a "simple" application like electronic prescribing. Peter Basch, an internist involved in a patient safety initiative, explained: "Once you begin to e-prescribe, you see that you're not just digitizing a prescription pad, but rather, entering patients' recent history, recalls, interaction and allergy checks, perhaps other indications such as patient weight, co-morbid conditions and such. You're actually spending time and effort creating better input. *So you're fundamentally changing what docs do.* [emphasis added]" (Hagland 2003).

1.2. Managing Change

It is this element of change that necessitates attention to human factors. Today, managing change is recognized as one of the four cornerstones of medical informatics that form the basis for developing a new information management paradigm, the critical challenge facing health care:

- "Producing **structures to represent data and knowledge** so that complex relationships may be visualized;
- "developing methods for **acquisition and presentation of data** so that overload can be avoided;
- "**managing change** among people, process, and IT so that the use of information is optimized;
- "**integrating information** from diverse sources to provide more than the sum of the parts, and information into work processes so that it can be acted on when it can have the largest effect." (Lorenzi 2000)

1.2.1. Core Principles

In 1995, working with Lorenzi and Riley, we outlined the core principles for effectively managing change (Lorenzi et al. 1995). Drawn from the social sciences and behavioral research, all are critical to successful technology implementations (see Table 6.1).

First among these core principles is the creation of a vision, a shared understanding of the changes and the outcomes a new paradigm can offer health care. Stead and Lorenzi (1999) suggest providing "a list of 'wins' that have been made possible by informatics and information technology" in support of the vision, detailing "cost, return on investment, critical success factors, and alternatives." This is especially important in health care, which as an industry has not yet linked information to financial outcomes. Visioning thus must "make the benefits of the proposed system clear and establish an explicit link between promised benefits on the one hand and informatics and information technology key enablers on the other."

Yet visioning is only the first step; making the vision real and moving theory into practice is a greater challenge. "Although health is an information-intensive industry," wrote Stead and Lorenzi (1999), "and most people agree that information is power, it is natural to resist information technology, because it changes roles and the social order." For the health providers who must bear the burden of change, technology must be seen as solving problems.

TABLE 6.1. Change management: core principles and manifestations.

Core principles	Manifestations
Vision	Clearly defined and effectively communicated to provide people within the organization with an understanding of the desired changes and the outcomes.
Respect	Making honesty and trust part of all interpersonal transactions, for example, in how information is presented and people are incorporated into the change process.
Involvement	Aggressively making people part of change by seeking inputs as early as possible and providing continuous feedback.
Empowerment	Enabling commitment, perhaps by flattening the organizational structure.
Teamwork	Involving people from all levels in the organization, always investing in skill development and often creating self-directed work teams.
Customer first	Calling upon the organization to refocus from internal concerns to external issues, specifically on how best to serve customers outside the organization.
Openness to change	Accepting intellectually and emotionally that complex systems "thrive only close to the edge of chaos."

Source: Extracted from Lorenzi et al. (1997).

At a September 2003 conference on wireless applications, consultant Peter de Jager warned that "IT professionals must stop selling solutions. Instead, they must work with others to identify problems" (Mobile Health Data 2002). His comments carry two key messages. First, as Max Planck stated, "In the formulation of the question, lies the key to the answer." Simply put, solutions cannot come first. Second, change must be collaborative, not imposed. According to de Jager, "Change is easily embraced when one personally makes the decision to change. But every single person resists being changed from without." He noted that the use of the term *buy in* is suggestive of the problem: "By definition, 'buy in' implies you've come up with an idea that you need people to accept, *an idea for which you did not allow input* (emphasis added) since they need to 'buy in.'" (Mobile Health Data 2002)

Allowing input is what the core principles of respect, involvement, empowerment, teamwork, and customer first are about. These five principles shown in Table 6.1 are critical to the adoption of technology and to the transformation it enables. The final principle, openness to change, is essential to visioning and implementing new systems, as Robert Kolodner explains in Chapter 2.

1.2.2. Visioning

In 1998, the American College of Medical Informatics (ACMI) brought together 32 of its elected fellows to develop "visions for the future of health care and biomedicine and a strategic agenda for health and biomedical informatics in support of those visions" (Greenes and Lorenzi 1998). These acknowledged leaders in the field of computers in medicine articulated three goals for 2008: a virtual healthcare databank, a national healthcare knowledge base, and a personal clinical health record. The goals include the same capabilities envisioned in HealthePeople's person-centered health systems. In short, "a standards-based, patient-oriented longitudinal database is implicit in every vision expressed by the informatics community" (Stead and Lorenzi 1999). Change of this magnitude is undeniably transformational. To realize this level of change, we must overcome the impediments posed by our current healthcare system and its orientation toward insurance, disease, and the bottom line (Stead and Lorenzi 1999).

In theory and in practice, person-centered health systems involve "a new relationship between people and the health system." This entails more than giving consumers access to information; information in and of itself does not change behavior. The new relationship means making consumers part of the decision-making process about their health care and giving them content to guide them through this process. The result of doing so will be profound changes in the "knowledge-as-power relationship" between provider and consumer (Stead and Lorenzi 1999).

1.2.3. Making Visions Reality

In the past, many of the successful systems implemented were stand alone. Set within specific areas, they involved relatively limited numbers of people and they provided visible and direct benefits. Lorenzi and Riley (2000) have commented on the growing importance of human factors as more complex systems affect "larger, more heterogeneous groups of people and more organizational areas." The behavioral changes effected in and by transformation of the sort envisioned in HealthePeople would be exponentially greater, stunning in their scale and significance.

2. Computerized Physician Order Entry

On a lesser but far from inconsequential scale, computer physician order entry (CPOE) illustrates some of the non-technical challenges facing person-centered systems. Although CPOE was "on everyone's radar screen" in 2002, and estimates called for over $10 billion to be spent on it the next few years, by March 2003 only 3% of urban hospitals had complete systems (Health Data Management 2003).

Through its Leapfrog coalition, the business sector continued to advocate the use of CPOE as a solution to the problem of medical errors, and leading informatics institutions, including the Vanderbilt Center for Better Health and the Oregon Health & Science University (JAMIA), hosted summits on CPOE implementation issues.

According to an article in the *Annals of Internal Medicine* (Kuperman and Gibson 2003), CPOE is "a relatively new technology and there is no consensus on the best approaches to many of the challenges it presents." The authors reviewed the growing body of research documenting the benefits CPOE can provide because it "fundamentally changes the ordering process." Thus, the costs are "substantial both in terms of technology and organizational process analysis and redesign, system implementation, and user training and support."

2.1. Lessons from Two Institutions

The experiences of two institutions that attempted, almost a decade apart, to implement CPOE underscore the risks involved in such undertakings. We relate them here for the lessons they teach us about human factors and managing change.

2.1.1. Brigham and Women's Hospital

More than a decade ago, in 1991 and 1992, Partners HealthCare developed one of the first computerized order entry systems at Brigham and Women's Hospital. By 1993, two pilots of the system had been conducted; physicians reported a number of problems, nurses fewer. Their input formed the basis for modifications to the interface and some data constructs (Teich et al. 1993). Initially, the system met with heavy opposition, according to Steve Flammini, the chief technology officer for Partners HealthCare, and "it took until 1996 to outfit the hospital with order entry and develop downstream processes" (Briggs 2003) Since then, Partners HealthCare has extended the system to Massachusetts General Hospital and Dana Farber Institute. In November 2002, it implemented a web-browser–based order entry system for its neonatal intensive care unit, where dosages are based on a baby's weight require complicated computations.

From the outset, the development team at Brigham and Women's Hospital acknowledged the problems inherent in "a radical cultural change" such as CPOE and took measures calculated to lessen resistance. A physician served as chief designer for the in-house system; the pilot systems elicited clinician input; and phased implementation allowed for process development. "At the end of the day," according to Flammini, "we smothered them with support. . . . We had knowledgeable, pleasant people available to hold their hand and get them through implementation. After six months, things settled down." And this support was available around the clock on the floors where clinicians worked. Above all, the Brigham and Women's Hospital and Partners HealthCare team did not consider order entry to be a technology solution: "It has to be a clinical initiative with an IT component" (Briggs 2003).

The Brigham and Women's Hospital initiative succeeded at a time when IT was "not that prevalent in medical schools, or even everyday consumer activity" (Briggs 2003). Given the changes in the IT landscape that have occurred since the mid-1990s, implementers today do not face the same obstacles, but there are other barriers to success.

2.1.2. Cedars-Sinai Medical Center

In October 2002, Cedars-Sinai Medical Center in Los Angeles rolled out the CPOE system it had developed in-house to support medical decision making (Wang et al. 2002). What happened next was not according to plan, and it happened remarkably quickly. A small group of physicians, primarily internists, protested the decision to make certification in CPOE mandatory. They also requested a medical staff meeting, where they expressed their "anger and frustration" that entering orders took longer with CPOE than with the previous method. In response to this physician resistance, Cedars-Sinai Medical Center turned the system off and went back to manual ordering by the end of January 2003 (Hagland 2003).

The experience at Cedars-Sinai Medical Center may seem a simple failure to address human factors, specifically, physician acceptance. The reality is more complex. First, the system was developed using a clinical rules taxonomy expressly to facilitate physician acceptance and approval (Wang et al. 2002). Second, the decision to make certification mandatory was made by the physician-led medical executive committee, not the administration, and fully 95% of the medical staff had been certified by October. Third, the state of California has mandated that all California hospitals have CPOE implemented by January 2005, meaning that Cedars-Sinai Medical Center will have to accept CPOE in less than two years. Their information officer was optimistic that the institution can learn from its first aborted implementation.

It is difficult to determine with certainty what lay at the heart of physician resistance at Cedars-Sinai Medical Center. It may have resulted from a lack of user ownership, perhaps compounded by communications deficiencies—factors repeatedly observed by Lorenzi and Riley as causes of implementation failure (2000, 2002).

The fact that the protesters were mostly internists may suggest that they were not included as a group during the planning process, or that Cedars-Sinai Medical Center and possibly even the internists themselves underestimated the impact of the system on their work flow. As primary care physicians, they treat a wider range of conditions than specialists (Hagland 2003) and therefore need more support when CPOE is introduced. The concern over the length of time to enter orders is often voiced by physicians (Ash, Stavri, Dykstra et al. 2003). Studies suggest that lost time spent may be recovered (Bates et al. 1994; Shu et al. 2001); better still, experienced users may become time-neutral (Overhage et al. 2001), taking no more time with CPOE than with paper-based processes.

3. Clinician Acceptance

Physician acceptance is only part of the human factors equation. Any clinical system, including CPOE, affects other hospital constitutencies, including "nursing staff, ward assistants, pharmacists, and staff in the laboratory and radiology departments" (Kuperman and Gibson 2003). Nurses in particular can be significantly affected by changes in clinical workflow. At one institution, their roles "as an integrator (or coordinator) of care and as a reviewer (or checker/editor) of orders" were significantly reduced. Although this freed up time for direct patient care, the nurses expressed dissatisfaction with their changed roles (Lorenzi et al. 1995). In addition, a 1996 study at Brigham and Women's Hospital of the CPOE system we discussed earlier found nurses less satisfied than staff physicians ($n = 200$ in each group). Using a scale of 1 to 7, with items assessing perceptions of the system's effect on productivity, ease of use, and speed, nurses ranked the system at 4.84 compared with 5.55 for medical house officers and 4.45 for surgical house officers (Lee et al. 1996).

In another implementation, this one of e-prescribing across an integrated health system with multiple sites and diverse legacy systems, one physician noted, "diffusion is slow, and technology is probably the least important reason among several. . . . E-prescribing is really the tip of the iceberg of knowledge-based medication management" (Hagland 2003).

According to a 2003 survey, physician resistance remains a concern. According to the Health Information Management and Systems Society (HIMSS), 45% of 247 senior executives and managers surveyed cited physician resistance as a "top barrier" to information technology implementation (iHealthBeat 2003b). (Also of interest: 43% found the technology immature and 79% cited budgetary issues.)

This continued focus on physician resistance is questionable. "Historically, people have looked at doctors' adoption of institutional technologies such as electronic medical records and e-prescribing and have been somewhat critical of them because they were not aggressive adopters. But most of the information technology that has been put forward to doctors over the last 20 years has been designed to improve the rest of the health care system a little bit at the expense of the doctor," said a Forrester analyst, who stated that the evidence shows physicians do adopt technology when it has "a clear business value" (Chin 2003).

According to Barry Chaiken, a physician who is vice president at a major software vendor, physicians are accustomed now to using a range of information tools, such as "a PDA [personal digital assistant], or a Blackberry with e-mail on it, or a slate, or a desktop. They see these tools as a part of their lives" (Hagland 2003).

TABLE 6.2. Physician and consumer adoption of technology.

Technology adoption	Physicians	Other consumers
Own any kind of mobile phone	88%	64%
Own any personal digital assistant	40%	8%
Have computer at home	88%	58%
Have broadband access at home	40%	23%
Use computer at or for work	88%	47%
Have broadband connection at work	43%	26%
Connect to the Internet from work	77%	41%
Online at least once a month	88%	64%

Source: Forrester Research, as reported by Chin (2003).

Two surveys published in September 2003 provide the evidence for this assertion. In one, Forrester Research reported that physicians are adopting technology tools at a "significantly higher rate" than the general public. Compared to other consumers, they are heavier users of computers at or for work and are five times more likely to own personal digital assistants (see Table 6.2). In a second study, conducted by PricewaterhouseCoopers, almost 8 out of 10 physician executives reported that doctors in their groups (median group size = 14 physicians) have high-speed Internet access in the office and were increasingly using it to read medical literature and to communicate with other physicians (see Table 6.3).

The fact that physicians are avid technology adopters bodes well for transformational efforts in health care. According to Brent James, a physician at Inter Mountain Healthcare in Salt Lake City and spokesman for the Institute of Medicine, "we're past the tipping point." He and a colleague listed 50 group practices using electronic medical records (EMRs), while "three years ago, we'd have been luck to have named five" (Chin 2003).

Nonetheless, technology adoption does not in itself ensure system acceptance. Other factors come into play. One of these involves cognitive issues in presenting knowledge in understandable ways. The value that the cognitive sciences bring to healthcare informatics is now being recognized, and meaningful work is being done in this area. For example, one study of two CPOE systems found user satisfaction correlated with the ability to perform tasks in a "straight-forward manner" (Murff and Kannry 2001). Such issues are indisputably significant and merit mention here; however, they fall outside the arena of behavioral issues addressed in this chapter.

In Chapter 2 of this book, Rob Kolodner spoke of the environmental characteristics that make it possible for transformation to occur and asserted that we are indeed at a moment of opportunity. And the HealthePeople concept is being implemented in an environment that is past the tipping point. According to the August 12, 2003, issue of iHealthBeat, the VA had "surpassed the private healthcare sector in terms of clinical

TABLE 6.3. Physician access to the Internet at group practice offices.

Internet access at office	
High-speed	80.0%
Dial-up	18.0%
No connection	2.1%

Source: HealthBeat (2003c).

IT adoption" and anticipated having 95% of all medication orders entered electronically by October 1, 2003 (iHealthBeat 2003a).

Earlier, in July 2002, Stephen Ross, a physician at the University of Colorado Health Sciences Center, stated that "I think they [the VA] will have a big impact in moving this forward. . . . The VA works with many teaching hospitals, and the program could familiarize more physicians with online records" (Chin 2003b). In fact, almost every medical student in the country rotates through a VA facility at some point during training. The weight of their VA experience—specifically with HealthePeople—will help to transform health care.

4. Mapping to the Tipping Point

In *The Tipping Point: How Little Things Make a Big Difference*, Malcolm Gladwell explains that "a number of relatively minor changes in our external environment can have a dramatic effect on how we behave and who we are. . . . That is the paradox of the epidemic: that in order to create one contagious movement, you often have to create many small movements first" (Gladwell 2000, p 182, 192).

As elaborated by Gladwell, three rules govern the creation of what he calls a social epidemic. Three laws affect the behavioral arena occupied by people and organizational issues: the Law of the Few, the Stickiness Factor, and the Power of Context.

In explaining the Law of the Few, Gladwell asserts that "the success of any kind of social epidemic is heavily dependent on the involvement of people with a particular and rare set of social gifts" and describes three specific types:

- Connectors know everybody and link up individuals whose needs and interests coincide.
- Mavens know everything about particular topic and share it with whoever wants to learn about it.
- Salesmen know how to communicate to others why a particular product or concept serves their needs. (Gladwell 2000, p 98)

This law is echoed in the taxonomy of Special People developed by Joan Ash and colleagues using data from interviews and field notes gathered in their study of successful CPOE implementations. Their taxonomy includes "administrative leaders, clinical leaders (champions, opinion leaders, and curmudgeons), and bridgers or support staff who interface directly with users." Ash and colleagues further conclude that "the recognition and nurturing of Special People should be among the highest priorities" for implementation (Ash et al. 2003, p 235).

Gladwell's second law, the Stickiness Factor, straddles the areas addressed by the cognitive and behavioral sciences. Gladwell holds that "there is a simple way to package information that, under the right circumstances, can make it irresistible. All you have to do is find it" (2000, p 132); "is the message—or the food, or the movie, or the product—memorable? Is it so memorable, in fact, that it can create change, that it can spur someone to action?" (2000, p 92). How information is structured and presented affects acceptance. For example, physicians appreciate being alerted to medication errors or drug allergies, but resent what they consider excessive interruptions and intrusions into the clinical decision making process.

The third law, the Power of Context, addresses how a social epidemic plays out. Gladwell asserts that context matters, that people behave differently in different settings, and cites evidence from research studies to support his assertion. In his judgment, "if you wanted to bring about a fundamental change in people's belief and behavior, a change that would persist and serve as an example to others, you needed to create a community around them, where those new beliefs could be practiced and expressed and nurtured" (2000, p 173).

For person-centered health systems to succeed, we need to create a community of practice that serves as an example. Today, we are seeing such communities created in many different places. Like outbreaks in an epidemic, there are small movements everywhere—in health systems, hospitals, and physician offices. In the town of Winona, Minnesota, Cerner Corporation is helping consumers link to their doctors and giving physicians electronic medical records (Chin 2002).

As more and more such projects surface and succeed, they bring the healthcare environment closer to the tipping point. With the help of Special People (connectors, mavens, and salesmen) and with the Stickiness Factor in play, we can successfully "get everybody on the same wavelength and introduce more common behaviors in the market," as Donald Berwick, of the Institute for Healthcare Improvement in Boston, hopes (Hagland 2003).

In all such efforts, there is complex interplay between information technology and the humans who use it. Now more than ever we must heed Postman's admonitions, all of which underscore the importance of human factors:

First, technology is not a neutral element in the practice of medicine: doctors do not merely use technologies but are used by them. Second, technology creates its own imperatives and, at the same time, creates a wide-ranging social system to reinforce its imperatives. And third, technology changes the practice of medicine by redefining what doctors are, redirecting where they focus their attention, and reconceptualizing how they view their patients and illness. (Postman 1992, p 105)

By mastering IT and the tools it provides, we can transform health care. Today, as we stand at the tipping point, we hold the power to fulfill the vision of HealthePeople.

Calling Attention to Human Factors

In 1993, Lorenzi organized a working conference under the auspices of the International Medical Informatics Association (IMIA). The meeting brought together, for the first time, individuals interested in the people and organizational issues of computer use in medicine. Following that meeting, IMIA approved a formal working group on the topic, and other related groups were established by medical and informatics associations in America, Europe, and Australia. All had as their charge "some variation of the following theme—applying knowledge of human behaviors to the implementation of informatics in a health care environment" (Lorenzi 1999). Under Lorenzi's leadership, the international and American groups launched a four-phase diffusion strategy.

The first two phases stressed building awareness about the topic and educating people about human factors research from other disciplines. The series of publications designed to achieve these goals began with *Organizational Aspects of Health Informatics: Managing Technological Change* (Lorenzi and Riley 1995); more books, articles, and conference presentations followed. In an article entitles "Antecedents of the People and Organizational Aspects of Medical Informatics: Review of the Literature" (1997), Lorenzi and an international team evaluated 156 publications to identify core knowledge from a wide range of fields and highlight implications for informatics.

The second two phases of diffusion were identified as applying established methods and models from other disciplines to medical informatics and, finally, developing new research methods and models specific to medical informatics. The working groups are actively encouraging activities in these areas, but "research in the area of human factors is just beginning to be applied to health care" (Institute of Medicine 2000, p 63).

Acknowledgment. In acknowledgement of their seminal work, we dedicate this chapter to Dr. Robert Riley and Dr. Nancy Lorenzi. Together, they led the health informatics community to appreciate the importance of human factors. The understanding they brought to us makes the transformation of healthcare systems possible, here in the United States and worldwide. We thank them for their insistence on a basic truth: People make things happen; technology is only the enabler.

References

Ash JS, Stavri PZ, Dykstra R, Fournier L. 2003. Implementing cmputerized physician order entry: the importance of special people. Int J Med Inf 69(2–3):235–250.

Ball MJ, Douglas JV. 2002. Redefining and improving patient safety. Methods Inf Med 41:271–276.

Bates DW, Boyle DL, Teich JM. 1994. Impact of computerized physician order entry on physician time. Proc Annu Symp Comput Appl Med Care 1994;996.

Briggs B. 2003 (February). CPOE: order from chaos. Health Data Management. Available from: http://www.healthdatamanagement.com. Accessed 2003 Aug 23. Stamford, CT: Thomson Media.

Chin T. 2002. The Winona project: developing an electronic link. AMNews. Available from: http://www.ama-assn.org/amednews/2002/03/11/bisa0311.htm. Accessed 2004 Jan 8.

Chin T. 2003. Doctors outpace consumers in embracing e-technologies. AMNews. http://www.ama-assn.org/sci-pubs/amnews. Accessed 2003 Oct 2. Chicago, IL: American Medical Association.

Gardner R. 1998. Davies keynote lecture. Proceedings of the Computer-Based Patient Record Institute Conference. Washington, DC: CPRI.

Gladwell M. 2000. The tipping point: how little things can make a big difference. Boston: Little, Brown and Company.

Greenes RA, Lorenzi NM. 1998. Audacious goals for health and biomedical informatics in the new millennium. J Ame Med Inform Assoc 5(5):395–400.

Hagland M. 2003. Reduced errors ahead. Healthcare Informatics. Available from: http://www.healthcare-informatics.com. Accessed 2003 Aug 28. Minneapolis, MN: McGraw-Hill.

Health Data Management. 2003. Report: CPOE market growing. Available from: http://www.healthdatamanagement.com. Accessed 2003 Aug 28.

iHealthBeat. 2003a. VA leads the pack in IT adoption. iHealthBeat: Reporting the Internet's Impact on Health Care. Available from: http://ihealthbeat.org. Accessed 2003 Aug 13. Washington, DC: The California Health Care Foundation.

iHealthBeat. 2003b. Doctors adopt certain technologies faster than consumers, survey finds. iHealthBeat: Reporting the Internet's Impact on Health Care. Vailable from: http://ihealthbeat.org. Accessed 2003 Sept 29.

iHealthBeat. 2003c. More physicians have high-speed Internet access. iHealthBeat: Reporting the Internet's Impact on Health Care. Available from: http://ihealthbeat.org. Accessed 2003 Sept 30.

Institute of Medicine. 1997. The computer-based patient record: an essential technology for health care, rev ed. Washington, DC: National Academy Press.

Institute of Medicine. 2000. To err is human: building a safer health system. Washington, DC: National Academy Press.

Institute of Medicine. 2001. Crossing the quality chasm: a new health system for the 21st century. Washington, DC: National Academy Press.

Kuperman GJ, Gibson RF. 2003. Computer physician order entry: benefits, costs, and issues. Ann Int Med 139(1):31–39.

Lee F, Teich JM, Spurr CD, Bates DW. 1996. Implementation of physician order entry: user satisfaction and self-reported usage patterns. J Am Med Inform Assoc 3:42 Institute of Medicine. 2000. To Err Is Human: Building a Safer Health System. Washington, DC: National Academy Press. 55.

Lorenzi NM. 2000. The Cornerstones of medical informatics. J Am Med Inform Assoc 7(2):204.

Lorenzi NM. 1999. IMIA Working Group 13: organizational impact of medical informatics. Int Med Inform 56(1–3):5–8.

Lorenzi NM, Riley RT. 2000. Managing change: an overview. J Am Med Inform Assoc 7(2):116–124.

Lorenzi NM, Riley RT. 1995. Organizational aspects of health informatics: managing technological change. New York: Springer-Verlag.

Lorenzi NM, Riley RT. 2002. Organizational aspects of implementing informatics change. In: Dewan NA, Lorenzi NM, Riley RT, Bhattacharya SR, editors. Behavioral healthcare informatics. New York: Springer-Verlag. p 156–170.

Lorenzi M, Riley R, Ball M, Douglas J. 1995. Involving health care professionals in technological change. Comments on case 9.1: Williams Memorial Hospital—nursing unit computerization, by Horak B & Turner M. In: Lorenzi M, Riley R, Ball M, Douglas J, editors. Transforming health care through information. New York: Springer-Verlag. P 233–246.

Lorenzi NM, Riley RT, Blyth AJC, Southon G, Dixon BJ. 1997. Antecedents of the people and organizational aspects of medical informatics: review of the literature. J Am Med Inform Assoc 4(2):79–93.

Mobile Health Data. 2003. If docs fear change, why do they marry? Press release dated 2003 Sept 8. Available from: http://www.mobilehealthdata.com

Murff HJ, Kannry. 2001. Physician satisfaction with two order entry systems. J Am Med Inform Assoc 8:499–509.

Overhage JM, Perkins S. Tierney WM, McDonald CJ. 2001. Controlled trial of direct physician order entry: effects on physicians' time utilization in ambulatory primary care internal medicine practice. J Am Med Inform Assoc 8:361–371.

Postman N. 1992. Technopoly: the surrender of culture to technology. New York: Alfred A. Knopf.

Shu K, Boyle D, Spurr C, Horsky J, Heiman H, O'Connor P, Lepore J, Bates DW. 2001. Comparison of time spent writing orders on paper with computerized physician order entry. Medinfo 2001;10:1207–1211.

Stead WW, Lorenzi NM. 1999. Health informatics: linking investment to value. J Am Med Inform Assoc 6(5):341–348.

Teich JM, Spurr CD, Flammini SJ, Schmiz J, Beckley RF, Hurley JF, Aranow M, Glaser JP. 1993. Response to a trial of physician-based inpatient order entry. Proc Annu Symp Appl Med Care 1993;316–320.

Vanderbilt Center for Better Health. 2002. CPOE Summit: capitalizing on the opportunity. Available from: http://www.mc.vanderbilt.edu/vcbh/summit. Accessed 2003 Oct 4.

Section 2
Building the Future: Essential Technologies and Methodologies

7
Laying the Foundations: Information Architecture for Health*e*People

James E. Demetriades

There is an endless variety of ways to implement a set of system requirements. We can approach Health*e*People in a traditional way and choose from a wide array of system designs. With diligence and effort, almost any design we select will meet surface requirements. But a more thoughtful look exposes a system that is anything but ordinary.

In the first section of this book, Kolodner, Christopherson, and others describe an uncommon opportunity to profoundly transform individual lives and community health. *If* it were somehow possible to design a system that in and of itself behaved as a transformational information system, then Health*e*People the health system *and* Health*e*People the information system taken together could leap beyond simply "punching the ticket." The approach could trigger a multiplier effect, shaping and then tipping the whole health delivery system, transforming it for the better. This is no ordinary opportunity.

Producing transformational systems is anything but traditional. These systems are not yet well understood or defined. There are no popular cookbook designs or industry standard methodologies for constructing them. Most transformational systems have come about by accident, not by the hand of man.

Fortunately, our knowledge of them is growing. Careful retrospective examinations have begun to identify qualities common to information systems that produce transformations.

Perhaps the most striking example is the World Wide Web. Clearly it has profoundly transformed our culture and done so with an utterly simple architecture comprised of just three technologies: IP, HTTP, and HTML. (That these technologies are recognized by their acronyms alone speaks to their pervasive acceptance; most Word Wide Web users are hard pressed to come up with their full names: Internet Protocol, Hypertext Transfer Protocol, and Hypertext Markup Language.)

Interestingly, the World Wide Web falls into a larger and better defined group called *complex adaptive systems*. Not limited to information systems, this group includes systems found throughout nature and everyday life. In areas as diverse as biology, economics, and astronomy, these systems share common patterns known to produce transformational behaviors.

We believe it possible to engineer into Health*e*People many of the desired principles and properties of complex adaptive systems. By deliberately not launching from today's requirements and technology but rather first laying a foundation of core principles, behaviors, and goals, we can maximize the value of Health*e*People. By thoughtfully balancing between new possibilities and best-of-breed traditional information architecture practices, we can craft a bold yet sensible approach.

Traditional and not-so-traditional designs and guidelines offer opposing choices. These can be viewed as a series of paradoxes or as paired issues that can severely tip the outcome of the system design. Tension between such concerns forms a turbulent mix. Stability–adaptability, uniqueness–universality, cooperation–competition, control–freedom, and homogeneity–heterogeneity all require trade-offs, not only within the pairing but also across pairings. If that is not enough, these paradoxes must all be considered simultaneously, not sequentially. To realize the full potential of HealthePeople, we must make wise system design choices early using novel approaches. We must at once deal with existing environmental constraints and a high degree of future uncertainty.

1. Architecture

Architecture serves as a language that allows individuals or communities to share an understanding of significant system components and their interrelationships. This is important for all but the most trivial of systems. The builders of the biblical Tower of Babel would have profited from good architecture.

The Software Engineering Institute defined systems architecture as the "structure of the components of a program/system, their interrelationships, and principles and guidelines governing their design and evolution over time" (Clements and Northrop 1996). The phrase *over time* is significant. Architecture needs to be more than the decomposition of a system into static viewpoints. HealthePeople's information architecture involves critical elements such as temporal considerations and abstract concepts such as principles. By describing component interrelationships and system processes capable of adapting over time, a healthier, more transparent architecture can evolve.

2. Goals

Above all else, formulation of the overall architecture and of required components within it—in other words, virtually all aspects of system activities—requires faithfulness to goals. For the person-centric health systems envisioned in the opening section of this book, there are five goals:

- individual empowerment;
- longitudinal composite health record;
- record accessibility;
- security and privacy of information and data;
- interoperability of records with shared semantic meaning.

2.1. Individual Empowerment

The goal of empowering individuals to manage their health information and data easily outdistances all other goals. Giving individuals the means to advocate for their own personal health or that of their dependants has dramatic implications for sustainable architectural design. As a goal, it gives rise to and is intertwined with other key goals for HealthePeople.

2.2. Longitudinal Composite Health Record

Empowering individuals requires life-long records of health-related information and data like that provided by electronic health records (EHRs) and personal health records (PHRs). Although the promise of such records is widely appreciated, there is limited understanding of their scope, attributes and behaviors, and their architectures. These remain volatile and are often passionately discussed within various shareholder communities.

2.3. Record Accessibility

The ability to access and contribute to their own health records allows individuals to become full partners with their care providers in fighting disease and fostering wellness. Such partnerships are strengthened by the ability of the individuals to grant record access to others as well, including multiple healthcare professionals, providers of other health-related services, and family and friends who support them in their care.

2.4. Security and Privacy of Information and Data

Accessibility intensifies the challenge to protect the security and privacy of health records. Cultural expectations change over time, but our laws, policies, and public attitudes are clear: Health information and data must be maintained with a high level of security and a pervasive respect for privacy. The intrinsic tension between record accessibility and security/privacy poses numerous architectural quandaries for person-centered health records. Recent advances in security standards and technology will aid in resolving these as we implement Health*e*People.

2.5. Interoperability of Records with Shared Semantic Meaning

Despite its massive economic scale and pervasiveness, health care has operated as a cottage industry for the past century. The traditional health record, whether paper or electronic, continues in virtually every case to be unique to the record keeper—what information architects call "organized and populated in native 'one-off' implementations." Over the last decade, we have seen considerable advances in the syntatic exchange of data. The challenge today is to ensure that multiple computers can read and semantically understand the data—that a medical term means the same thing in one system as it does in another.

These five goals collectively represent Health*e*People's first design consideration. They form the basis of a broader "fitness function" used to test the worthiness of the initial architectural design and all successor implementations. Each tangible design decision made in the production of Health*e*People is guided by the goals. The ability to trace back to these core drivers is essential and surpasses any detailed requirements specification. True system value requires fidelity of architectural design to the goals it serves.

3. Environment

A crucial consideration for any system is the environment in which it will be immersed. Health*e*People does not enjoy a clean-slate deployment. The as-is environment forms the starting point from which the system is cast. Recognizing and allowing for initial conditions are necessary for early survival. Accounting for both hostile and supportive elements to which the system will be exposed allows the architecture to better undergo early adaptation.

To minimize unnecessary risk, HealthePeople has avoided approaching its design from a clean-slate perspective in ignorance or defiance of environmental conditions. At best, this kind of blindness unduly stresses early deployment. Such an architectural approach is also prone to exhibit inherent built-in rigidity with blind design biases and lack of adaptability that position it for almost certain collapse.

3.1. Massive Scale

HealthePeople has immeasurable potential to grow in scale. Given the universal appeal of individual empowerment and the innate regard individuals have for their health, this architecture must thrive in an environment of massive scale. The expectation of health record accessibility and interoperability between individuals, caregivers, providers, and third-party institutions point to proportions of the same order of magnitude as the Internet. Indeed, closer examination reveals that the initial conditions calling for interoperability on a massive scale may be even greater than first expected.

Three communication laws help understand the potential pervasiveness of Healthe People and the architectural abilities it may require to succeed. The first, Sarnoff's Law, dates from the early days of radio and television, when David Sarnoff recognized that networks grow linearly with the number of recipients in a publishing or broadcasting environment. In the new HealthePeople environment, if an individual wanted to publish his health record for providers to have access to it, the value of the network would grow linearly with the number of providers (n) that can be reached on the network. More recently, Metcalfe's Law was formulated by the chief inventor of the Internet, Bob Metcalfe, who observed that a communications network grows with the square of the number (n^2) of nodes (people or devices) it connects. This was the case with Internet e-mail, and will be the case with HealthePeople, as it provides for two-way exchanges of information, such as requesting and receiving health appointments or ordering laboratory tests and receiving results. Designing for n^2 numbers begins to call into question the viability of centralized architectures and control structures such as master person indexes, yet the numbers do not stop here.

A third law is relevant and compelling in our design because we anticipate that HealthePeople will follow patterns similar to those now found on the Internet where collaborations have emerged. Known as Reed's Law, it identifies such "group-forming networks" and mathematically describes this growth potential as exponential (2^n) with respect to the number of persons communicating (Reed 1999). These community-forming networks often involve transactions among multiple combinations of groups of two and three. It is easy to imagine a HealthePeople environment where individuals engage communities of two and three to participate in health matters, such as third-party transactions or discussions with personal support groups or primary providers and specialists.

As a community environment, HealthePeople's design purposefully enables the ability of people to form new associations. The value of associations as "social capital" was recognized early in the 20th century. Much more recently, Francis Fukuyama (1995) described social capital to be "the ease in which people in a culture can form new associations." HealthePeople is engineered to foster this degree of connectedness. Robert Putnam (2000) underscores its importance in health care: "Of all the domains in which I have traced the consequences of social capital, in none is the importance of social connectedness so well established as in the case of health and well-being." Transformational efforts, like that envisioned in HealthePeople, cannot succeed without social capital. It is a highly desired emergent property of the new environment, and is accommodated and enabled by the architecture.

3.2. Functional Diversity

In the HealthePeople environment, system diversity is driven by the need to include a variety of functional capabilities. Not every node or end system within the larger HealthePeople system has or needs identical functional capabilities. A system for an individual will differ from a system for a family physician's office or a health provider institution or a commercial laboratory. One size does not fit all.

According to the Institute of Medicine (2003), there are four key settings for EHR systems: hospital, ambulatory care, nursing home, and care in community. And there are other settings, for example, home health agencies, pharmacies, and dental care. In these multiple settings, primary uses for EHRs include care delivery, care management, care support processes, financial and other administrative processes, and patient self-management. Recognition of these diverse functional settings has influenced HealthePeople to incorporate designs that support large numbers of systems that can have unique local interactions yet still interoperate.

Another aspect to functional diversity is maturity variation. Across like organizations, the maturity of information systems varies widely. For example, two long-term care facilities on the same platform with the same technical capabilities and same software application can differ widely. One may be running version 2, while the other uses version 4.5. Such variations characterize the HealthePeople environment now and will do so indefinitely. Even as the system evolves, different members will have varying abilities and/or motivations to obtain the most functionally rich or mature system attainable at any given time.

The functional needs of users are also diverse. At no time do all users have the same needs; over time, any one user's needs can be expected to change. Diversity exists even within a like-class of user. One architectural assumption should be made about the presence and use of specific functionality: both will be highly diverse in direct correlation to user needs.

3.3. System Diversity

A single healthcare institution or a small partnership can exert total control over its technical environment and specify detailed, uniform, technical platforms, often with significant gains in efficiency, performance, and simplicity. But large healthcare institutions and organizations [like the U.S. Department of Veterans Affairs (VA)] accept that multiple different systems can be in place at any given moment in time. In their view, tight system specifications in large settings are unrealistic, and therefore unacceptable. The HealthePeople philosophy does not embrace monolithic technology design, regardless of any niche features that may be attractive. The undeniable forces of evolutionary dynamics have influenced the design to be open and adaptive.

3.4. Loose Coupling

The massive scale of the HealthePeople community rules out any realistic opportunity for tightly coupled systems architecture. Its scale prohibits the use of command-and-control architecture and renders lock-step deployments of new functionality, technology, and design configurations far too complex to achieve. The distributed architecture reflects this. By design, the HealthePeople environment is and will remain loosely coupled.

Massive scale, functional and system diversity, and loose coupling—all are elements in the environment in which the HealthePeople system will function, and all require full consideration in framing the architecture.

4. Composition

As new technologies emerge and biomedicine translates genomics into patient care, HealthePeople will evolve to incorporate new domains like proteomics, nanotechnology, and neuroprostheses. The final composition of HealthePeople will not be set until its system life-cycle comes to closure.

Fortunately, we can see compositional components for the near future more clearly. Four elements are key: health records, content transport, semantic translation, and security. The HealthePeople architecture is sensitive to all four and capable of responding to them.

4.1. Health Records

Chief among the system's software components are health records, including both PHRs and EHRs. In the summer of 2003, definition of the health record and its functions witnessed intense activity and appeared close to a tipping point.

In one of the most promising efforts, the standards development organization known as Health Level Seven (HL7) is developing a functional model and standards for an EHR (Dickenson et al. 2003). With unprecedented participation from the broader health community, HL7 has incorporated the functionalities identified by the Institute of Medicine into the model. These include health information and data, results management, order entry/management, decision support, electronic communication and connectivity, patient support, administrative processes, reporting, and population health management (IOM 2003).

4.2. Content Transport

Because electronic communication and connectivity are core to HealthePeople, the network must be capable of moving health record content between systems that are both ubiquitous and diverse. In this role, individual EHRs function as health record nodes on a distributed information grid, serving as information appliances for the network. The grid then effects reliable secure transmission and receipt of entire health records, record segments, and transaction datagrams.

4.3. Semantic Translation

Simply delivering data payload is not enough; there must be shared meaning. Without an established terminology, there is only a string of characters forming free text and numbers, insufficient for decision support, research, or meaningful communication. As multiple EHRs interact across the grid, the data must be understood and computable.

The complexity of Western medicine and its historically insular documentation practices make shared meaning extraordinarily difficult. In his now classic Desiderata paper, James Cimino (1998) compiled a long list of medical vocabulary issues that impact the usability of health record content:

vocabulary content, concept orientation, concept permanence, nonsemantic concept identifiers, polyhierarchy, formal definitions, rejection of "not elsewhere classified" terms, multiple granularities, multiple consistent views, context representation, graceful evolution, and recognized redundancy.

Software design can also challenge shared meaning. One large healthcare organization found they had 30 different ways of computationally "getting to yes" (Brown 2003). Such designs clearly impact computer–computer interaction and possibly human–computer interaction as well. The resulting tension between rigid control and no control, between order and chaos, is particularly evident in the area of communications. Thus, how the architecture addresses semantic requirements can have dramatic and long-term effects. Brown, Lincoln, and Elkin discuss terminology issues in more detail in Chapter 9.

4.4. Security

The designation of security as a key compositional element of HealthePeople is a direct reflection of our culture. Health data protection and privacy have leapt to prominence in recent years, making security a top priority for all health information systems. Protection against threats is more difficult when distributed systems are involved, because their design makes them more vulnerable to unauthorized access, data tampering, or other intrusions.

We are designing the HealthePeople architecture to provide strong security from the beginning. The design allows us to achieve the target security model and implement its overall security policy. Interoperability with and between end system security domains is essential to the provision of services such as user identification, role management, access control, authentication, integrity, and audit control. Davis and Blobel discuss security and security architecture considerations more thoroughly in Chapter 10.

The core components comprising the initial overarching design form the basis of a starting point for delivering sought after functionality. HealthePeople's ability to deliver on this need can be characterized by a fitness function, or the measure of its potential to perform expected functions in a given setting. Such fitness functions are used in genetic algorithms to iteratively optimize the ability of an agent to succeed. Paying close attention to system characteristics and drivers that have significant effects can improve architectural performance. Providing components the facility to optimize their performance over time delivers two-fold advantage: capability to iteratively improve on providing initial functionality and capability to adapt as functional needs evolve.

5. System Characteristics

Classifying HealthePeople in terms of system type can help introduce a more complete set of design characteristics that we can leverage in establishing the initial architecture. The identification of desirable fitness signatures will aid in making choices as unanticipated events and opportunities arise far in the future.

According to Maier (1998), four characteristics distinguish true "system of systems" from very large, complex monolithic systems:

- **Operational independence of the elements.** This is the ability of an end system, for example, in a medical center, to "usefully operate independently."
- **Managerial independence from the elements.** The end system not only *can* operate independently from the overall system, it does.

- **Capacity for evolutionary development.** The overall system "does not appear fully formed. Its development and existence is evolutionary with functions and purposes added, removed, and modified with experience."
- **Emergent behavior.** The overall system "performs functions and carries out purposes that do not reside in any component system."

HealthePeople has the characteristics Maier describes, clearly distinguishing it as a system-of-systems: End systems operate independently and are managed independently; the overall system continuously evolves and supports emergent functions like community forming networks.

The type and extent of central management further defines systems (Maier 1998). In directed systems, it focuses on the specific purpose the system was built and is intended to perform. In collaborative systems, it relies on participants to collaborate voluntarily. In virtual systems, there is no central management authority. Instead, they rely on emergent behaviors similar to the swarming exhibited by bees, schools of fish, and other communities. At this point, we characterize HealthePeople as a collaborative system.

This has a strong impact on architectural design. We note, however, that the Internet, which Maier defines as a collaborative system, was developed almost three decades ago as a directed system in the Defense Department. Today, it has possesses elements of a virtual system. Over the long term, the same may be true for HealthePeople.

6. Future Proofing

In designing HealthePeople, we are also identifying architectural principles and designs that we hope will extend the system's life expectancy and prevent or delay its obsolescence—what some information architects have called *future proofing*.

In the information age, technology virtually always changes more rapidly than business requirements, making technology platforms obsolete long before the functional capabilities of the system. One of the ways to future proof is to use architectural designs that separate technology from the system it serves.

In one such model, Beale advocates using "archetypes" to maintain technology separation (Beale 2001a; Beale et al. 2001). Currently, most systems unify both information and knowledge within a single-level design. In Beale's approach, a two-level methodology is established that effectively de-couples the business domain from technology. The physical system design uses formal information models that are partitioned from content and functionality until run-time. As a direct and immediate benefit, this approach empowers health professionals, also known as *domain experts*, to control content and functionality without the involvement of intermediaries. Information architects call this *health domain extensibility*. Similarly, information technology (IT) professionals are free to design and mature the technology base without being constrained by changes, or "refreshes," made by domain experts (Beale 2001a, 2001b; Beale et al. 2001).

In a second formal model, Mailla describes using technology neutral adaptors to interface software components. He outlines a structure and semantic approach for both sharing and invoking services. The result allows for technology insertion, migration, and application evolution while minimizing impacts on running code. This is accomplished by establishing an abstraction layer model that draws upon interface patterns cataloged by the United Nations Center for Trade Facilitation and Electronic Business (UN/CEFACT). Standardizing component interfaces in this manor greatly minimizes complexity and is ideal for supporting multiple technologies simultaneously and using single technology versioning as it matures (Mailla 2002).

A third model has a history that goes back to the early 1990s and is called the Common Object Request Broker Architecture (CORBA). After a promising start for the approach, its designers in the Object Management Group (OMG) found they needed to produce an ever-expanding set of explicit technology specifications. At the same time, demands for the global integration of multiple diverse systems distributed across supply chains intensified. In response, OMG introduced Model Driven Architecture (MDA); this architecture makes it possible to specify a system independent of the implementation platform. Because the system is not technology-specific, it provides for changes after implementation, including selecting and moving to another platform (Soley and the OMG Staff Strategy Group 2000; Miller and Murkerji 2003). For a detailed explanation of how models work, see Chapter 10.

All three approaches advocate technology independent design through formal architecture models. Separating the business model from the technology platform model allows systems to protect their future and their ability to evolve. Achieving this type of separation functions as a measure of fitness for the envisioned virtual system.

The incorporation of future proofing techniques into HealthePeople is more than a technology consideration. According to the United Nations (2003), a child born in most developed countries at the beginning of this century will have a life expectancy of 75 to 80 years—for example, 78.0 in Germany, 79.0 in Australia, and 81.3 in Japan. In the United States, where the life expectancy is 76.9 years, requirements are to preserve health records for 75 years following a person's death. HealthePeople needs to provide for very long-term individual record persistence while maintaining meaning and security.

Clearly, the architecture of HealthePeople must adapt over time to endure.

7. Recognizing Core Behaviors

A transformation of the scale envisioned in HealthePeople is more than just technological. When we contemplate its foundations, there are core behaviors we should avoid and respect.

7.1. Reductionism and Determinism Are Not Realistic or Effective

In the 17th century, Isaac Newton brilliantly brought together astronomy, geometry, and algebra into what was then called "natural philosophy," known today as Newtonian physics. The centerpiece of Newton's revelation was a law for gravity that applied to all forms of matter from apples to planets. Combined with general laws of motion, the result was a set of physical laws that could be used to mechanically describe and predict the natural behavior of all objects in a "clockwork universe."

For centuries now, an accepted view has been if one could simply reduce the components of a system to its smallest particles and determine their complete initial conditions then this process of *reductionism* and *determinism* would allow one to predict the systems behavior in advance. In essence people believed the world around us and even the entire universe could be explained with the precision of a machine by simply using a single set of laws.

This belief profoundly influenced industrial age thinking to the extent it worked its way into business practices, organizational structures, military operations, and more. The term "a well-oiled machine" is still used to describe our organizations and operations, when in reality, the spell of Newton is simply unrealistic for all situations. Governments, stock markets, the Internet, and large-scale software projects are examples of systems that do not obey these rules. For systems of this complexity, there is no evidence supporting the effectiveness of these methods. No amount of control, standardization, planning, or measurement will cause them to be predictable. Despite repeated attempts of institutions and individuals to control large complex systems by chopping the system up into small isolated parts, the result is virtually always unexpected outcome. Highly non-linear and unpredictable systems obey a different set of laws.

For a system as intricate as HealthePeople, it would be futile to attempt to envision every possible condition imaginable. Further, we cannot infer information system behavior by simply tallying up the behavior of all its individual components. The architecture is sensitive to this and does not use wholesale reductionism and determinism in its design approach.

7.2. Closed-Ended Requirements Are Risky and Futile in Adaptive Systems

The association between initial requirements and future needs is similar to initial conditions and subsequent outcomes. For complex systems, articulating all requirements in advance is as equally unrealistic as predicting future system behavior. Whether functional, technical, or operational, such closed-end requirements are not practical. We could not have expected the early designers of graphical user interfaces in 1975 at Xerox's Palo Alto Research Center to anticipate all the windowing capabilities now seen in personal computers.

Data collected by Capers Jones show information system requirements change at an average rate of 2% per month. The requirements for an average large-scale system change completely over the life of the development effort (McKeeman personal communication). Moreover, according to McKeeman, the likelihood of software system project failure increases with project size. This can help explain why big-bang projects almost always fail. HealthePeople is using an incremental open-ended requirements approach.

7.3. Separation of Concerns Can Be Highly Leveraged at a Suitable Level of Abstraction

Cautioning against comprehensive, highly detailed specifications does not imply that complex systems should not be structured or have guiding mechanisms. Selective structure at the right level of abstraction is highly desirable.

In contemporary software design, decomposing systems into components (also called objects or modules) is widely accepted as good practice. Componentization can greatly improve the adaptability of a system and shorten development time. When done properly, it allows multiple components to be written simultaneously without knowledge of the details of the others. Further, components can be replaced by more improved versions or newer technology without needing to reassemble the entire application.

In addition, decomposition can make software systems more comprehensible. This is not a new idea: It dates back to at least 1972, when Parnas proposed identifying software modules not from a flowchart, but from a list of difficult or volatile design decisions. To achieve implementation efficiency, he stated, the most challenging design decisions need to be hidden from other modules, effectively separating concerns (Parnas 1972).

Although modern software formalisms recognize the benefits of separating concerns, problems persist, making systems less comprehensible and limiting the re-use of components. In an attempt to realize "the full potential of 'separation of concerns'" envisioned by Parnas (1972), Ossher and Tarr (1999) developed a modified model that identifies and encapsulates multiple concerns. They hypothesized using only one dimension to separate concerns—"the tyranny of the dominant decomposition"—is a common failing of software design compromising the goals of software engineering. Health information systems often fall into this trap and frequently suffer from limited separation or, even worse, from no decomposition. When this happens, it is much more likely to occur on the level of systems design and big picture concerns.

Fortunately, models exist to fill this void in the big picture. For example, the Reference Model for Open Distributed Processing (RM-ODP) provides a powerful framework for specifying distributed systems. (International Organization for Standarization/International Electrotechnical Commission 1995) The model is optimized for diverse systems distributed across organizational and technology boundaries, which makes it ideal for HealthePeople. By specifying viewpoints, the reference model delineates five primary axes of concern. This formalism embodies the same concerns critical to the larger HealthePeople environment in which our systems will function. These viewpoints include:

- Enterprise: Purpose, scope, policies and roles of the specified system/service.
- Information: Information semantics and information processing.
- Computational: Interaction patterns between system components (services).
- Engineering: Infrastructure required to support distribution.
- Technology. Hardware and software provisioning to support infrastructure.

The ODP also defines eight transparency requirements: access, failure, location, migration, relocation, replication, persistence, and transaction. These requirements all directly result from systems distribution. The solution may either be worked out by individual application designers (a nearly impossible task for HealthePeople) or through standard mechanisms. The value here is the application designer may then work in an environment transparent to the identified concerns provided they conform to the model. One further benefit accrues by providing this formalism for system specification: the ODP model provides a base for subsequent conformance assessment.

7.4. HealthePeople Is a Complex System Composed of Locally Interacting Components

In a complex system that is composed of independent agents—technically speaking, system nodes—capable of self-directed internal change, there is no hierarchy controlling system activities. The system interactions are driven by multi-directional causality. The many independent interactions between a heterarchy of agents produce unpredictable behavior that does not follow the top-down causality.

In these systems, small change will sometimes produce major shifts in system behavior, while seemingly large change may not have any discernable effect. Further, the behavior of components can differ in the collective system than when in isolation, producing an effect where the sum is greater than the parts. Moreover, as agents within the system adapt over time, so too does the system's overall behavior. In terms of HealthePeople, this allows the many and diverse organizations within health care to adapt and evolve; their evolution, in turn, causes the overall system to transform. The net result is a co-evolutionary process woven into the fabric of the system. Behavior emerges from the system as a whole. Accordingly, our process architecture for HealthePeople does not attempt to micro-control agent behavior.

7.5. Principle-Driven Design Can Guide and Inform Design Decisions for the Long Term

Because closed-end requirements do not work for complex adaptive systems, we must work at a more abstract level, using principles as "anchors" or "beacons" to guide system design over extended timeframes. Combined with goals and fitness functions such as those discussed earlier in this chapter, principles form a powerful method to guide and test system evolution when the future is unknown. As new technologies emerge in biomedicine and information science, principles offer a valuable way of informing and guiding design choices.

8. System Principles

System principles are fundamental truths that clarify and enrich a system's constitution. They nurture a shared vision among stakeholders and are invaluable when the design process requires difficult decisions and presents conflicting choices.

For HealthePeople, we have identified six over-arching system principles. Each interacts with the others to strengthen our strategies as we implement and evolve our vision of a person-centered health system.

8.1. Good Enough

Neither the HealthePeople architecture nor its implementation design needs to be perfect. It is more important to have running code deployed that is "good enough." This principal principle is intended to keep focus on the overall goal, so we can deliver value to the individuals HealthePeople serves as soon as possible.

8.2. Complexity at the Edge

Borrowing from the concept known as "end-to-end argument" (Saltzer et al. 1984) that guided Internet development, this principle calls for simplifying core functionality by pushing application-level functions as far out to the system edge as possible—to those "independent agents" or "system nodes."

In the case of HealthePeople, these edge systems are serving the highly diverse needs of medical centers, clinics, nursing homes, and other varied facilities—potentially, even the local fitness club. Concentrating too many functions in the core at the outset will present needless problems. For example, edge applications that may not need a particular function will have to manage it and pay for it. Light-weight applications or less mature ones may not have as much ability as higher level systems to do the job effectively. To avoid these problems, complex or specialty functions should be moved outward, as close as possible to the application that uses those functions.

According to Clark and Blumenthal (2001), reducing core complexity increases the generality of the network, thereby improving the chances that new applications will be fitting and the network reliable. Thus, the end-to-end approach fosters innovation and the social and economic benefits that follow. Moreover, as Sowa (2002) observes, a flexible modular framework can be tailored to an open-ended variety of architectures for different kinds of applications while a fixed architecture can do no more than simulate a single aspect of what is possible. The modular framework approach embraces the same goals as Clark and Blumenthal promote. In this case complexity is distributed across modules, reducing concentration points. HealthePeople uses this to establish easier access to common functions and avoidance of contact with unneeded module functions.

8.3. Degeneracy

As defined by biologists, degeneracy is "the ability of elements that are structurally different to perform the same function or yield the same output" (Edelman and Gally 2001). It is a ubiquitous property found at all biological levels (genetic, cellular, system, and population), and it is both necessary for, and an inevitable outcome of, natural selection. For example, two different food groups can provide the same nutritional values, or two different types of neural connections can send the brain the same signal in what is called *synaptic plasticity*. Degeneracy differs fundamentally from redundancy, in which two systems capable of performing the same function are identical in structure.

Drawing a parallel from biological to information systems, we posit that degeneracy can be extremely useful in the evolution of HealthePeople. There is not, nor can there be, an a priori plan on how to respond to agent/system co-evolution. In these circumstances, degeneracy can introduce, facilitate, and enrich a kind of natural selection process. Consider, for example, cable modem, high-speed dial-up, and direct Internet gateway technology. Despite their differences, all provide connectivity to HealthePeople system nodes; all perform the same function. Supporting and encouraging this kind of degeneracy strengthens the HealthePeople design and support its vision.

8.4. Free Extension

Articulated by Berners-Lee (1998), the "weaver" of the World Wide Web, the Rule of Free Extension promotes a system behavior where a receiving agent ignores what is not understood. This approach permits fast independent and parallel development. Those receiving agents that can process the emerging or novel extensions can take full advantage without waiting for a standard to propagate throughout the system. In a large-scale system like HealthePeople, individual systems can take advantage of new capabilities if they are ready, or bypass them if they are not. This approach comes with a tradeoff: it also permits duplication, confusion, and some level of chaos until standards emerge. One of the Internet architecture principles set forth by Carpenter (1996) is similar: systems should be strict when sending and tolerant when receiving, effectively ignoring what is not understood.

8.5. Least Power

Our sixth and last system principle also comes from Berners-Lee (1998). In his "Principle of Least Power," he advocates selecting the technology or approach that possesses the least power and avoids unnecessary over-kill. In making his point, he focuses on software programming languages, citing simpler design, implementation, and use as motivation for selecting the least powerful language suitable for the job.

Berners-Lee reports that this approach provided a huge windfall in the case of HTML. He deliberately chose the design of the hypertext markup language to not to be a programming language. Had he done so, the additional programming commands would have restricted the range of operations possible on the text. By applying the least power principle to satisfy his requirements, any and all applications in receipt of HTML files have full latitude including doing previously unimagined things with the text. This is a good example of pushing complexity to the edge.

9. Software Design Principles

Five software design principles are guiding us in the development of HealthePeople. All of them map to concepts and principles discussed throughout this chapter, and all are focused on the users of the system. Each is crucial to the success of HealthePeople.

9.1. User-Centered Design

This first principle places the user at the center of the software system. In designing the system, the intent must be to help users rapidly understand the range of choices and means available to achieve their goals. To achieve this, the design should provide interfaces that mask the underlying workings of the system. It should also provide forgiving interfaces that impart a sense of control to the user.

The next three principles are adapted from a more extensive set of "First Principles" put forth by designer Bruce Tognazzini in his discussion of human interfaces (1998). All three involve the development of interfaces to support the user.

9.2. User Autonomy

The first of these three principles calls for the creation of user autonomy by putting the user in charge of their personal computing environment. One technique to accomplish this is to keep users aware of relevant changes and supplied with actionable information. Technology tools like status dashboards can be effective and allow them to work independently.

9.3. Anticipation of User Need

This principle calls for a design that relieves the user of the burden of searching for needed information or tools. Working together with user automomy, this type of design provides for bringing the information and tools the users need directly to them.

9.4. User Efficiency

Software design must serve individual productivity as well as organizational efficiency. People are an essential, often scarce resource, and user efficiency must be considered when designing and judging overall system efficiency. One example of this is making software design decisions in favor of the user experience when tradeoffs between computer efficiency and users are involved. User productivity is more important. Another example is avoidance of unnecessary options and parameters. Users should not have to navigate through excessive choices; these should be minimized and configured or negotiated dynamically rather than manually.

9.5. Calm Technology

This final principle underlies the other four and centers around *how* technology engages the user. The concept of *calm technology* calls for it to remain unobtrusively on the sidelines until the user has need of it. Only then does it moves to the center of attention to more fully engage the user. Calm technology strives to avoid the chaotic bombardment so often associated with alert systems, pagers, e-mail, and other technology tools. Placing them off to the side until needed frees the user to manage more things. It also encourages the periphery to be informing without being overburdening (Weiser and Brown 1996).

10. Architecture and Evolution

Calm technology and the other principles we describe, like Berners-Lee's Least Power Principle, are key to creating complex adaptive systems. By engineering them into the architecture we develop, we can create the transformational information system envisioned in HealthePeople.

As we do so, we must focus on individual empowerment at the prime goal of HealthePeople. The other goals function as enablers by providing a lifelong, comprehensive health record; making it accessible while keeping its contents private and secure; and ensuring it can be shared and retain its meaning.

As a complex adaptive system, HealthePeople functions on the massive scale our health system requires. Loosely coupled, it accommodates the diverse needs inherent in health care while allowing for wide variation across uses and users. Non-deterministic, it does not attempt to reduce the intricacies of biomedicine, wellness, and health-care delivery to set requirements or to bring them under central management. Rather, its architecture is driven by principles that ensure long-term fitness.

Its parts operate independent of one another, each with the capacity to evolve and adapt to emergent behaviors in the healthcare environment. The technology that acts as its infrastructure is de-coupled from the content it carries, making it possible to update either one without invalidating the other. The system is extensible: it can incorporate newly discovered health domains and newly developed technologies.

In essence, it is future proofed. For HealthePeople, the architecture is not mechanist and fixed, like the drawing for a building made of concrete and steel. Rather, it mirrors the rules of cellular structures in living beings and behavioral constructs in social groups. For a system designed to empower individuals and by doing so enhance the health of entire populations, as HealthePeople will do, this new perspective provides the foundation.

References

Dickinson G, Fischetti L, Heard S, editors. 2003. ANSI/HL7 EHR system functional model and standard (DTSU), release 1.0. Health Level Seven, Inc.

Beale T. 2001a. Archetypes. Available from: http://www.deepthought.com.au. Accessed 2004 Mar 18.

Beale T. 2001b. Health information standards manifesto, revision 2.2. Available from: http://www.deepthought.com.au/health/HIS_manifesto/his_manifesto. Accessed 2004 Mar 18.

Beale T, Goodchild A, Heard S. 2001. EHR design principles, revision 2.2. Available from: http://www.gehr.org/openEHR. Accessed 2004 Mar 10.

Berners-Lee T. 1998. Evolvability. Available from: http://www.w3.org/DesignIssues/Evolution.html. Accessed 2004 Mar 18.

Brown S. 2003. VHA enterprise terminology. Presentation, June 12, Albany, NY. Department of Veterans Affairs, Enterprise Architecture Conference.

Carpenter B, editor. 1996. Architectural principles of the internet. Available from: http://ftp.isi.edu/in-notes/rfc1958.txt. Accessed 2004 Mar 17.

Cimino J. 1998. Desiderata for controlled medical vocabularies in the twenty-first century. Methods Inf Med 37:394–403.

Clark DD, Blumenthal MS. 2001. Rethinking the design of the Internet: the end to end arguments vs. the brave new world. ACM Trans Internet Technol 1(1):70–109.

Clements PC, Northrop LM. 1996. Software architecture: an executive overview. Technical Report CMU/SEI-96-TR-003, ESC-TR-96-003. Pittsburgh, PA: Carnegie Mellon University.

Edelman GM, Gally JA. 2001. Degeneracy and complexity in biological systems. Proc Natl Acad Sci 98(24):13763–13768.

Fukuyama F. 1995. Trust: the social virtues and the creation of prosperity. New York: The Free Press.

International Organization for Standardization/International Electrotechnical Commission (ISO/IEC). 1995. Open distributed processing reference model part 1: overview. ITU-T, International Standard Recommendation X.901; Standard Recommendation ISO/IEC 10746-1, ISO WG7 Committee. Geneva, Switzerland: ISO.

Institute of Medicine. 2003. Key capabilities of an electronic health record. Letter report. Washington, DC: The National Academies Press.

Maier MW. 1998. Architecting principles for systems-of-systems. Sys Eng 1(4):267–284.

Mailla T. 2002. VHA Deployment Architecture Framework. Unpublished report produced under VA contract.

Miller J, Mukerji J, editors. 2003. MDA guide version 1.0.1. Available from: http://www.omg.org/docs/omg/03-06-01.pdf. Accessed 2004 Mar 18.

Ossher H, Tarr P. 1999. Multi-dimensional separation of concerns in hyperspace. IBM Research Report 21452. Available from: http://www.research.ibm.com/papers/papers.html. Accessed 2004 Mar 18.

Parnas DL. 1972. On the criteria to be used in decomposing systems into modules Commun ACM 15(12):1053–1058.

Putnam RD. 2000. Bowling alone: the collapse and revival of American community. New York: Simon & Schuster. p 326–335.

Reed DP. 1999. That sneaky exponential: beyond Metcalfe's law to the power of community building. Available from: http://www.contextmag.com/archives/199903/digitalstrategyReedsLaw.asp. Accessed 2004 Feb 18.

Saltzer JH, Reed DP, Clark DD. 1984. End-to-end arguments in system design. ACM TOCS 2(4):277–288.

Soley R, OMG (Object Management Group) Staff Strategy Group. 2000. Model driven architecture: white paper, draft 3.2. Available from: http://www.omg.org/mda/papers.htm. Accessed 2004 Mar 18.

Sowa JF. 2002. Architectures for intelligent systems. IBM Sys J 41(3):331–349.

Institute of Medicine. 2003. Key capabilities of an electronic health record. Letter report. Washington, DC: The National Academies Press.

Tognazzini B. 1998. Interaction architecture solutions for the real world: first principles. Available from: http://www.asktog.com/basics/firstPrinciples.html. Accessed 2003 Mar 18.

United Nations. 2003. Human development indicators 2003. New York: United Nations Development Program. Available from: http://www.undp.org/hdr2003/indicator/indic_1_2_3. Accessed 2004 Mar 18.

Weiser M, Brown JS. 1996. The coming age of calm technology. Available from: http://www.ubiq.com/hypertext/weiser/acmfuture2endnote.htm. Accessed 2004 Mar 18.

8
Critical Areas of Standardization

Jeffrey S. Blair and Simon Cohn

To contain the rising costs of health care, respond quickly to national healthcare emergencies, improve the quality of care, and reduce medical errors, we need to move health care into the information age. This requires the development of a national health information infrastructure with electronic health record (EHR) systems as core components—in short, it requires a system like the HealthePeople concept. Healthcare information standards are absolutely essential to this effort.

The standards required to establish an information infrastructure for health care are generally referred to as healthcare information (or healthcare informatics) standards. Even the narrowest definition of standards includes message format standards. Broad definitions include other forms of information representation, such as identifiers, guidelines, federal regulations, and other types of standards.

While a broad definition of standards is useful as an academic observation, it is not the most understandable way to organize and discuss healthcare information standards. For this reason, we review the types of standards within the following categories: identifier, communication, terminology, quality of care, documentation, privacy and security, and supporting models. For each category, we identify what is required and describe how standards are currently addressing those needs. Finally, we give an overview of the organizations working to develop and coordinate standards.

Throughout our chapter, our frame of reference is the national health information infrastructure defined by the National Committee on Vital and Health Statistics (NCVHS), in its report, *Information for Health: A Strategy for Building the National Health Information Infrastructure* (2001). This is the infrastructure upon which HealthePeople is being built.

1. Types of Standards

1.1. Identifier Standards

Within health care, multiple entities require unique identifiers, including patients, healthcare providers (e.g., physicians, nurses, healthcare institutions), health plans (payers), and employers. The Health Insurance Portability and Accountability Act (HIPAA) addressed some of these needs under its Administrative Simplification Provisions when the legislation was passed in 1996 as Public Law 104–191. Others are being defined by the Secretary of Health and Human Services (HHS) under formal rule making procedures.

1.1.1. Patient Identifiers

For years, healthcare providers asked the federal government to establish and maintain unique patient identifiers (UPIs) to reduce medical errors and improve the efficiency of locating patient records. Although initially required under HIPAA in 1996, national patient identifiers became politically controversial, and the federal government postponed their development and issuance indefinitely. Today, the healthcare industry is forced to rely upon a less than perfect system of local and institutional patient identifiers and indices to map between these systems.

1.1.2. Provider Identifiers

The Health Insurance Portability and Accountability Act also recognized the need for provider identifiers that would cover physicians, other caregivers, and facilities where healthcare services are rendered. In May 1998, HHS proposed a national provider identifier (NPI); in January 2004, HHS issued the final rule for the National Provider System. It will go into effect May 2005, at which time providers can begin to apply for an identifier. The compliance date is May 2007. Until that time, current identifiers, such as the Unique Physician Identifier Number (UPIN), will continue to be used to identify physicians and certain other practitioners who provide Medicare services.

1.1.3. Health Plan Identifiers

Health and Human Services plans to publish a notice of proposed rule making for the HIPAA Health Plan Identifier in spring 2005.

1.1.4. Employer Identifiers

The HIPAA Employer Identifier was published as a final rule in May 2002. This identifier is the same as the Employer Identification Number (EIN) issued for tax purposes.

1.2. Communication Standards

Communication standards that send and receive information between healthcare entities are generally referred to as electronic data interchange (EDI) standards. These standards support activities such as verifying patient eligibility, enrolling/disenrolling patients in health plans, submitting healthcare claims, checking claim status, coordinating benefits, submitting health claim attachments, etc. Communication standards that define messages sent between computer systems within a healthcare institution are typically referred to as message format standards. These standards support functions such as patient registration, admission/discharge/transfer, order entry, results reporting, scheduling, patient care, etc.

TABLE 8.1. Transaction standards.

Transaction type	Standard
Patient eligibility verification	ASC X12N 270/271
Enrollment and disenrollment in a health plan	ASC X12N 834
Health care claims status/response	ASC X12N 276/277
Receipt of healthcare remittance	ASC X12N 835
Premium payment	ASC X12N 820
Referral certification and authorization	ASC X12N 278
Submission of health claims and coordination of benefits	ASC X12N 837
	NCPDP
Submission of claims from retail pharmacies	Telecommunication claim

Source: Health Insurance Reform (HIPAA) (2000).

Both EDI standards (healthcare entity to entity) and healthcare message format standards (between computer systems within a healthcare entity or facility) define the format of electronic messages. Both are therefore referred to by many as syntax standards.

1.2.1. Entity to Entity

Today, the EDI standards with the highest level of implementation are those that support communication of financial and administrative information among payers, providers, and clearinghouses. To encourage further implementation of these standards, the HIPAA Administrative Simplification Provisions mandate their use. Table 8.1 lists these standards.

When sending transactions electronically, healthcare providers and payers must comply with the standards adopted by HIPAA in October 2003. Detailed information about the HIPAA transaction standards is available at http://www.cms.hhs.gov/hipaa/hipaa2. Guidance with planning and implementation is provided by the Workgroup for Electronic Data Interchange (WEDI) at their website, http://www.wedi.org/.

The Health Insurance Portability and Accountability Act also called for adoption of a health claim attachment standard. This standard is being developed jointly by Health Level Seven (HL7) and the Accredited Standards Committee (ASC X12N) and the notice of proposed rule making (NPRM) is expected to be released in 2004. For more information about their work, consult http://www.x12.org/x12org/subcommittees and http://www.hhl7.org.

1.2.2. Within the Facility

The healthcare message format standards that have the greatest market acceptance today typically address administrative and clinical processes within a healthcare facility. As directed by HIPAA and in its role as statutory advisory committee to the Secretary of HHS, NCVHS (2000) published a framework and criteria for selection of standards for patient medical record information (PMRI). Using these criteria, the NCVHS recommended message format standards for administrative and clinical

TABLE 8.2. Clinical data standards for the consolidated health informatics (CHI) initiative.

Transaction type	Standard
Order entry	HL7 v2.x
Scheduling	HL7 v2.x
Medical record/image management	HL7 v2.x
Patient administration	HL7 v2.x
Observation reporting	HL7 v2.x
Financial management	HL7 v2.x
Patient care	HL7 v2.x
Public health notification	HL7 v2.x
Radiological imaging	DICOM
Prescription information between prescribers and pharmacies	NCPDP SCRIPT
Medical device communications	IEEE 1073

Source: http://www.whitehouse.gov/omb/egov/gtob/health_informatics.htm

processes (National Committee on Vital and Health Statistics 2002). In 2003, the federal government accepted these recommendations, setting forth what is known as the Public Health Notification Message Format Standard.

This was the first set of clinical data standards adopted by the Consolidated Health Informatics (CHI) initiative, a collaborative effort involving HHS, the Department of Defense (DoD), and the Veterans Administration (VA). For more information, visit http://www/whitehouse/gov/omb/egov/gtob/health_informatics.htm. Through CHI, the federal government acted to standardize the communication of healthcare information across all federal departments and agencies, and thereby provide an example to the private sector by serving as an early adopter of these standards. For a complete list of NCVHS/CHI clinical data standards, see Table 8.2.

While the message format standards listed in Table 8.2 enjoy some market acceptance today and significantly reduce the cost of interfacing between computer systems, they generally fall short of NCVHS criteria for complete interoperability. In the meantime, standards organizations have developed message format standards with greater degrees of interoperability. For this reason, the NCVHS and CHI have recommended that the government take steps to accelerate the development of emerging standards, such as the HL7 Version 3 Transaction Sets for administrative management, health and clinical management, and infrastructure management.

In one key step, the NCVHS recommended that the message format standards not be mandated. As a result, they do not need to go through the federal regulatory process required of HIPAA standards. Instead, the message format standards are set forth as guidance to the health industry (National Committee on Vital and Health Statistics 2002). In other steps, the federal government advanced these standards through announcements of support by the Secretary of HHS and of the intent of CHI to implement these standards within all federal agencies and departments.

1.3. Terminology Standards

An umbrella term, *terminology standards*, includes vocabularies, nomenclatures, classification systems, and code sets (National Committee on Vital and Health Statistics

2000). Within health care, terminologies have been developed to represent diseases, procedures, interventions, outcomes, medications, devices, anatomy, functional status, demographics, etc.

Today, several terminologies are in widespread use because they are required for reimbursement purposes. They are also often used by public health, clinical research institutions, and healthcare entities for a variety of secondary purposes.

1.3.1. International Classification of Diseases (ICD)

The current version of the ICD used in the United States is the Ninth Revision with Clinical Modification (ICD9-CM). Developed and maintained by the World Health Organization, it is based on codes originally developed to code and classify mortality data from death certificates. The National Center for Health Statistics made the clinical modifications, and the Center for Medicare and Medicaid Services (CMS) developed a separate classification for procedures (ICD9-CM Volume 3). Thus modified, ICD9 is the official system used for diagnoses at all sites of care and for coding procedures associated with hospital utilization in the United States. The Health Insurance Portability and Accountability Act transaction regulations require the use of ICD9-CM [Health Insurance Reform (HIPAA) 2000].

The new edition of this classification, ICD10, is not now in use in the United States. Recently, the National Center for Health Statistics completed the clinical modification (CM) and CMS developed the procedure classification system (PCS) for the new ICD10 codes. However, neither the federal government nor the private sector has begun to implement them. The NCVHS has recommended that the federal government begin the regulatory process that will lead to the adoption of ICD10-CM and ICD10-PCS codes.

1.3.2. Healthcare Common Procedure Coding System (HCPCS)

Historically, this system included three levels for reporting physician services and other healthcare services, medical supplies, orthotic and prosthetic devices, and durable medical equipment. Its Level I Code is synonymous with the Current Procedural Terminology (CPT) developed and maintained by the American Medical Association. Used to code physician and other healthcare provider services and procedures, CPT was recently expanded to include codes for new technologies and to support performance measurement.

Level II Code, also called alphanumeric HCPCS, is maintained by CMS; it identifies durable medical equipment, drugs, supplies, and services not covered by Level I. Level III includes local codes developed for Medicare carriers and fiscal intermediaries for specific local needs; other local codes were developed *ad hoc* by many different health plans and insurers across the healthcare industry.

The Health Insurance Portability and Accountability Act transaction regulations mandate the continued use of Level I and II codes, but eliminate the use of Level III (local) codes [Health Insurance Reform (HIPAA) 2000].

1.3.3. Current Dental Terminology (CDT)

The code on dental procedures and nomenclature, CDT, is maintained by the American Dental Association and is mandated for dental services under HIPAA.

1.3.4. National Drug Codes (NDC)

Developed by the Food and Drug Administration (FDA) for drug package labeling, these codes are required for that use under HIPAA. Drugs administered in healthcare settings may be reported using HCPCS Level II and/or NDC codes [Health Insurance Reform (HIPAA) 2002]. The National Library of Medicine (NLM) and the VA are working on new drug terminologies that will be more appropriate for use in clinical care and institutional and provider reporting.

1.3.5. Patient Medical Record Information (PMRI) Terminologies

Under the directive from HIPAA, the NCVHS (2000, 2003) is also responsible for evaluating and recommending terminologies for PMRI. As part of this selection process, the NCVHS identified a number of terminologies. In late 2003, NCVHS completed its initial recommendations for the core set of clinical data terminology standards for patient medical record information. They include the following:

- Systematized Nomenclature of Medicine Clinical Terms (SNOMED CT)
- the laboratory portion of Logical Observations Identifiers Names and Codes (LOINC);
- RxNorm;
- the representations of the mechanism of action and physiologic effect of drugs from the National Drug File Reference Terminology (NDF-RT);
- ingredient name, manufactured dosage form, and package type from the FDA.

This core set of PMRI terminologies will serve as reference terminologies and will be available to users from the NLM at no cost. The NLM will be responsible for integrating the terminologies into the core set within the context of the Unified Medical Language System (UMLS).

The NLM will also be responsible for mapping these terminologies to "important related terminologies" and for making these terminologies available to users. Two groups of important related terminologies will be mapped to/from the core set of PMRI terminologies. The first set of important related terminologies with the highest priority includes the terminologies previously designated to support the HIPAA financial and administrative transaction standards. They are:

- Current Procedural Terminology (CPT4) or (CPT)
- Current Dental Terminology (CDT)
- Level II Healthcare Common Procedure Coding System (HCPCS)
- International Classification of Diseases, Ninth Edition, Clinical Modification (ICD9-CM)
- National Drug Codes (NDC)

The second set of important related terminologies includes, but is not limited to:

- Diagnostic and Statistical Manual of Mental Disorders (DSM-IV)
- Terminologies in private sector drug information databases (e.g., FirstDatabank NDDF Plus, Medi-Span, Micromedex, Multum Lexicon)

- International Society of Blood Transfusion coding system for describing blood products and tissues (ISBT 128)
- Medcin© (codes for structured entry of clinical notes)
- Medical Dictionary for Regulatory Activities international code set for use by drug regulatory agencies (MedDRA)
- Nursing terminologies not otherwise included in SNOMED CT

Identifying a core set of PMRI terminologies encourages their use by healthcare providers and health information technology vendors in efforts to expand clinical decision support, move closer to semantic interoperability, and provide higher levels of specificity in outcomes measurement. These efforts are critical to achieving higher quality and fewer medical errors—to transforming the information technology (IT) environment in ways that enable continuous improvements in clinical processes.

1.4. Quality of Care Indicators, Data Sets, Guidelines, and Code Standards

Although there is no definitive national standard for quality of care, there are an array of indicators, data sets, guidelines, and code standards that are used to facilitate quality improvements.

1.4.1. Quality Indicators

The Joint Commission on Accreditation of Health Care Organizations (JCAHO) has developed a set of quality indicators referred to as the ORYX initiative. It includes quality indicators for acute myocardial infarction, heart failure, community-acquired pneumonia, and pregnancy and related conditions. For more information on ORYX, visit http://www.jcaho.org/.

The American Medical Association (AMA) has developed a set of clinical performance measurement tools to support physicians in their efforts to enhance the quality of patient care. The measurement tools are derived from evidence-based clinical guidelines. The performance measurement sets can be used by physicians to gather data from their own practice, measure their own level of performance, and ultimately enhance the care of their patients. Measurement sets are now available for chronic stable coronary artery disease, adult diabetes, heart failure, hypertension, major depressive disorder, osteoarthritis of the knee, and prenatal testing. To view the Physician Measurement Sets, visit www.ama-assn.org/ama/pub/category/4837.html.

1.4.2. Data Sets

The National Committee for Quality Assurance (NCQA) has developed the Health Plan Employer Data and Information Set (HEDIS). The 2004 data set includes quality performance measures for osteoporosis, urinary incontinence, colorectal cancer, appropriate use of antibiotics, and chemical dependency. For details, visit http://www.ncqa.org/Programs/HEDIS/.

1.4.3. Guidelines

Many organizations have developed practice guidelines/parameters during the last several years. These guidelines have been developed by national, regional, and local organizations, such as professional associations, government agencies, providers, consulting firms, and vendors. The Agency for Healthcare Research and Quality (AHRQ) maintains the National Guideline Clearinghouse™ (NCG™). Developed in partnership with the American Medical Association and the American Association of Health Plans, the Clearinghouse is a publicly available database of evidence-based clinical practice guidelines and related documents. It is updated weekly at http://www.guideline.gov/.

1.4.4. Bar Codes

To help reduce medical errors related to prescriptions and medication administration, the FDA proposed drug bar code regulation in March 2003 and finalized them in February 2004. These regulations would standardize and require the use of bar codes on prescription drugs, over-the-counter drugs packaged for hospital use, and biologic products used in the hospital. The regulation requires a linear bar code that meets Uniform Code Council (UCC) standards or Health Industry Business Communications Council (HIBCC) Standards. For details, visit http://www.fda.gov/oc/initiatives/barcode-sadr/.

1.5. Medical Record Content, Structure, and Documentation Standards

A first-generation standard has been developed for specifying clinical documents and will be proposed for use in claims attachments as part of HIPAA. Standards have also been developed for the content and structure of EHRs. Different standard development organizations are taking different approaches to this. There is no industry consensus, and the federal government has not formally sanctioned an approach or standard as of this writing.

The American Society for Testing and Materials (ASTM) Standards Committee on Healthcare Informatics (E31) has developed a standard guide for content and structure of the EHR. This guide, known as E1384, has assisted vendors and healthcare providers with implementation planning for EHRs, but has not been widely implemented by the healthcare community.

The HL7 Structured Documents Technical Committee has established a clinical document architecture (CDA) standard. It can be used to structure the format of clinical and administrative healthcare documents that are sent within an HL7 message. It uses the extensible markup language (XML) specification to standardize the formats for document headers, sections, and content. Health Level Seven is proposing the use of the CDA and XML for the HIPAA claim attachment standard.

The Healthcare Information and Management Systems Society (HIMSS), ASTM International, and the Massachusetts Medical Society have joined together to develop a national standard to facilitate continuity of care. The initiative is called the Continuity of Care Record (CCR). It will enable the sharing of clinical and administrative documents such as referrals, discharge summaries, history and physicals, and radiological reports in a technology neutral and standards neutral XML format. Unlike the CDA, which addresses this need from the perspective of the structure of messages from the top down, the CCR is focusing on the data content required for continuity of care and is developing the CCR standard from the bottom up. CCR documents can be sent within HL7 messages, shared via websites, or used in clinical settings that do not yet have electronic patient record systems.

American Society for Testing and Materials E31 has also developed a set of standards to support the documentation process of medical transcription. They include standard guides for medical transcription, proposals, amendments, quality assurance, and privacy and confidentiality.

1.6. Privacy and Security Standards

These standards have been set forth as federal regulations under the HIPAA Administrative Simplification Provisions (1996).

The privacy regulations specify that healthcare providers, payers, and clearinghouses are covered entities and must have complied with these regulations by April 2003 (Office of Civil Rights 2000). The regulations provide patients with mechanisms to protect the privacy of their healthcare information within the covered entities, define the responsibilities of the covered entities to protect the privacy of patient healthcare information, and specify constraints on the use of patient information for marketing and research purposes. For more information about the privacy regulations, visit the Office of Civil Rights website at http://www.hhs.gov/ocr/hipaa/.

The security regulations published in February 2003 require compliance by the healthcare industry by April 21, 2005. This regulation specifies a series of administrative, technical, and physical security procedures for covered entities to use to protect the privacy of electronic health information. For more information on the security regulations, visit http://www.cms.hhs.gov/hipaa/hipaa2/regulations/.

During the 1990s, the Computer-Based Patient Record Institute (CPRI) created a series of guidance documents to help healthcare institutions develop data security policies and practices (Blair 1995). In anticipation of the HIPAA security regulations, this set of documents was upgraded and formally balloted as ASTM standard guidelines. American Society for Testing and Materials publishes standardized security guides for authentication, access control, security frameworks, internet and intranet security, and security training. American Society for Testing and Materials has also developed standard specifications for digital signatures and audit and disclosure logs; these are available for viewing at http://www.astm.org. (While not part of the HIPAA Security Regulations and Standards, they can be helpful to organizations as they consider how to implement the regulations.)

The Workgroup for Electronic Data Interchange (WEDI) provides a set of white papers to assist with the implementation of the HIPAA privacy and security regulations. These white papers provide guidance for organizational change management, security risk assessment, security policies and procedures, etc. For more information, visit http://www.wedi.org.

1.7. *Supporting Models*

Typically, models support the development and use of standards, rather than serve as implementable standards in their own right. Standard development organizations develop models to promote consensus in complex areas and clarify conceptual ambiguities, facilitating and sometimes accelerating standards development. Examples of the types of supporting models include information models, functional models, ontologies, etc. These standards are necessary to support an information infrastructure for health care. Three models now being developed for specific purposes are likely to play an important role in the development of a national health information infrastructure.

1.7.1. The HL7 Reference Information Model (RIM)

Refined over six years, HL7 developed RIM primarily to generate Version 3 messages that are more interoperable. More recently, HL7 has realized that RIM may be a key foundation for EHR structure standards. Health Level Seven maintains an active website at http://www.hl7.org that provides up-to-date on their activities.

1.7.2. The EHR Functional Model

At the request of the federal government, including CMS, VA, and AHRQ, the Institute of Medicine (IOM) identified core capabilities of the EHR (Institute of Medicine 2003). Using the IOM's findings as a base, HL7 is now working to develop a functional EHR model. The purpose of this effort is to provide the definitions, functions, and framework that will support federal incentives to accelerate the implementation of EHR systems nationwide.

1.7.3. SNOMED CT

Now being developed by SNOMED International (http://www.snomed.org), this model is clinically specific and puts concepts within a hierarchical knowledge base, that is, an ontology. The purpose of this ontology is to provide a consistent, stable, and non-ambiguous collection of clinical concepts that can serve as a reference terminology for healthcare. SNOMED CT promises to facilitate the expansion of clinical decision support, improve the accuracy and precision of clinical outcomes measurement, and enable greater interoperability among healthcare information systems.

2. Organizations Involved in Standards

Today, there are standards capable of supporting the evolution toward a national health information infrastructure. But this evolution depends upon the continued commitment of organizations to develop, coordinate, support, and implement these standards.

In the United States, standards development activities typically take place within the private sector. For this reason most of the organizations that accredit, develop, and coordinate standards are within the private sector. Table 8.3 lists the private sector organizations involved in standards, along with a brief description of their roles.

TABLE 8.3. Private sector organizations involved in standards.

Acronym	Name	ANSI accredited	Organization role
ADA	American Dental Association		
ANSI	American National Standards Institute	n/a	Provides accreditation for standard development organizations (SDO)
ANSI-HISB	ANSI-Healthcare Informatics Standards Board	n/a	Provides a forum for the coordination of standards development organizations (SDOs) in the U.S.
ASC X12N	Accredited Standards Committee X12N	Yes	Develops electronic data interchange (EDI) message format standards for financial and administrative transactions between providers and payers
ASTM E31	American Society for Testing & Materials: Healthcare Information Standards Committee	Yes	Develops healthcare information standards for documentation, electronic health record (EHR) content and structure, policies and practices, and security
CFH	Connecting for Health Initiative	n/a	Promotes solutions to address HL7 implementation issues and lobbies to advance healthcare information standards
DICOM	Digital Image Communications	No	Develops message format standards and code sets for the communication of radiological images
HIMSS	Healthcare Information and Management Systems Society	n/a	Promotes and supports the development and implementation of healthcare information standards through work groups, initiatives and lobbying efforts; Secretariat for ISO TC 215 TAG
HL7	Health Level Seven	Yes	Develops message format and related standards to support the communication of administrative and clinical healthcare information
IEEE 1073	Institute of Electrical and Electronic Engineers	Yes	Develops message format standards and code sets to support the communication of healthcare information from medical devices to healthcare information systems
ISO TC 215	International Standards Organization: Technical Committee on Healthcare Informatics	n/a	Coordinates, develops, and publishes healthcare informatics standards for use worldwide
ISO US TAG	International Standards Organization: United States Technical Advisory Group	n/a	Coordinates the positions of U.S. healthcare informatics standards development organization for representation at ISO TC 215
JCAHO	Joint Commission for the Accreditation of Healthcare Organizations	n/a	Provides a set of quality of care and performance indicators and measures for healthcare institutions
NCPDP	National Council for Prescription Drug Programs	Yes	Develops message format standards to communicate prescriptions to retail pharmacies, and reimbursement information between pharmacies and payers
WEDI	Work Group for Electronic Data Interchange	n/a	Advocates for government support of healthcare EDI standards and provides support for implementation of these standards

* American National Standards Institute (ANSI).

In addition to the organizations involved in standards in the private sector, there are several important standards activities conducted by the federal government in addition to those discussed above in the section on terminologies. These activities include the following: the development and maintenance of federally mandated classification systems for reimbursement and statistical purposes; the development of message format standards and data sets necessary to support public health and government response to national emergencies; the selection and adoption of standards for HIPAA and for use within the federal government under the CHI initiative; and the provision of leadership and coordination for the national health information infrastructure. Table 8.4 lists government entities involved in standards.

TABLE 8.4. Government sector entities involved in standards.

Acronym	Name	ANSI accredited	Organization role
AHRQ	Agency for Health Research and Quality	n/a	Maintains a clearinghouse for clinical guidelines and supports the development of healthcare information and quality of care standards
CDC	Centers for Disease Control and Prevention	n/a	Working with healthcare informatics SDOs to develop the National Electronic Disease Surveillance System (NEDSS) and the Data Elements in Emergency Departments Systems (DEEDS)
CHI	Consolidated Health Informatics Initiative	n/a	Provides leadership and coordination for the adoption and implementation of healthcare information standards within the federal government, including CMS, DoD, VA, and IHS.
CMS	Centers for Medicare and Medicaid Services	n/a	Develops and maintains the project office for HIPAA standards; maintains the Level II HCPCS codes and develops and maintains ICD9-CM vol. 3
FDA	Food and Drug Administration	n/a	Develops and maintains the NDC and is supporting the efforts of the NLM and the VA to develop drug terminologies (Rx-Norm and NDF-RT) that will be more appropriate for patient care purposes
NCVHS	National Committee on Vital and Health Statistics	n/a	Studies, selects and recommends healthcare information standards to the Secretary of HHS for adoption as HIPAA and/or CHI standards. Also makes healthcare information policy recommendations such as for the national health information infrastructure
NCHS	National Center for Health Statistics	n/a	Develops and maintains the Clinical Modifications for ICD Codes and provides support for the NCVHS
NLM	National Library of Medicine	n/a	Develops and maintains the Unified Medical Language System (UMLS) which serves as a metathesaurus and mapping function among healthcare terminologies
VA	Veterans Administration— Health Affairs	n/a	Working with the NLM to develop NDF-RT, a Reference Terminology for medications

* American National Standards Institute (ANSI).

3. Enabling the National Health Information Infrastructure

This chapter has discussed why data standards are critical, the types of standards that will be required to facilitate a national health information infrastructure, the ability of current standards to meet these requirements, and the major organizations involved in healthcare information standards. Taken together these standards support and enable the national goals for health set forth by Gary Christopherson in his presentation to the NCVHS (Christopherson 2003):

- Maximize health/abilities
- Maximize satisfaction
- Maximize quality
- Maximize accessibility and portability
- Maximize affordability
- Maximize patient safety
- Minimize time between disability/illness and maximize function/health
- Minimize inconvenience
- Maximize security and privacy

Because these standards create an information infrastructure with many interdependent functions and components, it is not possible to relate individual types of standards exclusively to one goal and identify other types of standards exclusively to other goals. For example, the same standards that reduce medical errors also improve the quality of care and reduce cost. By extension, if we improve quality and reduce costs, we will probably improve patient satisfaction. Additionally, reducing costs will provide the nation opportunities to expand access to health care.

Tremendous progress has been made during the last decade to create and refine the standards necessary to facilitate the national health information infrastructure. These achievements include:

- The vision set forth by the IOM in 1990–1991 when it published the book *Computer-Based Patient Records: An Essential Technology for Healthcare.*
- The federal government provided a catalyst for the development and implementation for healthcare information standards with the passage of the Health Insurance Portability and Accountability Act of 1996 (HIPAA).
- The Consolidated Health Informatics (CHI) initiative has begun to focus and accelerate the acceptance of healthcare information standards by serving as an early adopter of these standards.
- The NCVHS has proposed the creation of a national health information infrastructure with EHR systems serving as core components and the federal government providing leadership and coordination.
- The healthcare industry has gone a long way to develop message format standards and terminologies to facilitate interoperability and data comparability.
- Additionally, the HIPAA regulations have also established higher standards for privacy and security of healthcare information.

However, there is much to be done.

- While there has been substantial market acceptance for current message format standards, there is a need to accelerate the development of new versions that will have higher levels of interoperability. Health Level Seven is attempting to address this by using its Reference Information Model (RIM) to help generate HL7 Version 3 Message Format Standards.
- Additional development is needed to create message format standards for health claim attachments, decision support, and clinical documents.
- A few leading healthcare institutions have adopted clinically specific terminologies to facilitate decision support and improve the measurement of clinical outcomes, but widespread adoption of these terminologies has not yet taken place.
- Standards for content and structure of patient records are in their infancy, and there are no nationally accepted standards for the exchange and communication of EHRs. More work in these areas is urgently needed.

The federal government is preparing to realign the incentives provided by our healthcare reimbursement system to move closer to a pay-for-performance model. The nation is fairly close to having the basic set of healthcare information standards to support this model. These standards will enable healthcare providers to routinely measure and improve patient safety, quality of care, and healthcare costs. A critical gap is the lack of a national standard that defines the functions of EHR systems that support these capabilities. The federal government is actively supporting the development of an EHR system functional model to address this critical gap.

References

Blair JS. 1995. Overview of healthcare information standards. Washington, DC: Computer-Based Patient Record Institute.

Christopherson G. 2003. Presentation to NCVHS: toward ideal health and health information systems. Arlington, VA.

Food and Drug Administration (FDA). 2003. FDA News: FDA proposes drug bar code regulation. Washington, DC: Food and Drug Administration.

Health Insurance Portability and Accountability Act (HIPAA). 1996. Public Law 104–191. H.R. 3103 21 Aug 1996.

Health Insurance Reform (HIPAA). 2000. Standards for electronic transactions. Final rule. Washington, DC: Department of Health and Human Services. Federal Register No.: 45 CFR Parts 160 and 162.

Health Insurance Reform (HIPAA). 2002. Modifications to electronic data transaction standards and code sets. Final rule. Washington, DC: Department of Health and Human Services. Federal Register No.: 45 CFR Part 162.

Health Insurance Reform (HIPAA). 2003. Security standards. Final rule. Washington, DC: Department of Health and Human Services. Federal Register No.: 45 CFR Parts 160, 162 and 164.

National Committee on Vital and Health Statistics (NCVHS). 2000. Report on uniform data standards for patient medical record information. Washington, DC: Department of Health and Human Services.

National Committee on Vital and Health Statistics (NCVHS). 2001. Information for health: a strategy for building the National Health Information Infrastructure (NHII). Final report. Washington, DC: Department of Health and Human Services.

National Committee on Vital and Health Statistics (NCVHS). 2002. Letter to Secretary Thompson recommending the selection of patient medical record information message format standards. Washington, DC: Department of Health and Human Services.

National Committee on Vital and Health Statistics (NCVHS). 2003. PMRI terminology analysis report. Version 4. Washington, DC: Department of Health and Human Services.

Office of Civil Rights. 2000. HIPAA. Standards for privacy of individually identifiable Health Information. Final Rule. Washington, DC: Department of Health and Human services. Federal Register No.: 45 CFR Parts 160 and 164.

9
The Role of Terminology in Future Health Information Systems

STEVEN H. BROWN, MICHAEL J. LINCOLN, and PETER L. ELKIN

The Health*e*People vision of an electronic health record (EHR) depends upon the meaningful sharing of health data within and between enterprises and across various computer systems. This kind of sharing requires terminologies that are technically advanced and universally implemented. In this chapter, we explain the role of terminology and outline the steps to be taken at the national level to build health information systems to serve us in the future.

1. Health Care in the Future

Future generations of clinicians will take the ability to share meaningful data for granted and wonder how anyone was ever safely cared for without such information. They will practice in a world where there is true data integration. Every health record will be encoded in interoperable controlled representation, making it possible to integrate information generated by disparate health organizations. Personal health information will be integrated in its own section within the health record. Decision support systems will have the ability to connect to the patient's lifelong clinical data (encounter, radiological, surgical, medication, allergy, and laboratory data), thus enabling real-time decision support at the point-of-care.

This level of interoperability will provide the basis for personalized medical care. Subspecialty advice will no longer be limited to individuals who can make it to an appointment with a scarce resource (e.g., a rheumatologist), but will be available online for all patients requiring expert advice. The transfer of information prior to subspecialty consults will facilitate the pre-scheduling of tests, making appointments more efficient. The packaging of information at the end of a consult will ensure more complete understanding by the referring physician of the results of the consultation. In addition to more streamlined subspecialty consultations, online decision aids will be able to be integrated into physicians' daily work processes. Decision support delivered to the point of care at the time of care has the ability to improve clinical practice and patient satisfaction with that practice (van't Riet et al. 2001; Garrison et al. 2002).

2. Two Illustrative Scenarios

Two scenarios illustrate the potential impact of widely deployed, standardized terminologies on healthcare delivery. For each scenario, we describe a series of events as is and how they could be in the future. (Names of the patients and facilities involved are fictional.)

2.1. Scenario 1

Millie Cooper, an elderly woman with occasional difficulty sleeping, takes a capsule of over-the-counter (OTC) diphenhydramine to help her fall to sleep. In the middle of the night, she awakens quite confused, slips while getting out of bed, and breaks her hip. In the emergency room (ER), she is evaluated for an acute confusional state of unknown etiology in addition to her hip fracture. It is eventually determined that her confusion was induced by diphenhydramine, and this adverse reaction is documented in the hospital's adverse event tracking system. Following hip repair surgery, she is transferred to a nursing home for additional care. One evening, Mrs. Cooper asks for a pill to help her sleep.

2.1.1. As Is

The cross-covering physician, unaware of Mrs. Cooper's previous adverse reaction, orders diphenhydramine. Within hours, she is markedly confused, and is transferred via ambulance to the hospital. The ER physician notes the workup performed for her recent episode of confusion and suspects a recurrent drug-induced event. The ER physician's suspicion is confirmed by a call to the nursing home where a supervisor reviews the medication administration record and documents a new adverse drug event in the nursing home's records.

2.1.2. Could Be

The cross-covering physician logs into the computerized order entry system and tries to enter an order for Benedryl. The order entry system "knows" that the active ingredient in Benedryl is diphenhydramine and also "knows" that Mrs. Cooper had a bad reaction to a generic medication containing the active ingredient diphenhydramine documented at the local hospital. An alert to this effect is presented to the cross-covering physician, who orders zolpidem instead. The computerized order entry system suggests that an appropriate starting dose of zolpidem for a patient of Mrs. Cooper's age is 5 mg. She sleeps soundly through the night and wakes up refreshed for another day of rehab therapy.

2.2. Scenario 2

Bill Kneivel is a 49-year-old male on vacation with his family in Florida. He is driving in wet conditions when a driver changing lanes cuts off his car. Mr. Kneivel swerves, but his car impacts an embankment. Unconscious, he is taken to the ER at the closest facility, Florida General Hospital (FGH). He routinely gets his care at the Northern Clinic, and the ER physician at FGH requests an online transfer of his health records. In moments, the text-based records come on the ER computer. His considerable health history includes several changes of medications in the past 18 months. Currently, Mr. Kneivel is taking metformin, aspirin, lisinopril, and hydrochlorthiazide, and it is clear that the patient has hypertension and diabetes. The patient was found to have had a myocardial infarction and his laboratory data included the following: Troponin-T of 0.42, a normal CBC, a creatinine of 2.7, normal electrolytes, and a glucose of 187.

2.2.1. As Is

The patient is continued on his prior medications. After two days, he has a serum potassium level (K+) of 7.2 and a bicarbonate of 14. Mr. Kneivel goes into ventricular tachycardia followed by cardiac arrest and death. Upon investigation of the cause of his metabolic acidosis, a diabetic etiology is ruled out. The acidosis is determined to be secondary to metformin, which should have been withheld when his creatinine was noted to be elevated.

2.2.2. Could Be

The admitting physician uses an order entry system that is able to integrate data from Northern Clinic into its decision support routines. The physician is alerted that the patient's renal function has declined since last measurement and that metformin, one of the active outpatient medications, is now contraindicated. The admitting physician elects to control the patient's blood glucose with insulin instead. Two days later, Mr. Knievel's K+ and bicarbonate are within normal limits, and his creatinine is returning back to its pre-accident state.

In the "as is" branch of the second scenario, FGH has a decision support system in place, but terminology incompatibity renders it incapable of using information from the northern clinic. The medication appears as metformin in the Northern system and as Glucophage at FGH. Because it is not coded, it cannot trigger the alert in the FGH decision support system that would save Mr. Knievel's life: "Prescribing Glucophage to patients with a creatinine of >2.0 risks the development of a serious metabolic acidosis." In the "could be" branch, the codes for metformin and the lab test for creatinine are included with Mr. Knievel's health records in a format that is compatible with the decision support module of the FGH physician order entry system. Thus, the alert appears and the physician prescribes insulin instead of metformin/Glucophage, averting a fatal medical adverse event.

3. A High Level View of Terminology

When we write, we typically form sentences and paragraphs that convey information to the reader. For example, the reader can easily interpret the sentence, "There is evidence to support the diagnosis of pneumonia." Computers, on the other hand, work primarily with data such as "482," the code for "Bacterial Pneumonia, Unspecified" according to the International Classification of Diseases Ninth Edition (ICD9). Computer-usable terminology bridges the two; it is accessible to both automated and human interpretation.

Computer-usable terminology provides a critical framework to support clinical and administrative data capture and reporting. Enterprises that use standard terminologies reap significant return on investment. For example, LDS Hospital in Salt Lake City, Utah, cut antibiotic charges 42% by implementing a computer-based Antibiotic Advisor that integrated coded terminology from various hospital systems (Pestotnik et al. 1996). It also reduced serious adverse drug events (ADE) three-fold with a clinical-terminology–driven computer-based screening and alerting tool (Evans et al. 1994). Research on the frequency of ADEs suggests the potential magnitude of such an intervention at the national level: they amount to about 6% of admissions (Bates et al. 1993) and cost between $3000 and $6000 per occurrence (Bates et al. 1997).

According to a recent Institute of Medicine (IOM) report, *To Err Is Human* (Kohn et al. 2000), institutions using standardized terminology are better able to link patient care information with administrative data. As a result, they enjoy reduced coding costs and fewer compliance errors. Recently, Kaiser Permanente estimated that $950 million of its Medicare revenues were dependent on improved encoding of patient diagnoses.

However, many highly successful computer-based approaches to improving health care depended on locally developed, minimally extendable, and non-sharable terminology solutions. For example, despite its own successes, LDS Hospital has encountered major impediments to disseminating their information systems to other sites within Intermountain Health Care, its parent group. Why might this be? We suggest that demands for interoperability were minimal in the earliest days of medical computing. As a result, systems designers solved the terminology problem in relatively simple ways.

Over the years, medical information systems have become more prevalent, and their architectures have evolved. The resulting growth in demand for data sharing and efficient maintenance has driven the development of increasingly sophisticated solutions for terminology content, data representation techniques, and deployment methodologies. However, until these advances and standards are broadly deployed in the field, we will continue to have islands of patient information that cannot be interchanged or compared algorithmically. To achieve benefits such as those accomplished at LDS at every healthcare institution in the country, we need a comprehensive, scientifically valid, well maintained, and highly integrated framework of interlocking terminologies.

Over the years, terminology users have changed. Initially, biologists and health workers used a common domain-specific language to share knowledge with one another. While this was effective for the care of individual patients, the rise of the statistical age of medicine demanded a different approach. The need to standardize and organize terminology emerged as analysts attempted to use medical records to establish facts about the patterns of disease in populations. In 1863, Florence Nightingale stated "I am fain to sum up with an urgent appeal for adopting this or some uniform system of publishing the statistical records of hospitals" (Nightingale 1863). Early attempts to achieve comparable data yielded lists of terms, organized to varying degrees. Today, printed tabular term lists, such as ICD9 coding manuals, are still used throughout health care.

The ways users access terminologies have also changed with the emergence of computer systems to manage health data. The ability to automate medical record entry and retrieval has created a need for ever more detailed content. Moreover, information system architecture has evolved over time, placing new demands on access to controlled terminology.

Early computer applications in health care operated in stand-alone mode. Because they did not interoperate with other systems, representing controlled terminology and its associated metadata in a hard coded manner within the application code was initially adequate. Gradually, as users asked for additional applications on the same hardware systems, the transition toward interoperation began, demanding new approaches to improve system maintainability as applications changed and evolved. One new method of terminology representation was the data dictionary, which makes terminology and its supporting metadata available to various applications on the same system, effectively removing them from being hard coded in any single application.

Today, information architectures provide for interoperation and maintenance between disparate systems that may not be physically co-located, placing new demands on terminology. As a result, terminology access is making the leap from being application bound to being system bound and, from there, evolving to become system and location independent. This is happening via the deployment of terminology services, functioning solely to provide access to terms and codes by way of what is called a standard application program interface (API).

TABLE 9.1. Terms about terms.

Terminologies come in different forms and formats. Often, people use terms about terminologies interchangeably when it is not appropriate to do so. Each of the terms listed below has been defined by the International Organization for Standardization (ISO) or other groups or individuals involved in standards development.

Terminology: An organized set of terms in a specific subject field whose meanings have been defined or are generally understood in the relevant field (ISO 5127-1:1983 clause 1.1.2-10). For example, a terminology for gender might include the terms "female," "male," "unknown," "not asked." It does not necessarily include definitions.

Vocabulary: A terminological dictionary that contains designations and definitions from one or more specific subject fields (ISO 1087-1 clause 3.5.1). According to this ISO definition, a terminology becomes a vocabulary via the addition of definitions.

Classification: Arrangement of concepts into classes and their subdivisions to express the semantic relations between them; the classes are represented by means of a notation (ISO 5127-6:1983 clause 3.4.1-02). Classifications are typically used to group similar items. For example, the ICD9 Clinical Modification (CM) groups acute rheumatic fever, chronic rheumatic heart disease, hypertensive disease, and ischemic heart disease into the class "diseases of the circulatory system." In turn, each of these four states is itself a class representing more than one clinical state. The class "Hypertensive Disease" contains the subclasses "Essential Hypertension," "Hypertensive Heart and Renal Disease," "Hypertensive Heart Disease," "Hypertensive Renal Disease," and "Secondary Hypertension."

Nomenclature: A terminology structured according to pre-established naming rules (ISO 1087-1 clause 3.5.2). The Logical Observation Identifiers Names and Codes (LOINC) is a good example of a nomenclature (Huff et al. 1998; McDonald 2003). LOINC terms are composed of one entry from each of five axes, much like ordering from a restaurant when you are allowed to select one item from column A and one item from column B. Another example of a nomenclature is the Document Naming Nomenclature (DNN) (Brown et al. 2001). In the DNN, a document title is composed of components describing characteristics of the author, the healthcare event, and the organizational unit providing the care, for example, "cardiology attending procedure note."

Reference Terminology: Reference terminologies are not simply terminologies to which people or computers refer. Instead, they have formal logic-based computer readable and processible definitions for each term (Campbell et al. 1996; Spackman et al. 1997; Rossi Mori et al. 1998) and are designed to facilitate data aggregation and data retrieval (Rector 1998). Figure 2 on page 112 offers an example of a formal definition.

4. A Terminologist's Perspective on Terminology

As the opening scenarios illustrate, terminology can empower computers and the people who use them. On first blush, implementing the advanced capabilities may seem simple, and the uninitiated may find it difficult to believe that health care has failed to establish and embrace standards for such common items as medications and laboratory test names. But what initially appears to be simple is in fact technically and politically complex. The path to greater functionality requires significant effort and resources—and it requires a common baseline of knowledge, as summarized in Table 9.1.

Without terminology, computer applications can represent only free-text and numbers. While this may be better than nothing, full interoperability of healthcare information requires much more. Although healthcare facilities could transmit most lab results as numbers only (e.g., 135), such numbers are useful only when they are accompanied by the name of the lab test and the units of measurement involved (e.g., serum sodium or mg/dL). Because the data used to provide day-to-day care are, in most cases, best represented by controlled terminology, the need for and use of terminology in healthcare applications are widespread. Simply using some/any controlled terminology is not a guaranteed solution. To be optimally effective, controlled terminologies must be properly designed, implemented, deployed, and maintained.

4.1. Good Terms Gone Bad

The sad fact is that controlled terminologies can create data and information problems rather than resolve them.

4.1.1. Getting to Yes

As part of the Government Computerized Patient Record (GCPR) project, the terminology team was tasked with gathering and mapping code sets used by the Department of Defense, the Department of Veterans Affairs, and the Indian Health Service for information that was to be shared between the agencies (Rowberg and York 1999; Forslund et al. 2000). This effort uncovered hundreds of different code sets used for thousands of different purposes. Code sets representing "yes" and "no" were particularly interesting. The team uncovered 3396 instances where yes-no code sets were used. Alarmingly, there were 30 different code sets used among the 3396 instances (e.g., Yes = 1 No = 2 and Yes = 0 No = 1). In this case, a lack of standardization of the controlled terminologies introduced considerable confusion in the interpretation of transmitted data.

4.1.2. National Drug Code Are Not Enough

The second example of good terms gone bad addresses medications, a more complex area than "yes" and "no." Figure 9.1 displays 160 unique National Drug Codes (NDCs)

NDC: 00686027720	NDC: 46193073801	NDC: 51285032190	NDC: 50053310901	NDC: 00615256113
NDC: 48695117305	NDC: 00555046506	NDC: 51285032160	NDC: 47679070204	NDC: 40039006001
NDC: 00047007032	NDC: 00555046505	NDC: 52985003606	NDC: 47679070201	NDC: 00025090152
NDC: 00047007024	NDC: 00555046502	NDC: 52985003601	NDC: 46703009410	NDC: 00025090131
NDC: 00223255002	NDC: 00054475833	NDC: 51285032112	NDC: 46703009401	NDC: 47202255103
NDC: 00223255001	NDC: 00054475831	NDC: 51285032109	NDC: 52584018410	NDC: 47202255101
NDC: 00364075690	NDC: 00054475825	NDC: 51285032105	NDC: 00363690810	NDC: 12027008902
NDC: 00364075602	NDC: 54441019750	NDC: 51285032102	NDC: 53489045101	NDC: 12027008902
NDC: 00364075601	NDC: 54441019725	NDC: 00555036505	NDC: 00157052610	NDC: 53487014510
NDC: 52953000304	NDC: 54441019715	NDC: 00555036502	NDC: 00157052601	NDC: 00781134413
NDC: 00378018210	NDC: 54441019711	NDC: 00308627099	NDC: 00054875825	NDC: 00781134410
NDC: 00378018201	NDC: 54441019710		NDC: 00005310931	NDC: 00781134401
NDC: 51432097106	NDC: 00182175_		NDC: 00005310923	NDC: 53978003410
NDC: 00677104110	NDC: 00182175_		NDC: 00071007024	NDC: 00117134405
NDC: 00677104105	NDC: 0022823_	*Propranolol*	NDC: 00046042191	NDC: 00117134401
NDC: 00677104101	NDC: 0022823_	*10Mg Tab*	NDC: 00046042181	NDC: 51316009004
NDC: 54569055650	NDC: 00046042_		NDC: 00046042180	NDC: 11146094210
NDC: 00102333502	NDC: 00046042_		NDC: 00046042162	NDC: 52544030551
NDC: 46193073810	NDC: 00046042_		NDC: 00046042161	NDC: 52544030510
NDC: 46193073805	NDC: 00603548_		NDC: 00046042160	NDC: 00839711416
NDC: 52544030505	NDC: 53258015_	NDC: 00894633104	NDC: 00814644630	NDC: 00536430910
NDC: 52544030501	NDC: 54269010901	NDC: 00894633103	NDC: 54697006305	NDC: 00536430905
NDC: 53633032116	NDC: 51813007299	NDC: 00894633102	NDC: 54697006304	NDC: 00536430901
NDC: 53633032110	NDC: 51813007290	NDC: 00894633101	NDC: 54697006303	NDC: 35470050801
NDC: 12071044010	NDC: 51813007260	NDC: 10647042101	NDC: 54697006302	NDC: 00143150225
NDC: 54441004350	NDC: 53492301303	NDC: 50111046707	NDC: 49884010601	NDC: 51608042104
NDC: 54441004325	NDC: 53492301302	NDC: 50111046703	NDC: 00686018201	NDC: 51608042102
NDC: 54441004310	NDC: 53492301301	NDC: 50111046701	NDC: 51079027760	NDC: 10465042109
NDC: 54441004305	NDC: 00591555404	NDC: 52555001010	NDC: 00349845190	NDC: 00721002301
NDC: 54441004301	NDC: 00591555401	NDC: 52555001001	NDC: 00349845110	NDC: 54421011001
NDC: 49884010610	NDC: 52493063960	NDC: 00093060010	NDC: 00349845101	NDC: 19458042007
NDC: 49884010605	NDC: 00839711420	NDC: 00093060001	NDC: 50053310902	NDC: 19458042001

FIGURE 9.1. National Drug Codes. These 160 codes were all extracted from a single hospital information system at one point in time; all are for the same generic medication: a 10 mg tablet of propranolol.

extracted from a single hospital information system at one point in time. These codes are used to identify packaged medication products distributed in the United States. To a computer system, each of the 160 NDCs is distinct. Most health providers would have a very different view, because each of the 160 codes shown represents the same generic medication, a 10-mg tablet of propranolol. Any order entry system that asks providers to order a 10-mg propranolol tablet from a 160-element pick list is certain to fail. Yet the distinct codes are useful to pharmacists who manage inventory and dispensing; they need to know that one NDC coded product is a bottle of 50 tablets and another contains 500 tablets.

There are several lessons here. First, terminologies designed for one particular use may not work well in other circumstances. Second, terminologies can uniquely identify elements that have different characteristics or group elements that share one or more similar characteristics.

4.2. Types of Interoperability

The HealthePeople vision requires meaningful sharing of health data within and between enterprises and across various computer systems. In short, this means interoperability, or exchanged data between a sending system and a receiving system that uses the exchanged data for some intended purpose. Interoperability is not a binary state, simply present or absent. It is a graded state. At one extreme, data are sufficiently different so as to be un-receivable. At the other, data can be used transparently by the receiving system for all the same functions as natively generated data, including display and decision support. This latter state is known as *semantic interoperability*; it is the state that HealthePeople aspires to attain.

The transition between these two extremes involves data that the receiving system can receive, parse, and enter as a value into its existing data model. To do so, the receiving system must have a data model to accommodate the transmitted data, and the data must come appropriately shaped to fit the data model, that is, be the right data type and in the right format. In addition, sufficient metadata must accompany the transmitted data to guide the integration. This is known as *syntactic interoperability*.

On occasion, the term *computable data* is used to imply semantic interoperability. Simply put, these data are or can be defined using symbolic logic so that a computer can reliably process and draw inferences from them. They differ from *comparable data*, data structured in a way that permits the computer to determine that two things are the same, for example, that the expression *"left foot"* is the same as the expression *"left"* + *"foot"*.

4.3. Tasks for Controlled Medical Terminologies

Some users of clinical systems and even some informatics experts expect that terminologies can be effectively applied to any task that comes up. For example, many system designers use ICD9 in applications intended to collect finely grained clinical information, and end users are frustrated because ICD9 does not permit them to express the details of a case adequately. The root problem is not that ICD9 is a bad terminology. The root problem is that ICD9 was designed to collect morbidity and mortality statistics, and systems designers have used the wrong terminology for the job they needed to accomplish.

The important point is that controlled medical terminologies, like software, must support selected tasks based on functional requirements. In essence, terminology is software and requires rigor in its design, creation, and deployment. However, terminology tasks are not unique to each application. According to Rector (1998), terminology tasks can be classified into six categories:

1. Human–Computer Interaction: To support quick, intuitive data entry and query formulation by clinical users.
2. Archiving and Retrieval: To record and retrieve clinical information in medical records.
3. Mediation, Sharing, and Reuse: To allow information to be shared between medical record, decision support, and information retrieval systems.
4. Indexing and Knowledge Organization: To make it easier to index and organize information for other uses.
5. Authoring and Maintenance: To make it possible to build, maintain, and extend the terminology itself.
6. Natural Language Processing: To make it easy to express and ultimately to understand concepts in the language users speak and write.

4.4. Desirable Characteristics of Controlled Medical Terminologies

In 1998, Cimino identified 12 desiderata for controlled medical terminologies based on his review of the literature that have since gained broad acceptance (Cimino 1998). We believe all new vocabulary development should adhere to these fundamental principles, listed briefly below.

4.4.1. Content

Adequate expressiveness, that is, what can be said using the terminology, is critical. Content must be added using a formal methodology in order to minimize content coverage gaps and organizational inconsistency.

4.4.2. Concept Orientation

Concepts and terms are not the same thing. Terms are strings of letters we use in order to communicate about concepts (Campbell et al. 1998). Terminologies, while obviously composed of terms, should be based on concepts. Terms must correspond to at least one meaning (non-vagueness) and no more than one meaning (non-ambiguity). Meanings must correspond to no more than one concept (non-redundancy). Each concept in the terminology must have a single, coherent meaning.

4.4.3. Concept Permanence

Once a concept has been created in a terminology, its meaning can not change. If the meaning does change, data coded using that concept may become impossible to interpret.

4.4.4. Non-Semantic Concept Identifier

A terminology must have unique concept identifiers that are free of hierarchical or other implicit meaning. Any meaning that might be implied in identifier should be represented explicitly in the concept's definition instead. For example, in ICD9, "Essential Hypertension" is given the concept identifier "401." The concept identifier "401.1"

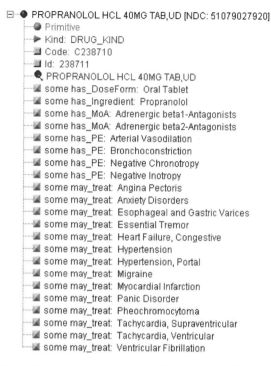

FIGURE 9.2. Description logic statements comprising a formal definition of propranolol.

is given to "Benign Hypertension." Paired together, these concept identifiers carry meaning, specifically that benign hypertension is a subtype of essential hypertension.

4.4.5. Polyhierarchy

Hierarchical arrangement of controlled medical terminologies is necessary to locate concepts, group concepts, and convey meaning. Multiple valid arrangements of concepts serving different purposes exist. Agreement on a single essential hierarchy is unlikely, and fortunately not necessary.

4.4.6. Formal Definitions

Formal definitions are represented in a form that can be manipulated with a computer, as opposed to narrative text definitions whose audience is human readers. Description logic is one of the most common ways to represent formal definitions. As Figure 9.2 illustrates, the term "propanolol hcl 40 mg tab ud (ndc 510790227920)" at the top of the figure is defined by the description logic statements such as "some_has_doseForm: Oral Tablet", and "some_has_MOA: andrenergic beta-1 antagonist." The total set of description logic statements, each starting with "some," comprises the complete formal definition.

4.4.7. Reject "Not Elsewhere Classified"

Sometimes terminologies include terms such as "Hypertension, Not Elsewhere Classified" (NEC) to collect concepts that do not fit well elsewhere in the terminology.

Unfortunately, catch-all terms are defined by exclusion. Each time a new concept is added to a terminology that uses NEC, the meaning of NEC may change. For instance, the concept "Hypertension NEC" has different meanings at different points in time if its parent terminology initially does not include the concept "Renovascular Hypertension" and subsequently adds it.

4.4.8. Multiple Granularities

The granularity of a term is a measure of its specificity and refinement. For example, "Congestive Heart Failure" is more coarsely granular than "Left Sided Congestive Heart Failure." Different users are likely to have needs for concepts with different granularities; terminologies should attempt to meet these varying needs.

4.4.9. Multiple Consistent Views

In a desideratum too complex to explain here, Cimino (1998) states that polyhierarchical terminologies with multiple levels of granularity must not permit inconsistent views of a concept. (For a full discussion of this principle, we refer the reader to Cimino's article.)

4.4.10. Context Representation

Controlled medical terminologies should include formal, explicit information about how concepts are to be used. Context has many dimensions, such as when it is appropriate or sensible to use a term. Most would agree that is sensible to use the term "fracture" in relation to the term "femur," but not to the term "eyebrow."

4.4.11. Graceful Evolution

The content and structure of controlled medical terminologies should change over time to reflect scientific advances, administrative changes, and other factors. Many changes, such as the addition of new concepts, are desirable. Other reasons, such as code reuse and changed codes, are undesirable. Whatever the case, any changes should be described and documented in detail.

4.4.12. Recognized Redundancy

Redundancy occurs when a terminology has more than one entry for the same concept. For example, in a fictitious terminology, the terms 1234 "Myocardial Infarction" and 3456 "Heart Attack" are redundant. If the terminology does not "recognize" that these terms represent the same concept, queries of encoded data (e.g., how many myocardial infarctions occurred in November) risk returning incomplete and inconsistent results. Synonymy is another name for recognized redundancy. Synonymy is desirable because it helps people recognize the terms they associate with a particular concept. Because synonyms map to a single concept, the coding is not redundant. In the previous example, if a terminology contains both terms "Myocardial Infarction" and "Heart Attack" but maps them to the same concept code, 1234, then the terms are synonymous within the terminology. Thus, a query for all myocardial infarctions in November would also return all data initially termed "heart attack."

Also in 1998, the ANSI Health Informatics Standards Board and the Computerized Patient Record Institute documented 11 desirable characteristics for controlled terminologies (Chute et al. 1998). More recently, standards development organizations have sanctioned technical specifications for terminology quality standards: the ASTM E 2087-00 (American Society for Testing and Materials 2000) and ISO TS17117 (International Standards Organization 2002). Additional publications advance our understanding of terminology quality indicators even further (Elkin et al. 2001; Elkin, Brown et al. 2002).

4.5. Rossi Mori Classification of Terminological Systems

Angelo Rossi Mori and colleagues evaluated the state-of-the-art in terminology format and representation and developed a three-part classification scheme, as shown in Table 9.2 (Rossi Mori et al. 1998). The Rossi Mori framework is a useful way to understand terminology at a high level.

4.5.1. First Generation

Traditional paper-based terminological systems are considered first generation in the Rossi Mori classification.

4.5.2. Second Generation

Compositional terminological systems built according to a categorical structure and a cross-thesaurus with predefined values for each category. Terms are defined by creating semantic links (e.g., "has-component, performs") to target categories (body part, health care procedure) and using predefined descriptors (colon, hemi-colectomy) to instantiate the target category.

TABLE 9.2. Comparison of terminological generations in the Rossi Mori classification.

	First generation	Second generation	Third generation
Presentation	Systematic list Alphabetic index	Categorical structure + cross thesaurus + lists + knowledge base of dissections	Universal Model engine by combinatorial rules
Organization	Fixed, typically single hierarchy	Dynamic, multiple hierarchical	Dynamic, multiple hierarchical
Purposes	Devoted to single application	Multiple	Multiple
Flexibility & extension	No, predefined list of allowable expressions	New atoms can be added, new compositions can be made	New combinations validated by computer by pre-validated rules
Processing on semantics	No, only storage, transmission, and retrieval of strings and codes	Clustering of phrases according to criteria Structured extension of lists Extract and rearrange details Structured input interfaces	Complete formal processing

Source: Rossi Mori et al. (1998).

4.5.3. Third Generation

Formal terminological systems represent concepts with a set of symbols and rules that create a structured and coded system that is computable. A unique canonical form made up of one or more symbols represents each concept. Models with formal rules are designed to allow an engine to manipulate symbols in a formal way. The symbols behave in ways that correspond to methods that humans use for represented concepts. Such formal and structured rules enhance internal consistency of a terminology system, and facilitate language evolution and maintenance. Formal techniques include, but are not limited to, description logics and higher order logics such as conceptual graphs.

5. A National Agenda for Terminology

New and evolving concepts of terminology content, representation, and delivery are necessary to realize the full potential of interoperation envisioned by HealthePeople. There are five steps we must take to achieve semantic interoperability on the scale envisioned by HealthePeople and other virtual health systems.

5.1. Step One. Content Coverage

The first step is to develop a series of terminologies to cover content in areas where the need for interoperation has been established. Work on content coverage is addressing at least three subtleties: setting priorities, granularity, and creation and curation.

5.1.1. Setting Priorities

The content coverage step implies that we set priorities for areas needing interoperation, and significant work has been performed to date. Organizations working to set priorities for terminology coverage include the Institute of Medicine, the National Committee on Vital and Health Statistics, the federal Consolidated Health Informatics Council, and the private sector eHealth Initiative, among others. Recommendation from these groups most commonly focus on the following areas, or domains: medical problems, laboratory test results, medications, and allergies. Other areas considered to be of primary importance are procedures, document titles, vaccinations, and anatomy.

5.1.2. Granularity

Content coverage must be at a level of detail, or granularity, sufficient for the intended task. We offer ICD9-CM as an illustrative example: because it was designed to group diseases for statistical evaluation of patterns of morbidity and mortality, it does not provide the more detailed terms necessary for day-to-day clinical care processes (Chute et al. 1996). However, other terminologies appear to provide content coverage with the extent of detail clinical care requires. Standardized Nomenclature in Medicine-Clinical Terms (SNOMED-CT) covers over 90% concepts contained within problem statements (Penz et al. 2004). The National Drug File Reference Terminology (NDFRT) covers all medications used in the VA, 97% of drug-related concepts in FDA oncology drug indications, 99% of medication physiologic effects (Rosenbloom et al. 2003), and 99% of concepts found on dictated medication lists (Brown et al. 2004). Formal content coverage studies of Logical Observation Identifiers Names and Codes (LOINC) for laboratory test names are lacking, but several publications informally confirm that its coverage is extensive (Lau et al. 2000; Dykes et al. 2003; Khan et al. 2003; McDonald et al. 2003).

5.1.3. Creation and Curation

Numerous domains do not yet have controlled terminologies that cover their content. Work must be done to address their creation, including how to identify the areas, how to create the content using the input of subject matter experts in the domain, how to integrate the new terminologies with existing terminologies, and how to keep the new terminology up to date once it is created. One possible approach is to solicit professional societies to be the content experts and curators of terms in their areas. Whatever approach is taken, terminologies should undergo content coverage studies performed by independent objective reviewers in accordance with established guidelines. Assertions by the terminology developers should be viewed as advertisements.

5.2. Step Two. Integrate and Interlock Terminologies

Two types of integration are necessary to create an interlocking system of terminologies to cover the depth and breadth of health care.

First, there needs to be organization and integration of content creation efforts. To date, groups have created terminologies without regard for the efforts (or lack thereof) of other groups. Terminology creation efforts should be orchestrated to ensure that important areas are addressed once, no more and no less. A directed approach will help ensure that terminologies for the breadth of biomedicine are available all the sooner. It is counterproductive for content development teams to duplicate or overlap in their efforts.

Second, there needs to be integration between terminologies covering different domains. For example, a particular medication, taken from a medication terminology, is used to treat a disease taken from a terminology for diseases. This is a special case of compositionality, covered in Step Four below.

5.3. Step Three. Timely Distribution

For terminology to be effectively deployed in production clinical applications, timely distribution is essential. The language of medicine is continually changing, making maintenance and evolution critical to clinical terminologies. New medical discoveries or simply new ways of categorizing known disease states constantly change the landscape. Nowhere in medicine, however, is the rate of change as rapid and visible as in the area of medications. While pharmaceutical companies introduce only around 20 new molecular entities, they launch tens of thousands of new packaged products. Thus, timely distribution means different things in different domains. Yearly or quarterly updates are sufficient for domains with relatively low rates of change; daily updates are essential in areas, such as medications, with rapid rates of change.

There are costs to a slow update process. If end users cannot find an appropriate term to accurately represent a particular fact, they may refuse to use the system or they may complain. To respond to user complaints and solve their immediate problems, local technical support staff may add a "new" term into a local version of the terminology. But the addition of new terms by local staff who are not subject matter experts familiar with the structure of the underlying terminology may create new problems—including the introduction of unrecognized synonymy and ambiguity, the misplacement of valid terms, and the mis- or under-definition of the new term. Even if the new term is properly formed and sent on to the terminology's official curators for review and inclusion, problems can arise. It may not be included in the next national release, putting it at risk of being lost when the local site updates their files. Or it may be included in a form different than that created locally. In both instances, the local update penalty applies: Data stored using the local term are not comparable to data stored using the nationally approved term and code. These data are potentially lost to research studies and decision support applications.

A rapid national terminology update system can address this problem. If the first local site to discover a missing term promptly reports the need to the national curators, and the national curators respond promptly, it is likely that the deficit can be corrected on a national scale before most users even realize there is a deficit. If turnaround times lag, multiple local versions of the new concept will exist, and the new update penalty price will be high. Patient records using different versions of the terminology will store different data, even when they are recorded at the same point in time.

To address this problem, the VA is evaluating two processes to improve the responsiveness of the missing term update problem. In the first, a pilot project named New Term Rapid Turnaround, a common interface for new terms helps end users place, document, and track their requests; it also helps curators with request intake, assessment, tracking, and end user feedback. In the second, a transactional update mechanism expedites updates for rapidly changing terminologies by permitting small changes to be made and efficiently distributed. For example, the mechanism may send out daily updates for new packaged drug products, rather than sent out monthly or quarterly versions of the entire terminology. Used in tandem, the two processes form the basis for responsive national scale terminology updates, as shown in Figure 9.3.

5.4. Step Four. Compositionality

Vocabulary construction and organization are an essential part of a functional electronic health record (McDonald 1997). Virtual health record systems require robust clinically relevant large-scale vocabularies with structures that support the construction of new terms. This functionality, known as compositionality, permits the creation of new terms via the combination of existing terms and appropriate linkages. For example, the new complex term "Cellulitis of the Left Foot" might be "post-coordinated" by using the following terms now available in SNOMED-CT:

Cellulitis (disorder) (128045006)
(has Finding Site)
Entire foot (body structure) (302545001)
(has Laterality)
Left (qualifier value) (7771000)

Compositional terminologies are one potential solution to the problem of content completeness. Post-coordinations are novel concepts constructed by users or applications that have not been included in the terminology but are entirely composed of concepts from the terminology. Pre-coordinations are concepts existing in a terminology that can also be expressed as a compositional expression using two or more concepts. For example, "Lung Cancer" can be represented as a "Malignant Neoplasm" of the "Lung."

If improperly executed, compositional terminologies can render data incomparable. A complete and explicit representational structure is needed to ensure that composi-

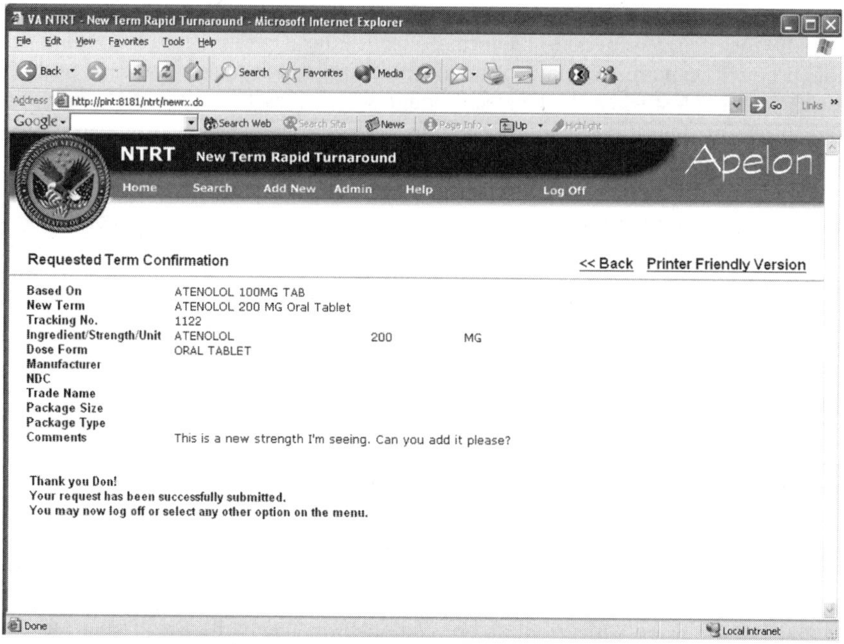

FIGURE 9.3. New term rapid turnaround request. This is a screenshot of a finished new term request. The process permits users from around the country to submit and track requests for new terms. To reduce data entry, the system permits users to use the closest existing concept in the terminology as the basis for a new term request.

tional data are comparable. Both pre-coordinate and post-coordinated expressions should use the same or a semantically translatable representational structure to be comparable.

Although compositionality is rigorous, it is necessary, as a recent usability trial at the Mayo Clinic made clear (Elkin et al. 1998, 1999). Users need to be able to form problem statements that represent the concepts of their practice, yet it is impossible to anticipate everything a clinician might wish to say about a patient. With the ability to form compositional expressions using well formed controlled vocabularies, we can represent the vast majority of clinical medicine (Elkin et al. 2003).

5.5. Step Five. Intellectual Property Issues

Intellectual property issues must be understood and addressed prior to the deployment of any controlled health terminology. This caveat applies to national standard terminologies as well any other terminologies that an institution may select and acquire on its own. Terminology users must acknowledge data as their most valuable information system asset and protect its value. Enterprises should read and understand licensing agreements for national standard terminologies such as SNOMED-CT, LOINC, and the federal drug terminologies. Pre-negotiated licensing agreements for these terminologies should be in effect and carefully reviewed prior to use.

For other terminologies, licensing terms must be negotiated. Prudent organizations will develop, implement, and test realistic plans to access coded data after license expiration or cancellation. The plan must respect legal data retention requirements and give practical consideration to the useful lifespan of specific data elements.

Another intellectual property issue to reconcile is ownership of new terms. Inevitably, sites need terms not found in the licensed vocabulary and may wish them to be included in subsequent releases. During initial deployment, legacy term sets may need wholesale inclusion; in releases that follow, missing terms may be discovered upon occasion. To address these issues, clear processes and ownership rights must be established for the inclusion and subsequent re-use of legacy term sets.

A third issue is derivative works. An organization that develops and maintains in-house terminologies in addition to using licensed materials should carefully explore the implications of content overlap upon future development. Finally, the issue of sending coded data beyond the licensing institution should be examined. Circumstances that may require this include mandatory reporting, management and research data "roll ups," and publications.

5.6. Step Six. Terminology Services

Getting terminology to end users and applications is critically important. As we discussed earlier, the emergence of new uses and system architectures drives access. Initially, terminology was stored as paper lists. Increasing demands for interoperation and standardization have driven terminology access toward broader availability, first across applications within the same system, and currently toward availability between different systems that may be geographically separate.

Having a single repository of terminology for more than one application or system makes sense. It facilitates data standardization and the creation of comparable data by eliminating multiple unrecognized ways to represent the same concept and implementing approaches to compositionality that cannot be formally normalized. It also reduces maintenance costs and conflicts. Obviously, updating terminology on one system is easier than on many. Less obvious is the cost of having different versions of the same terminologies in use across applications and systems at a single point in time. This situation is almost guaranteed with a multiplicity of terminology sources.

Terminology servers and services are a current approach to the problem of terminology access, maintenance, and data standardization. A terminology server, much like a web server, is a special purpose computer that waits for terminology requests from other computer systems and answers them. For example, a billing system might ask the terminology server for the ICD9-CM code for the term "hypertension." A more complicated example is the case that a provider order entry system needs to present a list of beta blocking agents to a clinician. The order entry system would request a list of medications from a terminology server that have in common the value "beta blocker" for the "mechanism of action" property.

At first it seems a daunting task to provide terminology services that can accommodate all possible requests. Fortunately, terminologies have enough common structural features (e.g., they all have terms and associated codes and many have hierarchical links) that it is possible to make terminology services that are largely independent of the terminology content being served. In fact, several specifications for terminology services have been developed. One of the first was the Common Object Request Broker Architecture (CORBA)-MED lexicon query service specification, now renamed the terminology query service. Other efforts in this arena include the Health

Level Seven (HL7) centralized terminology service specification, and the terminology query language developed at the University of California at Davis.

Adoption of terminology services has been slow. Perhaps too few organizations are sufficiently advanced in their implementation of electronic medical records to fully understand the power and importance of this approach. We hold that a service-based architecture for terminology access is a critical step within the national terminology agenda.

6. Preparing for the Future

6.1. *The Evolving Role of the Unified Medical Language System*

The National Library of Medicine's (NLM's) Unified Medical Language System (UMLS) project, begun in 1986, represents a long-term research and development effort to design, build, and maintain knowledge representations and data contents useful in facilitating electronic biomedical information retrieval (Lindberg et al. 1993; National Library of Medicine 2002). (Information about obtaining the UMLS Metathesaurus may be accessed at www.nlm.nih.gov/research/umls.) For example, the UMLS represents with one identification code the same concept from multiple disparate "standard" vocabulary sources, such as NLM's Medical Subject Headings (MeSH) and the World Health Organization's ICD9. The UMLS-based mapping from ICD9 to MeSH can facilitate electronic medical record based, quasi-automated, literature retrieval relevant to a patient case whose diagnoses are coded in ICD9 by submitting a MeSH-based query to NLM Pub Med (McEntyre and Lipman 2001; Sequeira et al. 2001; Macleod 2002). Annual editions of the Metathesaurus have been distributed since 1990. National Library of Medicine moved to quarterly updates in 2002. The November 2003AC edition includes 975,354 concepts and 2.4 million concept names in over 100 biomedical source vocabularies, some in multiple languages (National Library of Medicine 2003b).

The NLM has played a central role in the development, acquisition, and/or distribution of many of the 2003 PMRI core terminologies. For example, the NLM led the recent U.S. government-wide contract process for SNOMED-CT, and plans to incorporate CT into the UMLS in 2004 (National Library of Medicine 2003a). Further, NLM will be distributing the Federal Drug Terminologies including NLM's RxNorm, VA's NDF-RT, and three terminologies from the Food and Drug Administration (FDA) in upcoming versions of the UMLS.

National Library of Medicine's role in clinical terminology will be increasing in the future. In a letter to the Secretary of Health and Human Services dated November 5, 2003, the National Committee on Vital and Health Statistics recommended that the Secretary "designate the National Library of Medicine (NLM) as the central coordinating body to manage this terminology resource and coordinate its ongoing maintenance and distribution." While it remains to be seen exactly how this recommendation will be put into operation, the NLM has a long track record of successfully meeting its mandates.

6.2. *Facilities and Health Systems: Steps to Take*

To take advantage of data standardization at present and to be prepared for the change that will occur in the near future, facilities and health systems can take some additional steps.

6.2.1. Step One

Have clinical and administrative stakeholders assess institutional needs and priorities for comparable data and interoperation. The assessment should also include the institution's current and projected ability to use that type of data in their systems. For example, all stakeholders may agree that allergy information from other care sites is the single most important data they want, but there may be no current system to track and communicate this information within the facility. At the end of this process, a prioritized list of data types and timelines should be created. As new systems are contemplated, the list should be "evergreened."

6.2.2. Step Two

Review current systems and determine if, or how, they employ current standards for patient medical record information (PMRI) set by the National Committee on Vital and Health Statistics (NCVHS) and code sets required by the Health Insurance Portability and Accountability Act (HIPAA). This inventory should then be compared to the data priority list (created in Step 1) and an evaluation of conversion risks and benefits made. From this, a plan should be created for repairs that considers how to represent new data coming into the system and whether or not or how to convert old data already stored in the system.

6.2.3. Step Three

Monitor NCVHS PMRI standards on a routine basis. These recommendations are likely to evolve over time.

6.2.4. Step Four

Insist on the use of standard terminologies for all system purchases. In addition to the obvious effect of improving standardization at the purchasing site, the message communicated to system vendors will be loud and clear. As a result, the systems offered to other prospective clients will become increasingly compliant with emerging standards.

6.2.5. Step Five

Become involved with standards organizations such as HL7 and LOINC. While this step is not mandatory, contributing to the development of standards will help accelerate interoperability.

7. A Final Scenario

The increasing globalization of our economies and relative ease of international transportation underlies our opinion that interoperability of medical record information should not end at national borders. We offer a brief final scenario that illustrates this concept.

While on a business trip to Europe, Bill Kneivel becomes weak and notices his heart racing. He is treated for atrial fibrillation via an increase in the dosage of his blood pressure medicine. A new medication, ximelagatran (Exanta), is prescribed to reduce the risk of blood clots. Mr. Kneivel is sent out of hospital with his heart rate controlled, one week's worth of ximelagatran, and the advice to continue his care with his U.S.

physician. He cuts short his trip and returns home. On the way home, his heart rhythm silently changes between atrial fibrillation and normal several times. In his doctor's office the next week, Mr. Kneivel reports that he had some kind of heart problem but "they didn't explain it to me." Testing shows his heart rhythm to be normal, and a moderate inflammation of the liver.

7.1. *As Is*

Staff are unable to identify Mr. Kneivel's new pills, which he has repacked with his other medications in a single bottle for convenient transport. The doctor, uncertain what transpired in Europe, suspects that some cardiac event may have occurred but has no real idea what exactly that may have been. The doctor elects to further evaluate his status with non-invasive tests including an exercise tolerance test followed by 24-hour heart rhythm monitoring. Hepatitis is considered a possible explanation for fatigue and liver inflammation, and appropriate tests are sent. Four days later, while at home during the 24-hour heart-monitoring test, he notes the acute onset of left sided weakness. Emergency room doctors find that he has suffered a thromboembolic stroke, a known complication of the atrial fibrillation documented on his rhythm-monitoring device.

7.2. *Could Be*

The medical staff identifies Mr. Kneivel's new medications by typing in the imprint codes into a database at the NLM. Relevant articles and the European product labels are printed out for his doctor in the United States to review. The hospital summary is requested and delivered electronically. Although the record is written in French, the diagnoses, procedures, and medications are coded using standard terminologies and are automatically translated into English. The doctor is able to determine that Mr. Kneivel is suffering from intermittent atrial fibrillation, and that he has been placed on an anticoagulant available only in Europe that may account for the elevation in liver enzymes. The doctor starts an anticoagulant available in the United States and begins an evaluation of the rhythm disturbance. One week later, Mr. Kneivel's liver has returned to normal, and his rhythm is controlled on medications.

8. Closing Thoughts

Much of the promise of electronic health records lies in their ability to reach between sites and across time to meaningfully share and act upon health information. Fully realizing this vision demands that we meet the terminology challenges we have set forth in this chapter, including complete content coverage, the development and implementation of methodologies that create unambiguous compositional expressions, and the emergence of some workable system of coordinating and integrating various terminologies. Active work is underway in each of these areas, and we believe that future results will build upon past successes.

Much benefit can be derived from stepwise solutions. We can meet the terminology challenge in a series of small steps, rather than with a big bang. Prudent institutions will stay abreast of emerging national standards and implement them expeditiously. Benefits from deploying standards will be immediate at many sites and will accrue on a national scale as market penetration increases. The process will be speeded dramatically if systems purchasers *demand* products that adhere to standards.

We believe that the implementation of terminology standards and the concomitant accrual of clinical and business benefits will snowball at some point in the mid-range future. Only after a critical mass of institutions adhering to terminology standards is achieved will we be able to reap the full benefits of the Health*e*People vision.

References

American Society for Testing and Materials. 2000. E2087-00 Standard specification for quality indicators for controlled health vocabularies. Conshohocken, PA: American Society for Testing and Materials.

Bates DW, Leape LL, Petrycki S. 1993. Incidence and preventability of adverse drug events in hospitalized adults. J Gen Intern Med 8(6):289–294.

Bates DW, Spell N, Cullen DJ, Burdick E, Laird N, Petersen LA, et al. 1997. The costs of adverse drug events in hospitalized patients. Adverse Drug Events Prevention Study Group. JAMA 277(4):307–311.

Brown S, Elkin P, Rosenbloom S, Husser C, Bauer B, Lincoln M, et al. 2004. VA National Drug File Reference Terminology: a cross-institutional content coverage study. Medinfo 2004, in press.

Brown SH, Lincoln M, Hardenbrook S, Petukhova ON, Rosenbloom ST, Carpenter P, et al. 2001. Derivation and evaluation of a document-naming nomenclature. J Am Med Inform Assoc 8(4): 379–390.

Campbell KE, Cohn SP, Chute CG, Rennels G, Shortliffe EH. 1996. Galapagos: computer-based support for evolution of a convergent medical terminology. Proc AMIA Symp 1996; 269–273.

Campbell KE, Oliver DE, Spackman KA, Shortliffe EH. 1998. Representing thoughts, words, and things in the UMLS. J Am Med Inform Assoc 5(5):421–431.

Chute CG, Cohn SP, Campbell JR. 1998. A framework for comprehensive health terminology systems in the United States: development guidelines, criteria for selection, and public policy implications. ANSI Healthcare Informatics Standards Board Vocabulary Working Group and the Computer-Based Patient Records Institute Working Group on Codes and Structures. J Am Med Inform Assoc 5(6):503–510.

Chute CG, Cohn SP, Campbell KE, Oliver DE, Campbell JR. 1996. The content coverage of clinical classifications. For The Computer-Based Patient Record Institute's Work Group on Codes & Structures. J Am Med Inform Assoc 3(3):224–233.

Cimino JJ. 1998. Desiderata for controlled medical vocabularies in the twenty-first century. Methods Inf Med 37(4–5):394–403.

Dykes PC, Currie LM, Cimino JJ. 2003. Adequacy of evolving national standardized terminologies for interdisciplinary coded concepts in an automated clinical pathway. J Biomed Inform 36(4–5):313–325.

Elkin PL, Bailey KR, Chute CG. 1998. A randomized controlled trial of automated term composition. Proc AMIA Symp 1998:765–769.

Elkin PL, Bailey KR, Ogren PV, Bauer BA, Chute CG. 1999. A randomized double-blind controlled trial of automated term dissection. Proc AMIA Symp 1999:62–606.

Elkin PL, Brown SH, Carter J, Bauer BA, Wahner-Roedler D, Bergstrom L, et al. 2002. Guideline and quality indicators for development, purchase and use of controlled health vocabularies. Int J Med Inf 68(1–3):175–186.

Elkin PL, Brown SH, Lincoln MJ, Hogarth M, Rector A. 2003. A formal representation for messages containing compositional expressions. Int J Med Inf 71(2–3):89–102.

Evans RS, Pestotnik SL, Classen DC, Horn SD, Bass SB, Burke JP. 1994. Preventing adverse drug events in hospitalized patients. Ann Pharmacother 28(4):523–527.

Forslund DW, Smith RK, Culpepper TC. 2000. Federation of the person identification service between enterprises. Proc AMIA Symp 2000:240–244.

Garrison GM, Bernard ME, Rasmussen NH. 2002. 21st-century health care: the effect of computer use by physicians on patient satisfaction at a family medicine clinic. Fam Med 34(5):362–368.

Huff SM, Rocha RA, McDonald CJ, De Moor GJ, Fiers T, Bidgood WD, Jr., et al. 1998. Development of the logical observation identifier names and codes (LOINC) vocabulary. J Am Med Inform Assoc 5(3):276–292.

International Standards Organization. 2002. ISO 17117 Health informatics—controlled health terminology—structure and high-level indicators. ISO Technical Specification 2002;2002–02–15:32.

Kohn LT, Corrigan J, Donaldson MS, Institute of Medicine Committee on Quality of Healthcare in America. 2000. To err is human: building a safer health system. Washington DC: National Academy Press.

Khan AN, Russell D, Moore C, Rosario Jr AC, Griffith SP, Bertolli J. The map to LOINC project. Proc AMIA Symp 2003:890.

Lau LM, Johnson K, Monson K, Lam SH, Huff SM. A method for the automated mapping of laboratory results to LOINC. Proc AMIA Symp 2000:472–476.

Lindberg DA. Internet access to the National Library of Medicine. Eff Clin Pract 2000; 3(5):256–260.

Lindberg DA, Humphreys BL, McCray AT. 1993. The Unified Medical Language System. Methods Inf Med 1993;32(4):281–291.

Macleod MR. PubMed: http://www.pubmed.org. J Neurol Neurosurg Psychiatry 2002;73(6):746.

McDonald CJ. The barriers to electronic medical record systems and how to overcome them. J Am Med Inform Assoc 1997;4(3):213–221.

McDonald CJ, Huff SM, Suico JG, Hill G, Leavelle D, Aller R, et al. LOINC, a universal standard for identifying laboratory observations: a 5-year update. Clin Chem 2003;49(4):624–633.

McEntyre J, Lipman D. PubMed: bridging the information gap. CMAJ 2001;164(9):1317–1319.

National Library of Medicine. 2002. Fact Sheet Unified Medical Language System. Available from: http://www.nlm.nih.gov/pubs/factsheets/umls.html. Accessed 2002 Oct 24.

National Library of Medicine. 2003a. Fact Sheet Unified Medical Language System. Available from: http://www.nlm.nih.gov/pubs/factsheets/umls.html. Accessed: 2003 Dec 8.

National Library of Medicine. 2003b. SNOMED Clinical Terms® To Be Added To UMLS® Metathesaurus®. Available from: http://www.nlm.nih.gov/research/umls/Snomed/snomed_announcement.html. Accessed 2003 Dec 8.

Nightingale F. 1863. Notes on hospitals. 3rd ed. London: Green, Longman, Roberts, and Green.

Penz J, Lincoln M, Nguyen V, Brown S, Carter J, Elkin P. 2004. Evaluation of SNOMED coverage of Veterans Health Administration Terms. Medinfo 2004; 540–544.

Pestotnik SL, Classen DC, Evans RS, Burke JP. 1996. Implementing antibiotic practice guidelines through computer-assisted decision support: clinical and financial outcomes. Annals Int Med 124(10): 884–890.

Rector AL. Thesauri and formal classifications: terminologies for people and machines. Methods Inf Med 1998;37(4–5):501–509.

Rosenbloom ST, Awad J, Speroff T, Elkin PL, Rothman R, Spickard IA, et al. 2003. Adequacy of representation of the national drug file reference terminology physiologic effects reference hierarchy for commonly prescribed medications. Proc AMIA Symp 2003:569–578.

Rossi Mori A, Consorti F, Galeazzi E. 1998. Standards to support development of terminological systems for healthcare telematics. Methods Inf Med 37(4–5):551–563.

Rowberg AH, York WB Jr. 1999. Developing a framework for worldwide image communication. J Digit Imaging 12(2 Suppl 1):189–190.

Sequeira E, McEntyre J, Lipman D. 2001. PubMed Central decentralized. Nature 410(6830):740.

Spackman KA, Campbell KE, Cote RA. 1997. SNOMED RT: a reference terminology for health care. Proc AMIA Symp 1997:640–644.

van't Riet A, Beog M, Hiddema F, Sol K. 2001. Meeting patients' heads with patient information systems: potential benefits of qualitative research methods. Int J Med Inform 64(1):1–14.

10
Modeling for Health Care

Kenneth S. Rubin, Thomas Beale, and Bernd Blobel

1. Making the Case: The Rationale for Modeling

1.1. Why Model?

The world is complex. Health information systems are complex, and their interaction even more so. Differences in technologies, software, policies, and practices of care all converge to create an environment that is particularly complex. Modeling is a vehicle for managing complexity, allowing us to focus on areas of interest while intentionally concealing details not germane to the purpose.

Models add clarity to our understanding. Much like tools—for that is what they are—models exist for a purpose and within a context. Producing a model for the sake of doing so, or because some methodology dictates that it is "the way things should be done" delivers little or no returned value. Alternatively, using models to sharpen our understanding allows us to better navigate through difficult problems and situations and select what to include and exclude. The entire process is about determining the best way to express what is of interest while ignoring what is not.

Models allow us to formalize our understanding of a problem, and enable effective communication by sharing that understanding with a broad community. Using formal expressions to communicate is nothing new. Both mathematics and music have long relied upon specialized notation. Although these languages have little in common at the surface, they share an ability to capture, document, and communicate meaning to their target audiences clearly and concisely.

Health care is a uniquely complex domain. It is the confluence of so many things: the biological intricacies of the human organism, disease states, the social dimensions of care delivery in a finite-resource economy, and the consequences of world events such as epidemics and war. Not surprisingly, the discipline of health informatics is complex. It attempts to provide solutions at numerous levels and in multiple disciplines—real-time monitoring of intensive care unit patients, clinical decision support, and distributed interoperable health records, to mention a few. Modeling is a cornerstone to understanding these complexities.

1.2. All Models Are Wrong . . .

To quote the statistician George Box, "All models are wrong. Some are useful."

If this is true, why invest in modeling at all? We do every day. The entire software industry is nothing more than a set of models that happen to be executable. In the broadest sense, every information technology (IT) solution is a model of some sort, performing a set of functions perceived to be of added business value to an organization. A program is nothing more than a model running on a computer.

Given that models exist to increase our understanding and ability to manage complex subjects, we can recognize the value that the modeling process itself brings. The act of modeling—the discipline of parsing apart complex and intertwined concerns—often enables us to understand the true nature of a problem domain and leads us to a formal expression of solutions.

To use a medical analogy, surgeons do not train on cadavers to heal the cadaver. The end state of the cadaver is not the issue. The understanding of the practice and the subject is. This is certainly not to say that we should strive to create models of limited value, but we need to realize that the practice of modeling itself has inherent value. Failed modeling attempts often result in significantly increased understanding that results in a much stronger end result. Because of this, iterative modeling and, in fact, iterative development have taken such a stronghold in the marketplace.

1.3. Models as Formal Artifacts

Industry consensus as to the proper role of models over the lifetime of systems has been elusive. Experience has shown that good projects not only use models as implementation specifications, but also continue to maintain those models over time, using them for maintenance, enhancement, and training. Unfortunately, many projects still consider modeling exclusively as an analysis and design activity. Designs are given to programmers and used as static input documents. They are not seen as deliverables that provide ongoing value in a holistic process.

This approach results in the loss of value of the models over time: Code is maintained, but models and documents are not. This leads to the well-known programmer's complaint that software is inadequately or entirely undocumented (Brooks 1975).

Many software developers and methodologies fail to recognize that various expressions of a system—requirements, analysis models, design models, and code—are each representations of the same thing at varying levels of abstraction. Thus, software engineering management does not always embrace a culture where all deliverables are maintained throughout the life of the product. As IT expenditures come under increasing pressure, IT management in the development and procurement environments is finally beginning to see the business value of methodology and models, and the ongoing maintenance of the latter.

1.4. Modeling in Health

Certain legacy efforts within health care provide a good foundation from which the next generation of models are emerging. Healthcare models, like perhaps all models, may never be complete. After initial development, models often undergo revision and harmonization cycles as efforts continue to improve and adjust them. In addition to changes to the models themselves, there are changes to the modeling practices, improving and morphing along with our understanding of how to best capture our knowledge.

Early works in this space that went on to influence future activity include the Good European Health Record (GEHR), 1992–1995; Patient Oriented Management Architecture (POMA), 1995; Comité Européen de Normalisation (CEN) ENV 12265 Electronic Health Record (EHR) standard, which emerged in 1993; RICHE, a European project which developed reference models for the cooperative act management concept; CEN ENV 12967 Health Informatics—Health Information Systems Architecture (HISA).

Many health jurisdictions, including localities, federal governments, and nations, have embarked upon modeling efforts as part of their attempts to understand and manage their healthcare needs. Prominent examples include the Australian National Health Information Model (http://www.aihw.gov.au/knowledgebase/index.html), the U.S. Department of Defense Functional Area Model-Data—FAM-D, the United Kingdom's National Health Service Healthcare Model (http://www.standards.nhsia.nhs.uk/hcm/index.htm), and the Canadian Conceptual Health Data Model (http://www.cihi.ca/).

Several industry efforts are making inroads into modeling architectural services to support health informatics. Comité Européen de Normalisation is revising its ENV 13606 EHR standard and ENV 12967 HISA service specifications on the basis of technical and knowledge models.

The Object Management Group Healthcare Domain Task Force (OMG HDTF) expressed its specifications using the object-oriented interface definition language (IDL) and included models as supportive knowledge (Object Management Group Healthcare Domain Task Force 2000). Health Level Seven (HL7) was among the first healthcare organizations to embrace a model-based development approach in messaging standards, manifested in its Model Development Framework (MDF) to manage what had been growing inconsistency, variability, and optionality (Health Level Seven Modeling and Methodology Committee 2003) Today, this approach is at the core of current work on Version 3 of their standard. Models play an important role in the Open Source and *open*EHR initiatives as well.

2. A Framework for Modeling

Modeling has inherent value as a step toward interoperable health systems. An analytical framework allows us to understand existing modeling products and to develop new ones. Without a framework, it is difficult or even impossible to understand what models are needed, what each model's role and purpose are, and what means of expression are capable of creating and integrating them.

The framework we present is based on widely accepted industry approaches. It describes the structure of the *modeling landscape* and serves to remind us that a multiple models are required to specify a complex system or standard.

2.1. Performance Criteria for Good Models

What constitutes a good model? Like good software, good models are based upon requirements, criteria that can be specified and ultimately evaluated to assess the value of the work product. Good models represent good business value. Unbridled, unconstrained, resource-intensive effort does not result in a good model. Quite the contrary: good models are almost never attainable without clearly defined purpose, objectives, quality controls, and expectations.

These strategically important qualities of good models are described via performance criteria of the models over their lifetime. Quality models remain relevant and economic over time. Creating a good model requires modeling efforts that:

- **Effectively support complex requirements**. Real world systems are complex, as are the requirements that drive them. The formal expression of these complexities can easily be logic defying. For instance, a condition like diabetes becomes incredibly complicated when the cause, diagnosis, treatment, and social implications are formally and rigorously captured. A good model can capture information of import effectively and accurately, while managing complexities by obscuring unnecessary detail.

- **Cope with continual change in requirements.** There are many sources of change, such as research, best-practice clinical protocols, economic factors, legislation, and epidemics. Good models result in adaptable systems that are economic and reasonable to maintain and enhance over time.
- **Create models that are economically implementable.** Many projects have spent significant resources (people and money) the yielded results of limited value, often in the form of domain models or data sets. Such failures tend to lack purpose or a coherent view. Without a clear use, modeling activities proceed uncontrolled. A model has little value if it does not affect an implementation directly or indirectly.
- **Promote information and knowledge longevity.** History teaches us that IT investments are long-term capital investments. In some instances, they last years beyond even optimistic projections. The impetus to hang on to legacy platforms arises in part from the fact they often contain institutional knowledge that resides nowhere else.

It takes conscientious effort and practice maturity to extract this business knowledge, both rules and information semantics, and maintain it separate from the code base of systems. Mining existing systems for business rules is painful, as is making the business case to incur the upfront investment to not repeat this tragic mistake. Embedded enterprise knowledge ultimately adds significant maintenance burdens (e.g., time and cost) to systems development.

To avoid such burdens, business rules and information content must be captured and described in a place physically separate from the executable code base itself. These rules may be templates upon which the code base relies, but the separation of them as distinct first-order artifacts is significant and promotes longevity beyond the technologies upon which systems are built. In sum, models are the vehicles to capture and communicate this content.

2.1.1. Design Future-Proof Software

Longevity of software is achievable by designing systems with future-proofness in mind from the outset. Through modeling, projects may achieve this objective by creating logical separations in areas that are particularly prone to aging, such as foundational technologies, implementation techniques, etc.

2.1.2. Connect with the Targeted Community

Whether represented on paper or within tools, models must be comprehensible to succeed in their basic intent, that is, to effectively communicate with those for whom they are intended. The selection of approach and formalism are crucial to ensuring that models are useful for their relevant communities. If models are written by a select few in an inappropriate formalism and interpreted by those few for the rest, the community is put at risk. This inner-circle mentality serves primarily to exclude, positioning the broader community either to agree blindly or disagree with that which they do not understand.

3. The Modeling Landscape

The naïve approach to modeling—the selection of a formalism and then jumping in—is the modeling equivalent of hacking. It inevitably results in issues: the chosen formalism is not well suited to the subject matter; the modeling activity explodes exponentially or suffers analysis paralysis; the effort loses sight of its original objectives or requirements; and so on.

Success demands discipline and structure. Concepts of separation allow for partitioning a problem space in support of real-world solutions. They include:

- Separation of Interests: breaks a subject domain into recognized areas of responsibility
- Separation of Technical and Knowledge Spaces: differentiates the worlds of IT and domain knowledge
- Separation of Viewpoints: views the problem space from multiple formally specified perspectives

3.1. *Separation of Interests*

Separation of the modeling space on the basis of interests (such as subject domains—clinical, financial, administrative, etc.) brings several benefits: it limits the size and scope of models, it allows incremental delivery of systems, and it enables cohesive information gathering and validation through coherent user community engagement. Simply put, separating interests allows for a narrower focus on a more precise topic which itself has inherent value in understanding and capturing what is of interest in that topic.

Multiple criteria influence the selection of sub- or super-domains. Probably the most important indicator is that the area of interest has already been identified in literature, research, and by the industry. This is often based upon items such as common semantics, shared communities of interest, strong cohesion within a subject area, and minimal codependence with another subject area.

It is in this subdivision of complex spaces that better understanding can be gleaned. Though there is no absolute rule for separating interests, several qualities should be considered as such decisions are being made. Organizational, logical, and technical properties are broad-based domains and often best separated. For instance, multiple organizations working within one enterprise may have differing policies that need to be understood and manifested in models and systems. A policy domain model describing requirements and solutions of a system beyond technology is a powerful and tremendously useful concept.

Domain specialties are also used as categories for separation: laboratory, radiology, histopathology, endocrinology, oncology, and so on. At a systems level, different separations become evident, with categories such as the EHR, decision support, terminology, and messaging as lead contenders.

Ultimately, the purpose of separation is to differentiate those concerns with significant value in a way that they can be comprehended and managed, while limited efforts in those that do not. There are no absolutes, and the rationale by which these decisions are made must be germane to the effort underway. If a particular domain separation does not add value to the overall effort, there is no need to do it.

3.2. *Separation of Knowledge and Technical Spaces*

The next area that requires distinction during modeling lies between the knowledge space (where domain knowledge is captured and structured by content experts) and the technical space (focused on and used by information system developers). As this division has not achieved widespread industry adoption, it merits a bit of explanation.

In this approach, domain experts directly create and maintain specifications of their information and workflows. Domain experts are not asked to become expert modelers, though training on approach and tools is required. Contrary to most methodologies, this approach does not require IT staff to become domain experts—a real strength. By setting the stage for well-architected software—embodied by a separation between business knowledge and technical infrastructure—more flexibility exists to respond to changing business needs and the requirements gap between subject matter experts and IT staff is effectively eliminated.

Known as two-level modeling (Beale 2000), it has been successful in health care. For example, computerized clinical guidelines such as Prodigy (Purves et al. 1999) are defined in object models built from clinical subject matter experts using knowledge tools and executed by systems at runtime. Ontologies and terminologies such as Galen (Rector et al. 1995) and SNOMED-CT (Spackman 1999), used directly within information systems, also exist in the knowledge space and are maintained by clinical specialists using dedicated tools.

In two-level modeling, generic models of information and services are defined in the technical space, while formal configurations of these technical models are defined in the knowledge space. It is these configurations that comprise the second level. The knowledge describes the principles and methodologies at meta-level, which are applied (or "instantiated" in the GEHR terminology) at the technical level.

Each level is focused on one community (functional or technical), and the project team composition must reflect this. The approach allows the project team to maximize available resources by playing to the experience and strengths of its members rather than forcing them into unfamiliar paradigms. Further, the approach exploits such key principles as clear role identification, targeted purpose for the models, and effective communication with designated audiences.

3.3. *Separation of Viewpoints*

The third paradigm involves the recognition different roles result in differing points of view that come together to provide a more complete picture of a problem space. The quip that "all of us are smarter than any of us" is a coy reference to the value of viewpoints: the more points of view considered for any given thing, the more insight we have.

Thus, a standard that can provide us with a set of viewpoints is tremendously valuable. The International Organization for Standardization (ISO) gives us that standard in its Reference Model for Open Distributed Processing (RM-ODP), which specifies five viewpoints and provides the criteria and language for differentiating them (International Organization for Standardization 1995)

Fundamental to understanding the value of viewpoints is realizing that they are not derivative, duplicative, or competitive; indeed, ISO asserts all five viewpoints are needed to describe a complex distributed system. Thus, RM-ODP provides a more robust set of tools allowing us to make educated decisions and achieve maximum value as we strive to meet the objectives of our modeling.

The viewpoints identified below are based upon the RM-ODP standard, thus they have clear names and precise definitions. In effect, the standard can serve as the arbiter of the complexity. Project teams working without this insight often resort to phrases like "in my experience," "it is best if . . . ," and "professional opinion," indicative of subjective measures for decision making. The RM-ODP viewpoints provide a technical, repeatable underpinning to objectively separate problem spaces. The RM-ODP viewpoints are:

- **Enterprise**: concerned with the business activities—the purpose, scope, and policies of the specified system. This viewpoint describes the real world as it interacts with the system or subject in question, irrespective of technology. It is concerned with the forces affecting the business (rules, regulations, constraints, etc.) and how they interact, not how they are represented in an IT system.
- **Information**: concerned with the meaning, semantics, and structure of information that needs to be stored and processed in the system—what the system provides in terms of information. This view captures attributes of interest, relationships to other types of information, information constraints, and so on. Information viewpoint models are commonly expressed using the static class models of the Unified Modeling Language (UML) (Object Management Group 2003).
- **Computational**: focused on how a system will do its activities—concerned with the description of the system as a collection of parts and interfaces that must coordinate to meet its objective of a logical design. This view addresses the capabilities, responsibilities, and behaviors of each major component. Unified Modeling Language can be used to capture this view through diagrams such as functionally oriented class diagrams, state diagrams, sequence diagrams, and collaboration diagrams.
- **Engineering**: concerned with the construction of the system—how the subject is to be built. Is the implementation of this component to be federated? How will that federation be implemented? What is the targeted deployment architecture? How will the different components communicate? What role will middleware play? This view focuses on the pragmatics of implementation, ultimately including information specified by the information view and behaviors from the computational view.
- **Technology**: concerned with the detail of the parts from which the system is to be constructed. This bill of materials lists all the technologies and products that make up the system platform. For instance, it could describe a system as a Java implementation supporting J2EE on Linux platform residing on *XYZ* servers across a wide-area network connecting 300 workstations. The engineering view describes how the pieces fit; the technology view identifies what those pieces are.

Armed with this knowledge, let's apply the RM-ODP viewpoints to an example to illustrate their utility:

Mr. John Smith presents at a community clinic with his wife, who has taken ill [use case described in the Enterprise View]. They have never been to this clinic before. Mrs. Smith has a personal electronic health record "vault" on the web, containing her medical information [Information View] to which she has granted consent. She is asked to provide her smart card [Technology View] and identifying information: her date of birth, health plan identifier, and address [Information View]. Using this information to identify her, the clinic system calls an Identity Management System [Computational View] to verify her identity, and then retrieves her record from the EHR vault.

3.4. A Synthesis

Applying the RM-ODP viewpoints, we are better equipped to parse this scenario to determine how and where it influences the system that we are designing. Yet parsing a problem space results in a significant quantity of models being produced. This gives rise to the question whether maintaining multiple small models is more effective than maintaining just one larger model.

The answer is yes, for a variety of reasons. Harkening back to our principles, the "one larger model" approach inevitably means that the model is multi-purpose, trying to meet the needs of varying audiences and objectives. In health care, there is a need for general practitioners, but they are not a replacement for specialists. To cover the breadth necessary to provide quality care, both have their place and result in optimal treatment when properly used.

So it is with models. Broader models have utility if they have uniformity of purpose, internal integrity, and other characteristics of good models. Models parsed according to the views and separations described here are more focused, smaller, and more manageable. The separation techniques provide a modeling tool kit for dissecting complex problem spaces into manageable chunks.

The process of modeling is more art than science. Methodologies that prescribe absolute steps inevitably fail if they are not adaptable to project-specific needs and concerns. The concepts presented here are intended to provide alternatives that can be applied to navigate complexities or to complement other methodologies in use.

Although professional opinion differs on how to apply these techniques to result in the best product, there is little controversy about the value of the techniques themselves. Each has its strengths and an ability to add insight into the problem space.

4. Putting Models to Work

Discussions of modeling may be interesting and perhaps even compelling, but they are academic without a practical approach that uses them to guide systems development. Effective models are not only artifacts; they are tools used in the process of system engineering, development, and maintenance to formally and unambiguously communicate.

Putting models to work requires understanding the principles that form the basis for best practice. These principles are fundamental to any effort that involves modeling.

4.1. Getting Started

First, consider the problem space as a whole. Begin to understand the complexities of the problem. As you develop an approach to address them, you can start to understand where models may be of benefit. Questions to raise include the following:

What parts of the project definition are simply not understood?
What aspects of the effort are particularly unclear or subject to misunderstanding?
How do you plan to capture knowledge from your subject matter experts?
How do you plan to communicate specifications with project technical staff?
From what pieces and technologies will the system be constructed?

Each of these questions helps to estimate the overall number, purpose, and role of models within a project. The better you understand each modeling product and the value it brings, the better prepared you become to make decisions about the level of effort, semantics, and rigor required—and the complexity of activities to produce them.

4.2. Determine What Models Are Needed

Once the project begins and you start to understand its demands, it is time to apply the modeling framework. The framework separates out the problem space into manageable pieces and outlines what can be a very broad and complete coverage. Pragmatism dictates that you do *just enough* of the framework to address your needs without expending efforts on models that do not add value.

When applying the modeling framework, remember that the models you choose must cover the intended and necessary breadth. The Modeling Landscape is intended to be broadly based. Do not demand equal treatment across all the interests and viewpoints for a given activity. Despite the natural human tendency to seek consistency, do not seek or expect equal depth and coverage across the model. Always keep in mind the purpose you are trying to achieve with the model. Modeling to detail beyond the model's purpose is merely wasted effort.

As an exemplar, let's apply this approach in a context of the communication and management of patient information. This example focuses on clinical computing, but is easily applicable to other genres.

4.2.1. Identify Area(s) of Interest

The first step is to identify those areas of the problem space the model will address. Consider the match based upon required functionality and recognized areas of interest within the domain. For our project, these might include the EHR, workflow, laboratory investigations, prescribing, and patient administration. The Object Management Group's Healthcare Domain Task Force (OMG HDTF) has provided a useful partitioning of the clinical computing space that merits consideration here.

4.2.2. Locate the Project in Knowledge and/or Technical Space

The next step is to determine how knowledge engineering fits in the overall fabric of the effort. In clinical computing, knowledge artifacts play a significant role, particularly because terminologies are prevalently used. The key issue then becomes the decision whether it is more appropriate to create our own knowledge definitions (special terminologies or vocabularies, archetypes, templates, computerized clinical guidelines, or other ontological specifications) or to use standard ones.

Projects need two kinds of models: knowledge models and technical models. Knowledge artifacts rely upon a formalism (and ultimately a language to express that formalism) to be sufficiently expressed and satisfy the needs of the software engineering community. The languages used for this knowledge expression can be elusive, particularly because they are usually embedded within tools. Several alternatives exist to support building and maintenance of terminologies, clinical guidelines, archetypes, and templates (Beale 2003).[1]

This activity of knowledge content selection and representation is the backbone for the future proofing needed for HealthePeople to be successful. Ultimately, the instances

---

[1] Note that within the HL7 Standards organization, a number of specialized constructs to support that organization's methodology are consistent with this theme. HL7 Refined Message Information Models (RMIMs) and Common Message Element Types (CMETs) are examples.

supporting this knowledge must be collected and used directly (instances being the vocabularies, guidelines, message models, and archetypes representing that knowledge). The source of the ontology development tools and languages is important, but merely an enabler to this ultimate need.

This set of activities must be carefully planned, as it is the stepping stone toward empowering the domain community to being knowledge providers while separating the technical community from trying to embed that knowledge in source code.

4.2.3. Determine Required Viewpoints

In the technical space, some viewpoints will play more significant roles than others. In our experience, the information and computational viewpoints have been absolutely essential, and should be considered the primary focus areas. The role played by the other viewpoints depends greatly upon the purpose of the activity. For example, a standards development organization (SDO) working on functional specifications would be far less interested in the engineering and technology views than would a project focused on deployment.

Every viewpoint to be used requires production of a distinct model in each area of interest from the project's list of desired artifacts. This combinational effect, plus the presence of knowledge languages and models, defines the model space for the project.

As a result, no single diagram can effectively *model* multiple viewpoints (though multiple viewpoints may be cross-walked on a common diagram to show relationships). It is from this basis that we assess which models may be drawn from existing sources (standards, public domain, procured) and which must be built. It is risky to underestimate the effort involved in adapting another model to our purposes, particularly if it is being even slightly re-purposed as a result.

Examples of distinct models required due to the use of viewpoints in multiple areas of interest include the EHR information model, EHR service model (or API), demographic business rules, demographic information model, demographic service model, terminology service interface, and so on.

4.3. A Picture Is Worth a Thousand Words . . .

The old adage may be true, but does that mean that a picture is a model? There is a common misconception that any diagram depicting technical content constitutes modeling. It probably does not. If that picture is an abstraction of a problem space absent of unwanted detail, it may satisfy the most basic definition of a model. If that same picture can also clearly and concisely capture and communicate knowledge, then we are getting closer. It is more likely, though, that the picture is just a picture. Here's why.

Have you ever attended a great brainstorming session? The group convenes and hashes out a number of complex and difficult issues, around a whiteboard, and emerges with what everyone agrees is *the solution*. The whiteboard diagram grows and grows to encompass this perfect solution. A willing volunteer captures the diagram and agrees to distribute it out. Is this a model?

Yes and no. If we were part of that meeting, the diagram is crystal clear and depicts the understanding that was reached. It is a meaningful communication of what happened. Now let's change the example. Most of us have received such a diagram from a meeting that we did not attend. Did it make sense? Did it unambiguously communicate? Did we understand it before someone who had attended walked us through?

It is unlikely, because such diagrams have no semantics, no meaning. Until meaning is attributed to the symbols, they are merely boxes and lines, and subject to interpretation. This is the difference between diagrams and models. Formalisms have both a depiction and a meaning. Use of a symbol means something, and that meaning is conveyed to anyone with a knowledge of that formalism. Without an underlying semantic model, the result is merely a diagram of boxes or lines or whatever that have no inherent meaning (or interpretation).[2]

Models, then, are capable of standing on their own. If the outcome of that same meeting was a model, the need to communicate the diagram to those conversant in the modeling language is minimal. This is not to say that a brainstorming session must be conducted using rigorous notation. In fact, there are good reasons not to.

What we are asserting, however, is that it is not sufficient to capture the knowledge gleaned from the event exclusively in the informal diagram. It is far more powerful to rework the picture into a formal model, reconvene the group, talk through the formal representation, and ultimately validate both the model and the understanding that will persist beyond the meeting. The diagram is useful, but primarily as a stepping stone.

This leads us to our first principle of modeling: *Not all pictures are models.*

4.4. Choice of Formalism for Each Model

So, if we are to do modeling and not merely drawing, there is a need for us to select a formalism. As used here, a *formalism* is simply the language, notation, or semantically meaningful expression—graphical or textual—in which to express a model. Models may be formal or informal. Informal models are based upon expressions that are limited or no semantic rigor.

For informal models, their strength is also their weakness. Lack of semantic rigor makes informal models easy to create and easy to use—so long as everyone consuming them really understands what the model is saying. One question remains that cannot be overlooked: how can the author be sure that the reader really understands if the symbology being used has no inherent meaning? Informal models have intrinsic value, but tend to fall short at their ability to unambiguously communicate—one of our asserted objectives.

In the end, projects with non-trivial objectives are best served using formal models. The project is left with selecting a formalism to meet its needs, and that is best done through a formalism that is a semantic match to the purpose and types of models needed. For example, knowledge models might require a constraint language; an information model could be modeled in UML; a service model could be modeled in UML, IDL, or WSDL; business rules might need their own syntax.

Even in this small example, different formalisms are used for different models, each of which is part of the modeling landscape. Semantic fit is not the only factor. Other issues must also be considered:

Who is the primary audience of the artifact?

Are there de facto representations familiar to that audience?

Are the de facto representations adequate/sufficient to unambiguously express what is trying to be captured?

---

[2] An excellent critique of meaningless diagramming and how to add meaning to diagrams is given by Clements et al. (2003) in "Documenting Software Architectures: Views and Beyond." Boston, MA: Addison-Wesley.

Are there multiple audiences?
How rigorous an expression is required?

First, we must decide how precise our communication must be. For example, if we are targeting a very broad audience, pretty pictures with less semantic rigor are a good fit. Alternatively, if a knowledgeable, skilled, and focused audience is our target, we are better served using formal notation with little ambiguity. This leads us to our second principle: *Choose a formalism based upon its ability to accurately represent the semantics you are trying to capture. When alternatives exist, use the formalism best suited to each audience.*

In each case, the purpose and formalism must be married. Industry experience has shown little success with business users when they are shown technical models. This should come as no surprise. The very specificity that speaks well to a technical audience is too detailed, obtrusive, and cumbersome for non-technical audiences. What results is the basis for our next principle: *Technical models do not speak to non-technical audiences.*

Formal models use textual or graphical notation in which the meaning of every utterance in the language is defined. Further, because the rules of such notations generally distinguish proper for improper representations, expressions in such a notation are testable to determine if they are well formed and syntactically accurate. In much the same way that a syntax checker parses computer code, so too may rigorously expressed models can be parsed to determine if they are well formed. When selecting a formalism, the following questions can help determine how rigorous it is:

Is there a set of symbols (or reserved words) identified within the notation?
Do the symbols/words have defined meanings?
Are the rules for applying the notation clear?
Can they be applied consistently and repeatably?
Is the notation robust enough to express what needs to be captured for its intended purpose?
Would two skilled readers of the model come away with the same understanding?

Does this make a difference? We know it does. Several years ago, one of the authors attended an industry seminar on data warehousing and security where the creator and zealot of a new methodology presented his work. He introduced his symbology via loose descriptions of symbols and his intentions behind them. We were then asked to perform exercises to demonstrate what we had learned. When our work was evaluated, we were informed that our representation was wrong. When we asked why, we were told "because you didn't use the symbols right." The symbols had no underlying definitions. The symbols had no objective criteria upon which their use could be assessed. We were wrong "just because." No one wants to be the business owner, manager, technical director, or chief architect of a large-scale expensive project that failed as the result of a miscommunication of a key requirement between technical staff "just because."

Models, like other languages, require definitions that others beside their inventors understand. This gives us our next principle: *Select formalisms capable of rigorously expressing content and capable of communicating to your target audience.*

Where practical, leveraging accepted industry notations and semantics offers benefits. Usually such languages have identified meanings, rules, and conformance criteria to determine whether a particular model is well formed. Notations accepted by industry have been embraced by at least some community. If that community is our target audience, then the formalism is a good one (for them anyway).

Finally, caution requires that we live within the rules of an industry formalism. If we re-purpose a standard to meet our needs, we may alienate everyone conversant in that formalism. In the realm of language, for example, if we changed the meaning of "no" to mean affirmative, no one reading that word would understand its meaning. Good formalisms provide mechanisms to extend themselves to meet these types of needs. Limiting customization to these accepted extensions ensures that we reap the benefits of using the industry formalism in the first place.

4.5. *Tooling*

Tooling is an important consideration when choosing formalisms. Although idealists assert that tools are non-essential when conducting modeling activities, pragmatists realize that software and systems are built with tools, models that cannot easily foster this environment are much less likely to be used.

This is not to imply that tooling should overshadow the value of the models expressed in those tools. The tooling exists to support the overall modeling and development process, and not vice versa. It is amazing how many projects lose sight of this—focusing on tooling for its own sake and sacrificing product and methodology as a result. This forms our first principle of tooling: *Those formalisms that are truly open, well accepted within a community, and portable will have a marketplace of off-the-shelf products to support them.*

The investment in the modeling effort far exceeds the investment in tooling. It is the models that are the organizational asset, ultimately a knowledge asset. Thus, it is important to ensure that the expression of those knowledge assets remains portable. Locking-in to tools devoid of open access to knowledge assets presents incredible long-term risk. How will that knowledge be retrieved if there is a change in products, either by choice or by default?

There are products that import and export knowledge freely. Many alternatives may be acceptable: industry-accepted open APIs [such as XML Metadata Interchange (XMI)], persistence of information in an open data format [such as Structured Query Language (SQL) tables], and non-proprietary content export option [such as eXtensible Markup Language (XML)] are among reasonable choices. It is for this reason that we add the second principle of tooling: *Ensure that your tooling selection supports free exchange of information. The content of the model must outlast today's tooling.*

4.6. *Executable Models and Model-Driven Architecture*

In some cases, formal models can be converted directly to executable systems using sophisticated tools. In fact, there are products available at the time of this writing that support this, both in terms of formalisms and products capable of reading and executing those formalisms. When conditions support their use, choosing to use such products can be advantageous.

However, this option is not ideal for every situation. It requires a project team experienced in models, use of formalisms capable of supporting the capability, advanced tooling, and organizational interest and commitment to this as a path. But for those willing to make this commitment, significant benefits are realized by narrowing or eliminating the gap between models and executable code.

Within a framework such as the OMG Model Drive Architecture (MDA), UML is one formalism from which executable systems can be automatically generated. In brief, the MDA describes a set of related models, some of which are independent of platform and computational concern, adding technology details in supporting models to provide for code generation.

A UML component diagram describes software components and their dependencies in a structural form, ultimately defining rules of implementation and specifying a physical architecture. This content, coupled with tools capable of understanding and mapping the formalism into code, produces a set of implementation files. In addition, the UML deployment diagram describes hardware and software component of the run-time architecture.

Using a rigorous process such as the Rational Unified Process (Kruchten 1999), executable code is directly derived from the verified set of UML models. To develop flexible, scalable, portable, future-proof systems, the logical and physical views expressed in UML should be developed separately.

The notion of model-driven architecture is realized by generalizing key underlying concepts and representing them as a platform, separate from environmental concerns such as conditions and constraints. In this sense, a platform is not limited to hardware, but includes characteristics of technology, organization, function, etc., that classify and distinguish one platform from another. This is how platforms may be abstracted, resulting in specifications that are platform independent and open.

Described in the OMG's MDA specification (Object Management Group 2003), platform independent models (PIMs) are represented using UML as a formal semantic expression. Using UML as a rigorous formalism, a rich model is developed and matured, containing the subjects, behavior, and constraints of the information and system being modeled. It is important to recognize that PIMs are exactly what their name denotes: models that are free of specific hardware or computing platform requirements and constraints. This is essential to the approach.

The use of model-driven architectural approaches in health care is not unprecedented. Efforts such as the Harmonization of Web-based Applications (HARP) have employed this technique to produce executable systems derived almost entirely from model with minor manual augmentation (Blobel et al. 2003).

Ultimately, a PIM requires a platform specific model (PSM) as its counterpart. There are two aspects to using PSMs. They must be conformant to an officially adapted platform specific profile—fitting within a template for a platform whose qualities are known. Diagrams must be expressed appropriately using the formalism in order for the platform specific bindings to work correctly.

They must also include interface definitions in a concrete implementation technology (such as Java, the XML Metadata Interchange Standard, or the OMG Interface Definition Language). In both cases, additional description—primarily behavior and constraints—may be specified in either UML or natural language.

4.6.1. Implementing Model-Driven Architecture

Implementing health information systems using MDA may be done using either of two approaches: a tool-supported rigorous development process, or a heterogeneous application development environment. Irrespective of which approach is used toward an MDA-based implementation, MDA itself offers advantages in enabling system lifecycle support that is model based.

The first approach is supported by comprehensive tool suites, such as Rational Suite®. Using MDA-capable products, modelers are able to express their content in the tool and then use bindings to PSMs, allowing providing rigorous and complete modeling expressions (based upon a targeted platform) that may ultimately enable a run-time version to result.

Model-driven architecture–based solutions better position projects to manage scalability, flexibility, and portability of the ultimate system. Because the PIM is separated from the PSM, new platforms can be supported as necessary, adding longevity to the content. Further, the intellectual property of the domain being modeled is captured in the PIM, offering it longevity beyond the implementation technologies that are represented in the PSM. Today, these activities are not entirely seamless. Several subsystems must be implemented to provide an application development environment, such as Metamodel and model repositories, data warehouse metamodel repositories, component management and assembly tools, mapping tools, and IDEs.

Despite these additional requirements, MDA systems provide the ability to separate out evolution of business needs from technologies, allowing each to evolve with minimum dependency. As an approach, it is wholly consistent with what we consider to be best practices in the modeling space.

5. Modeling for HealthePeople

5.1. The Paradigm Shift

Realizing the benefits of model-driven system development begins with applying the principles we describe in a fashion that is sensible for system development. A primary shift in the development culture toward the separation of knowledge and technical modeling spaces allows for the construction of quantifiably better systems, better resource planning, and better project management.

The fundamental feature of such environments is the nearly total separation of technical developers from knowledge authors, and the emergence of systems based solely on technical infrastructures that consume formal knowledge models during operation. This approach leverages the significant investment in knowledge engineering that has already been made in the health domain: terminologies, controlled vocabularies, ontologies, and clinical guidelines, as well as newer methods of operational knowledge representation of templates, archetypes, and message models. Knowledge engineering also provides a proper home for the formal expression of enterprise rules and workflow models.

All kinds of knowledge assets require tools for authoring and sharing, navigation and reuse. One example of such tooling is the use of online knowledge registries that allow for open community participation. These registries encourage standardization of formalisms and approaches in knowledge creation and maintenance. The use (and reuse) of tools that observe such principles as the separation of interests and of viewpoints provides us with a viable technical approach for selecting and applying models that result in usable, tractable, maintainable systems.

5.2. Using Standards

An organization with total autonomy would have no need for standards. It could declare exactly how things would work; systems would interface and build or integrate products to meet the organization's needs. Unfortunately, no organization has this luxury.

We live in a global economy, and health care by its very nature is an integrated domain. There are dependencies among every facet of the industry. Care providers, public health, research, suppliers, and, ultimately, patients, all play a role and all need to interact. It is this community interaction requirement that underscores the importance and value of standards.

When we consider the flow of information across organizational lines, it becomes clear why organizational policies such as standardizing upon a particular product or platform have achieved limited success at best. Ultimately, that success extends solely within the sphere of control of that organization, but many factors are not under control: government/legislative drivers, business partners, and so on.

It is from this understanding that we cull our next two principles:

- *Use standards where they support the needs of your enterprise.*
- *Diverging from a standard sets your organization apart and makes it an island— choose instead to work within the standards community to have your needs met.*

Standards provide a basis—a common ground—to further communication between organizations and systems. We must carefully consider which standards to include in our organizational portfolio, and understand that the selection of a standard is not enough. Because standards often overlap and have ambiguities, the organization must decide exactly what role a given standard will play.

Standards have limitations that can be truly problematic: insufficient or incomplete coverage, inconsistencies, omissions, errors, and so on. As these are discovered, many organizations opt for the easy path, coding around the standard to make up for shortcomings. The result can be troubling, because the implications are not discovered in the short term.

In the short term, these workarounds are often successful, addressing an immediate point of pain and solving that problem. However, when the organization needs to integrate with a new system or business partner, it finds it is now incompatible and incurs maintenance rework costs at that point. In addition, any existing interfaces built upon the proprietary extensions may have to be reworked.

The alternative strategy is not without pain. It requires involvement within the standards community itself, working within that realm to make the case for proposed changes to the standard. This approach comes at a price, for there is the expense involved in such engagement: time, travel, and commitment. Further, changes in such communities do not come quickly or easily—a particular problem for smaller organizations.

That said, even a single individual can significantly influence thinking with a demonstrable need and a firm resolve to have that need addressed. Standards work is increasingly becoming an asynchronous, distributed activity. Active participation online, thoughtful review of draft and pre-adopted work, and commitment are often enough to see that concerns are addressed.

Perhaps most importantly, members of the community working on standards have significant experience and vested interest in subject areas of concern, and often bring knowledge and insight not available elsewhere, at any price. For instance, the co-authors of this and several other chapters in this book might never have met (much less collaborated) were it not for their standards involvement. Table 10.1 lists health-care-oriented standards bodies that merit ongoing attention.

TABLE 10.1. Standards bodies by name and subject area.

Standards body	Name	Subject area
HL7	Health Level Seven	Electronic health record standards, healthcare messaging standards, context management standards
ISO TC 215	ISO Work Group on Health Informatics	
ANSI HISB	ANSI Health Informatics Standards Board	Coordination among ANSI healthcare standards development organizations
OMG	Object Management Group	Unified Modeling Language (modeling and constraint language expression) Healthcare services interface specifications
CEN TC/251	Comité Européen de Normalisation—Technical Committee for Health Telematics	ENVI3606 EHR pre-standard HISA
W3C	World Wide Web Consortium	XML Semantic web activity

5.3. Recommendations

So what is a reasonable approach toward the consumption of standards? We have attempted to parse the standards space to provide some practical guidance and principles to govern the use of standards. Our work is by no means exhaustive, and there is quality work we have not cited here. However, our short list includes some critical resources that time and time again have proven themselves useful, in many organizations and even countries. We offer our recommendations as a launch-point into further exploring this exciting space.

5.3.1. Requirements-Oriented Standards

Significant work has been done in the requirements area relating to EHRs across a variety of venues. Although you may ask why you should look to the standards community for requirements when you have enough of your own, there are benefits. Perhaps most importantly, they serve as a completeness check. The standard may include something of interest that you may have overlooked. Further, the expression of the requirements may be useful and/or more mature that what you captured. Ultimately, requirements that are well expressed and testable are better.

5.3.1.1. Health Level Seven

Right now, the pinnacle of energy in this area lies within HL7 and its Electronic Health Record (HL7 EHR) committee (Health Level Seven Modeling and Methodology Committee 2003). The group has developed a Draft Standard for Trial Use (DSTU) in the form of a functional model that describes the key functions of an EHR system. The standard includes a superset of functions potentially applicable in any setting of care. For a specific setting, the standard specifies how a *profile* may be created specific to that support the needs of that setting, and may be used to specify system requirements, aid in procurements, or for regulation. The HL7 group has based much of their work on existing industry literature, with a particular emphasis on an Institute of Medicine Letter Report on the same subject (Institute of Medicine 2003).

5.3.1.2. *International Organization for Standardization*

International Organization for Standardization TC215 has developed TS 18308, which is ". . . a set of clinical and technical requirements for a record architecture that supports using, sharing, and exchanging electronic health records across different health sectors, different countries, and different models of healthcare delivery" (ISO 2004). The primary users of this requirements standard will be developers of EHR standards (e.g., CEN 13606) and other specifications such as the *open*EHR.

This work should be monitored for acceptance and regulatory requirements. Given sufficient momentum in the marketplace, this effort could emerge as the lingua franca for describing EHR system functionality, providing more comparability between expressed EHR system needs and product offerings.

5.3.1.3. *Other Initiatives*

The work done by the European Community's 3rd Framework Good European Health Record (GEHR) included requirements for clinical EHR information architecture, medico-legal requirements, and secondary uses such as education and population studies (Ingram 1995). This project was followed in the fourth framework by the Electronic Health Care Record Support Action (EHCR-SupA) project, which further developed these requirements.

The current synthesis of EHR information architecture requirements is the ISO Technical Specification (TS) 18308, which draws heavily on the work of GEHR, EHCR-SupA, CEN/TC 251, and ASTM as well as various U.S., European, Canadian, and other sources. TS 18308 defines over 120 requirements condensed from hundreds described by its sources. It has already been used as a benchmark to validate completeness for many emerging activities, such as the HL7 EHR Functional Model and Standard and *open*EHR specifications. The TS 18308 requirements focus primarily on the information viewpoint of the EHR, and secondarily on the communication and enterprise viewpoints.

From this rich content source, we distill our next principle: *Leverage existing requirements work to the extent possible.*

5.3.2. Semantic Specifications

Numerous health information specifications are available that formally describe aspects of the health domain, using various models and languages. As we consider the representation of semantics in models, there are three components to be addressed: the structure, datatype representation, and instance representations. The structure by which semantics are captured determines the utility and flexibility of that content. The following short list merits consideration when working in this space.

5.3.2.1. *Structure*

In the software field, the notion of patterns has emerged as a best practice that benefits this particular purpose. Patterns are abstract models that can be used as a semantic basis for concrete models that reflect the needs of the pattern. Fowler's Analysis Patterns (Fowler 1997) are effectively a set of abstracted best practices documented in a consistent way so that a consumer understands the benefits and implications of using such an approach. A number of efforts in the healthcare space are such patterns, even if they are not so named.

One is the HL7 Reference Information Model (RIM). The RIM consists of a backbone set of classes defining the semantic rules into which all HL7 content representations must comply. The RIM acts as a pattern language, expressing both the abstract semantics (such as Acts, Participations, and Roles) and their interdependencies. All HL7 knowledge artifacts within their Version 3 methodology are based upon the backbone foundation of the RIM.

Fowler's demographic patterns describe the semantics of parties and their relationships. This work has influenced the HL7 RIM and the *open*EHR demographic model. Other patterns developed for healthcare include the *open*EHR patterns configuration management used to model the versioning in the EHR and the data/protocol/state pattern relating the information elements of a clinical or scientific observation.

Two other important structural standard are the CEN ENV 13606 Electronic Healthcare Record Architecture standard and the HL7 Clinical Document Architecture (CDA). The former defines structure and rules for EHR extracts and communication, while the latter defines an XML-schema for the representation of clinical documents. Both identify the same levels of granularity, key components, and approximately the same inter-component relationships.

5.3.2.2. *Data Type Representation*

Although specifications for data types and data structures for clinical computing may seem a trivial engineering concern, all other standards (and hence systems and data) rely upon them. Thus, their standardization is critically important. Current specifications include the HL7 Version 3 messaging data types, the CEN/TC 251 data types (partly based on the HL7 ones), and the *open*EHR clinical data types for the EHR. Efforts to harmonize these specifications are underway within HL7 and CEN. Specifications for clinical data structures include some basic data structures included in the HL7 Version 3 Data Types and the *open*EHR Data Structures.

5.3.2.3. *Instance Representations*

Beyond the patterns themselves, there must be constructs to capture information of interest against which we may compute. These instance representations occur at two levels of abstraction. The more abstract level describes the generic case: "what does a blood pressure look like." The detailed level is an instantiated version of the abstraction as appears in a specific case: "Mr. Jones' blood pressure as taken today." The former represents the clinical concepts, their representations, constraints, normal ranges, and so forth describing the compositional makeup of a blood pressure. The latter, the actual readings taken at specific points in time, are based upon the real-world knowledge such as the cuff position and systolic/diastolic readings. This is a representative example of the manifestation two-level modeling concept we introduced earlier.

The use of archetypes and templates as formal representations of information in a usable and computable way is gaining ground. *open*EHR's significant use of archetypes and HL7's emerging archetype and template work both reflect early indicators of the value of this approach.[3] These constructs represent the confluence of structure, representation, and terminology and address all these aspects. Consequently, they are rea-

---

[3] As of May 2004, the HL7 Archetype and Template Architecture work had been accepted and passed the formal balloting of that working committee. This reflects a significant milestone en route toward formal adoption of this work as a standard.

sonable components that can be used and shared among organizations while retaining meaning and business value. Plans are emerging to collect, register, and maintain such constructs in registries; these will allow organizations to reuse content that is publicly available and to describe how their proprietary instances relate to public versions.

5.3.3. Functional and Service Specifications

Standards exist for numerous functional areas in clinical information; here we mention only the key specifications required to support an EHR environment. One approach to addressing these functional areas is to model common services to support the functions desired. Taken collectively, these common services create a service-based architecture.

A service-based approach offers substantial benefits. It minimizes the need to duplicate functionality as services are more generic and re-usable. This allows the development of specialized teams, each focused in a narrower area, ultimately resulting in code that is better developed and more optimized to perform its function. It also promotes consistency in processing practices. For example, a business rule implemented once in a shared service will be in effect for all consumers of that service.

A pioneering developer of functional healthcare specifications was the OMG Healthcare Domain Task Force (formerly CORBAmed). The HDTF deliverables included specifications for person identification (PIDS), access control (RAD), terminology access (TQS), and clinical observation access (COAS). This work is a foundation for describing key functional behaviors for several components required to successfully implement an EHR. Current efforts in the functional interface area in Europe include the CEN Standard Architecture for Healthcare Information Systems (ENV 12967, commonly known as HISA), which builds on the OMG experience, and which is under major revision in 2004.

5.3.3.1. Identity Management (OMG)

A service providing the ability to uniquely identify a person based upon a set of qualifying traits. For example, the OMG Person Identification Service (PIDS) receives a set of identifying traits to describe a person and returns the identity (or candidates) matching those traits. Personal Identification Service also provides a mechanism to correlate multiple indices, as would be needed for cross-organizational queries.

5.3.3.2. Terminology Mediation(HL7, OMG)

A service that manages one or many terminologies and controlled vocabularies, providing navigation between and among them. For example, there are many representations of a given drug that, from a provider view, are medically equivalent (e.g., equivalent dosage, route, clinical use) but may vary by manufacturer. Services such as Terminology Mediation enable support of computer-based drug–drug interaction checking across facilities where formularies may differ. Standards in this space include the HL7 Common Terminology Services (CTS) and the older OMG Terminology Query Service (TQS).

5.3.3.3. Access Control (OMG)

The ability to allow or disallow access to information based upon contextual information. Legislation, notably the Health Insurance Portability and Accountability Act (HIPAA), makes this service increasingly important. No longer is it sufficient to authenticate a user and grant him access to all information. Patient–provider relationships, consent, need-to-know, and business partner relationships all influence access to information. Services such as Resource Access Decision (RAD) provide the ability to control and grant situationally dependent information access.

5.3.3.4. The EHR (HL7, CEN)

The central service of interest is that of the EHR itself. The EHR has responsibility to collect, manage, maintain, and share semantically meaningful information about all subjects of care. It does this within, between, and across institutions and points of care, including personal health settings and direct patient interaction. Sources such as CEN ENV 13606, the *open*EHR EHR models, the HL7 CDA clinical document XML-schema specification, and emerging HL7 EHR SIG work are all valuable resources in this space.

6. Conclusion

Healthcare information systems, particularly electronic health records, are very complex and must be simplified if a reasonable understanding of the problem space is to be ascertained and ultimately managed. Modeling is an indispensable mechanism allowing a project team to gain clarity and insight that would not be discovered otherwise.

To be successful in Health*e*People, we must understand the value brought by modeling activities and sharpen our understanding of the information and knowledge necessary to support the functionality we seek. We must capture formally our business understanding and mature that understanding into rigorous expressions. We must recognize the variety of stakeholders impacting this work and identify products suitable to clearly and concisely communicate with them, ensuring that their requirements have been met and that our designs are sufficient.

Cognizant that Health*e*People cannot exist within a vacuum—we must ensure that it is capable of interoperation among a potential myriad of organizations. This is achieved through standards alignment, where standards are selected based upon fitness for purpose and not necessarily best of breed. This standards alignment requires more than just their adoption, as no standard will be a perfect fit. It requires commitment to work within the standards community to evolve and mature that work to reflect our needs.

Our solution must embrace information modeling and formal knowledge representations, ensuring the ultimate manifestation of Health*e*People allows for maturation of knowledge without the maintenance of code, (e.g., employing two-level modeling).

The Health*e*People design and development process must recognize that models that sit on shelves unreferenced are not useful. By seeking to produce models that are directly usable in system development, we can narrow the gap between our understanding and system implementation. Using technologies such as executable modes and the model-driven architecture, models themselves form the direct foundation and even instantiate executable code.

Perhaps most important is the recognition that there are very few original ideas in this world. We must steer clear of hyped solutions that promise the world but have not demonstrated their ability to deliver. Conversely, we cannot afford to dwell in the past, merely repackaging older solutions in newer technologies. Success lies along the path of judicious choice, melding the latest advances with the long-evolved foundation of existing work. Through careful analysis and understanding of our scope, identification of relevant products, rigorous expression and formalization, and the practical application of the results, HealthePeople is poised to achieve new heights in health informatics.

References

Beale T. 2000. Archetypes: constraint-based domain models for future-proof information systems. Available from: http://www.deepthought.com.au/it/archetypes.html. Accessed 2003 Aug 10.

Beale T, Heard S. 2004. The archetype definition language (ADL). Available from: http://www.openEHR.org/repositories/spec/latest/publishing/architecture/archetypes/language/ADL/REV_HIST.html. Accessed 2004 Apr.

Blobel B, Stassinopoulos G, Pharow P. 2003. Model-based design and implementation of secure, interoperable EHR systems. In: Musen MA, Friedman CP, Teich JM, editors. AMIA 2003 Symposium: Biomedical and health informatics: from foundations to applications. Bethesda, MD: American Medical Informatics Association. p 96–100.

Brooks FP. 1975. The mythical man month. Philippines: Addison-Wesley.

Fowler M. 1997. Analysis patterns: reusable object models. Reading, MA: Addison-Wesley.

Health Level Seven Modeling and Methodology Committee. 2003. Health Level Seven development framework. Available from: http://www.hl7.org. Accessed 2003 Aug.

Health Level Seven Special Interest Group. 2003. HL7 EHR system functional model and standard, draft standard for Trial Use Release 1.0. Available from: http://www.hl7.org/ehr. Accessed 2003 Aug.

Ingram D. 1995. The Good European Health Record project. In: Laires MF, Laderia MJ, Christensen JP, editors. Health in the new communications age. Amsterdam: IOS Press. p 66–74.

Institute of Medicine. 2003. Key capabilities of an electronic health record system letter report. Available from: http://www.nap.edu/books/NI000427/html/. Accessed 2003 Aug.

International Organization for Standardization (ISO). 1995. Basic reference model of open distributed processing, ITU-T X.900 series and ISO/IEC 10746 series. Available from: http://www.itu.int/ITU-T/com7/index.html. Accessed 2003 Aug.

International Organization for Standardization (ISO). 2004. ISO Technical Specification (TS) 18308. Health Informatics-requirements for an electronic health record architecture. Available from http://www.iso.org/iso/en. Accessed 2004 Nov.

Kruchten P. 1999. The rational unified process. Reading, MA: Addison-Wesley.

Object Management Group. 2003. The OMG unified modeling language specification, version 1.5. Available from: http://www.uml.org. 2003 Jul.

Object Management Group. 2003. MDA guide version 1.0. In: Miller J, Mukerji J, editors. Available from: http://www.omg.org/mda/specs.htm#MDAitself. Accessed 2003 Aug 23.

Object Management Group Healthcare Domain Task Force. 2000. The CORBAMed roadmap. In: Nicklin P, editor. Available from: http://healthcare.omg.org. Accessed 2003 Aug 5.

Purves IN, Sugden B, Booth N, Sowerby M. 1999. The PRODIGY project—the iterative development of the release one model. Proc AMIA Symp 1999:359–363.

Rector AL, Zanstra P, Solomon WD, and the GALEN Consortium. 1995. GALEN: terminology services for clinical information systems. Laires MF, Laderia MJ, Christensen JP, editors. Health in the new communications age. Amsterdam: IOS Press. p 90–100.

Spackman KA. 1999. Terminology convergence: SNOMED gets a boost. MD Comput 16(5):23–25.

11
Health*e*People Security Architecture

Bernd Blobel and John M. Davis

Patient medical information is needed by both individuals and communities for care and treatment, to advance the public health, provide research and educational services, and facilitate reimbursement.

By law, custom, and patient expectation, private health information is protected. Beyond this, there are also significant healthcare motivations to protect private health information. To instill trust, patient personal health information must be treated as confidential and private. To be useable, patient medical information must be protected from unauthorized modification. To be relevant, it must be available when needed.

Health*e*People meets these needs by providing security services through a practical service-capability infrastructure approach. The Health*e*People security infrastructure also facilitates sharing of security information in a way that decouples security mechanisms previously tightly integrated with specific applications.

Health*e*People provides essential open, modular confidentiality, integrity, and availability security services protecting health information systems and data. While not ignoring the importance of other services, this chapter will generally focus on Health*e*People's crucial identity and access management services and the models and methods necessary to develop and implement such services.

1. Global Trends and Challenges

Protecting patient medical information presents special difficulties in Health*e*People's world-wide interoperability context. In addition to increasing patient numbers, ever more mobile and longer-living populations, complexities of modern technology, and cost constraints, it is also clear that healthcare security architectures face major challenges in providing technical solutions for confidentiality, integrity, and availability stemming from:

- Complexity: Multiple different systems, protocols and implementations, changing over time
- Scalability: Hundreds to thousands of systems and tens of thousands of users, millions of people
- Adaptability: New policies and practices, local, national, trans-border (international), and an ever-growing array of new technologies

- Assurance: Testing and maintaining confidence in security functions over the system life cycle and the life of the electronic health record
- Interoperability: World-wide inter- and intra-agency health information sharing

2. Boundaries

The HealthePeople security boundary includes all participating organizations with a primary mission of providing health care, research, and education as well as supporting development, management, maintenance, finance, and vendor interactions.

The HealthePeople security boundary includes various domains of people and systems coupled by security policies that are, by nature, compound, complex, and overlapping. Where we rely upon local boundaries such as operating system, operators, and organizations to operate properly, we will continue to do so. At the same time, within HealthePeople, single enterprise boundaries inevitably interact with whole communities of independent organizations. By defining boundaries, participating organizations can establish models of trust to protect current and local as well as the long-term and integrated patient medical information bases.

3. Assumptions

HealthePeople access to patient medical information and healthcare workflows is based upon the following assumptions:

- Personal health information resides in multiple institutions in electronic form.
- Individuals will have significant control over the organizational access to their personal information.
- Patient acceptance of the health system requires an environment whose security policies and activities are trusted and understood.
- People want to carry on private patient/provider communications in a secure, trusted framework.
- There must be accountability built into the system.
- There must be access to emergency services when and where the need arises.
- Access to medical information is critical even in remote locations (possibly international).
- Trustworthy agents are needed to guide and protect healthcare processes in a person's health space.

4. Security as a Service

The HealthePeople information security strategy is to enable security service migration from platform-focused to distributed open systems. This requires a framework providing security services that are themselves distributed and security application program interfaces (APIs) that are independent of underlying security mechanisms. HealthePeople will provide security services that allow for sharing of security information bases and that decouple security mechanisms tightly integrated with specific applications.

The security framework strategy must involve a standards-based security architecture promoting the *interoperability* and *openness* needs of the HealthePeople participants. This includes secure information linking, meaning the need to link separate data from various health information service sites as well as hospitals, practitioner offices and clinics, nursing facilities, and home health agencies. Without a distributed security framework, the distributed environment adds yet another layer of complexity.

Fundamental technical security services implemented in the layers of communicating open systems ensure security of systems and data transfers. The security services of International Organization for Standardization (ISO) 7498–2 include authentication, access control, data confidentiality, data integrity, and non-repudiation (International Organization for Standardization 1989). These are extended in their definitions for use in the Health*e*People security framework beyond communications alone to include end systems as well. The Health*e*People security framework also includes availability and accountability among its fundamental security services. Security management is described in relation to the proper configuration and technical management of each of the security services.

The following security services, along with each associated security management service, form the basis for implementing the Health*e*People security model:

- Identification and authentication
- Access control and authorization
- Data confidentiality
- Data integrity
- Non-repudiation
- Availability
- Accountability
- Security management

The Health*e*People environment for secure and reliable communication and co-operation requires participants to analyze and define their security needs and requirements. This is done in reference to a well-defined security service model. Figure 11.1 illustrates a generic service-based security architecture where applications address local and distributed security services either directly or through middleware.

Using a layered service approach, Health*e*People security is mapped onto a set of reusable building-block services separated into increasingly granular tiers. Using security tiers provides Health*e*People robust, extensible infrastructure making it capable of providing either á la carte implementation or a full menu for those organizations wishing to use it to its maximum capability.

Alternatively, Comité Européen de Normalisation (CEN) ENV 13608, *Health Informatics: Security for Healthcare Communication*, provides a security concept and terminology approach which enables a checklist-type analysis and definition phase (Comité Européen de Normalisation 2000). A brief overview of such a narrative approach appears below. Later in this chapter, component-based modeling is discussed, consistent with Chapter 10 of this book.

As shown in Figure 11.1, the CEN ENV 13608 names the services as availability, integrity, confidentiality, and accountability. At the next layer, conceptual security needs are defined in terms of security objects, security subjects, and security policy. These conceptual security needs include object availability, subject availability, object integrity, subject integrity, transport confidentiality, and clearance, sending, delivery as well as exchange accountability.

Each one of the four global security needs is further refined into a set of conceptual security needs. This refinement process helps to clarify the security needs in terms of

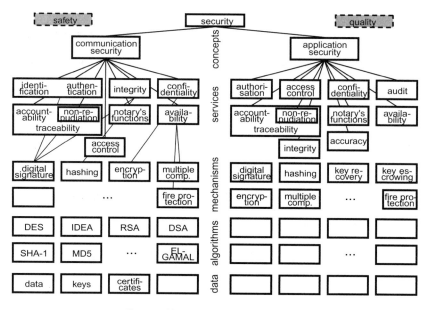

FIGURE 11.1. Layered security model.

a security policy, expressed in terms of security objects, security subjects, and the constraints placed upon them as expressed in the security policy.

These concepts represent a series of infrastructure services whose capabilities are summarized in Table 11.1. Capabilities can be reused across all segment applications within HealthePeople.

4.1. Approach

The HealthePeople information protection approach includes all the traditional security services. What is new is the realization of distributed identity and access management as infrastructure services. Infrastructure services are directly accessible by applications services and replace individual application functions with authoritative network-based functions.

Authentication and authorization stand out among all of the security services. Authentication is a core service on which all others rely. When authentication must be individually implemented in each of an enterprise's many applications, it becomes more and more unmanageable as the number of installations increases. In an organization with tens of thousands of systems, just reliably verifying that user accounts of departing employees have been removed becomes a daunting task. A service-oriented approach overcomes issues of scale, complexity, adaptability, assurance, and interoperability by centralizing and simplifying user management and provisioning.

Accordingly, HealthePeople Security Service and authorization infrastructure capabilities will include the following:

- Users will be authenticated in a centralized way and their permissions and roles (authorizations) will be validated across the enterprise.

- Users will be authenticated once and centrally, with centralized authorization and security management information bases supporting distributed access control decision function architectures.
- Based upon flexible access decision rules, user authorizations to multiple systems will be managed, negotiated, and decided without the need to modify individual system account information.
- Sign-on and access to network resources will be available from any workstation across cooperating security domains.
- Security policies will be capable of dynamic implementation, revocation, or suspension of user permissions and accounts as determined by proper authority.
- Uniform enterprise-wide fine-grained access control decisions will be maintainable without requiring time consuming and costly modification to individual application systems.
- People will be authenticated and authorized in a HealthePeople security domain supporting custom and personalized health care as well as individual privacy decisions (as permitted by policy).

By implementing a service-oriented architecture and the capabilities above, HealthePeople will:

TABLE 11.1. Summary of HealthePeople high-level security service capabilities.

Capability	Description	Security service
• Enterprise-wide distributed authentication • Medical sign-on/single sign-on • Healthcare identifiers	• Strong authentication for all users and systems/persistent clinical sessions • Fewer logons with a goal of achieving single sign-on to all applications • Enterprise-wide person identifiers	• Identification and authentication
• Enterprise-wide distributed authorization • RBAC and role engineering • Break-glass access • Federated authorizations • Distributed/local access control	• Enterprise-wide hierarchical security policies, business oriented least privilege and need-to-know access, business partner access, centralized user profiles, policy based access control • Static roles and functional roles	• Access control and authorization
• Health information system audit • Monitoring security function • Application audit	• Centralized auditing, processing and reporting	• Accountability

• Security management information base protection/integrity
  ○ At rest
  ○ In transit
	• End-to-end confidentiality and integrity for security control, messaging and management data
	• Digitally signed security credentials
		• Confidentiality
		• Data integrity
		• Digital signature

• Centralized user and system security management	• Configuration management, provisioning, test and operations • Enterprise-wide Security Management Information Bases/ Operation Centers	• Security management • Availability
• Software/hardware trust • Common secure software development environments	• Secure software development life cycles • Certification • Standard interfaces to security function	• Assurance

- Improve enterprise management of security configuration.
- Manage user security information centrally for all applications.
- Reduce complexity of managing many systems and interfaces.
- Speed ability to apply change.
- Reduce administrative burden on limited resources.
- Allow rapid re-configuration to meet unexpected conditions/ threats.
- Simplify provisioning of user security configuration.
- Provide better assurance of security function through certifying services once and centrally.

4.2. Definitions

We establish the following definitions:

- **Access Control Information (ACI).** Any information used for access control purposes, including contextual information.
- **Access Control Decision Function (ADF).** A specialized function that makes access control decisions by applying access control policy rules to a requested action, ACI (of initiators, targets, actions, or that retained from prior actions), and the context in which the request is made.
- **Access Control Decision Information (ADI).** The portion (possibly all) of the ACI made available to the ADF in making a particular access control decision.
- **Access Control Enforcement Function (AEF).** Access control enforcement allows or denies use of a protected resource. Decisions are made on the basis of whether or not the authenticated user possesses permissions equal to or greater than those required to access the resource as well as other potential access control information (ACI) such as time-of-day, strength of authentication used, etc.

5. HealthePeople Reference Framework

Implementing the HealthePeople service-oriented security architecture framework starts with the task of documenting security requirements and scenarios. This includes risk assessment descriptions of the threat to the organization's data, business case analysis, and establishing the expected gains/value emerging from a distributed security environment.

Traditionally, user authentication/authorization is vested in individual applications that maintain their own hard-wired set of user accounts, authentication, and authorization information/services. Each application supports a single application-centric security policy view. As a consequence, support requirements grow proportionally to the number of supported enterprise systems and as more and more users (including business partners) are redundantly added to these systems.

To improve upon this, a network-aware end system approach allows applications to communicate directly with distributed security services and networked access control decision functions. Such service-aware applications natively parse and process security server messages, credentials, and user requests. Service-aware applications do not need to maintain permanent user accounts (though they may); instead, they accept user ACI from network security services. Security-aware applications perform their own access control enforcement.

Network application agents act to bridge the gap for non-service-aware end systems. The agent interfaces (bridges) the application access control enforcement functions with access control decision functions provided by the network. The agent optionally performs access control enforcement functions for the application. Agents are either custom software components or product specific APIs.

In this environment, network-based policy evaluators use access control information and pre-programmed rules to make authorization decisions while a distributed enforcement function controls access. World Wide Web–based and N-Tier systems in particular may take advantage of having both access control decision and access control enforcement functions delegated as network security services.

5.1. A Practical HealthePeople Architecture

In the HealthePeople practical security service reference architecture, some authorization decisions may continue to be made directly by rules in the application software (e.g., fine-grained application specific functions, local security policies, security management requiring direct access via a terminal). High-level role-groups (slow-changing enterprise roles)[1] are used by the distributed authentication (sign on/single sign on) and authorization infrastructure to provide connect access to the protected end system resources. Once connected, it will be necessary to assert/verify the application-level permissions (functional roles) owned by the user in order to access the application data and functions. Functional roles grant privileges to the user needed to perform work. Access Control Decision Information may be used by both the network and end system ADF to make access control (permissions) decisions. This allows for policies not in the original application to be part of access enforcement. It also allows for standard roles that are valid across the enterprise to be centrally managed, which could provide significant economy in large organizations.

In today's application-oriented systems, support becomes increasingly difficult or fails as the number of users and requirements for increasingly complex policies increase. HealthePeople's service-oriented security architecture gains scale by making authentication and authorization network services instead of in being placed in each application. A service-oriented security architecture allows Access Control Decision Functions (ADF) to be separated from Access Control Enforcement Functions (AEF). A Control Decision Functions on the network can then be centrally managed.

5.2. HealthePeople Security Components

Figure 11.2 illustrates the identity and access management components of the HealthePeople security architecture framework. In the figure, HealthePeople implements the distributed practical security services architecture. HealthePeople's service-oriented security provides centralized user authentication as well as permission and role validation as an enterprise-provided security infrastructure. Users are centrally authenticated by any number of authentication methods (based upon policy). Their status as authenticated users is passed to supported applications, providing a capability for single sign-on, eliminating user needs to remember passwords, or to authenticate to individual systems. Such authentication approaches also can be integrated with clinical context switching methods such as those provided by Health Level Seven's (HL7) Clinical Context (CCOW) standard.

---

[1] American Society for Testing and Materials (ASTM) E1986 lists healthcare roles for which access controls are warranted. These enterprise roles are referred here as static roles.

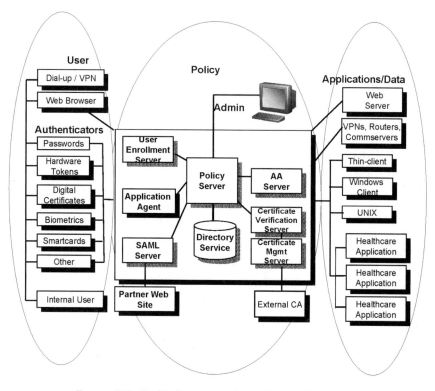

FIGURE 11.2. HealthePeople security architecture framework.

Based upon flexible access decision rules, user authorizations to multiple systems are managed, negotiated, and decided without the need to modify individual system account information. New authorizations can be dynamically implemented, revoked, or suspended as necessary.

HealthePeople's service-oriented security allows uniform enterprise-wide fine-grain access control decisions to be made without requiring time consuming and costly modification to individual application systems. In addition, HealthePeople provides people (patients/members) with their own authorizations supporting custom and personalized health care as well as enforcing individual privacy decisions (as permitted by policy). HealthePeople distributed security services give people secure access to their own personal information and select information services.

The outcome of all of this is that HealthePeople offers security interoperability among its membership while still supporting organizational autonomy. Participants have flexibility to deploy HealthePeople within their organization (so long as they honor the community constraints) while remaining shielded from the minutia of deployment detail of their brethren organizations, all the while retaining the ability to interoperate among the community. This distributed service-oriented infrastructure provides the primary means by which HealthePeople is being integrated across organizational boundaries.

6. Security Models

Privilege management and authorization may be assigned to individual actors or to groups of individual actors playing the same role. Actors interacting with system components are called Principals, which can be a human user, a system, a device, an application, a component, or even an object.

Regarding privilege management and access control management, two basic class types must be dealt with:

- Entities
  - Principals
  - Policies
  - Documents
  - Roles
- Acts
  - Policy management
  - Principal management
  - Privilege management
  - Authentication
  - Authorization
  - Access control management
  - Audit

In order to obtain the above described structure and functionality there are a number of models, mechanisms, processes, objects, etc., that are needed. This chapter considers the following security models:

- Domain model
- Delegation model
- Control model
- Document model
- Policy model
- Role model
- Information distance model
- Authorization model
- Access control models

For enabling future-proof electronic health record (EHR) systems, all specifications made must be kept open, platform-independent, portable, and scalable. Therefore, the models provided will be described a meta-meta-model level, and at the model level keeping the instance level out of consideration. For expressing systems in such a way, specific languages and meta-languages are used such as Unified Modeling Language (UML) and eXtensible Markup Language (XML) including means for transfer from one vocabulary to another one.

For UML, UML itself, UML profiles, and all different diagrams needed have been deployed. As to XML, several specifications within the XML standard set will be used.

All models being used establish a specific kind of constraint, forming constraint models. This concerns any thinkable services or view on systems. A model is a simplified view at the reality according to special concepts. The language to be used for graphical models is UML and the Meta Object Facility (MOF). The language for verbal models is the XML standard set.

It is expected that many documents will be expressed using XML. The structure for such a document is defined in a document type definition (DTD) or an XML schema instance. A privilege policy may act directly on the XML elements (e.g., by comparing attributes in an authorization certificate to elements in the document).

6.1. Domain Model

To keep (complex) information systems that support shared care manageable and operating, principal-related components of the system are grouped by common organizational, logical, and technical properties into domains. Following OMG (Object Management Group) definitions, this could be done for common policies (policy domains), for common environments (environment domains), or common technology (technology domains). Any kind of interoperability internally to a domain is called an *intradomain* communication and co-operation, whereas interoperability between domains is called an *interdomain* communication and co-operation. For example, communication could be realized between departments of a hospital internally to the domain hospital (intradomain communication), but externally to the domain of a special department (interdomain communication). Regarding security requirements, security policy domains are of special interest. Real-world systems are most likely composed of multi-domain information objects that cut across different information contexts.

As used here, an information domain consists of a set of data, users, and an information security policy linking the two. A domain is characterized by a domain identifier, a domain name, a domain authority, a domain qualifier. Within an information domain, all information objects exist at the same level of sensitivity. Members of a domain may have different security attributes, such as read, write, or execute permissions on information objects. Systems or networks of systems do not bound information domains. An information domain's objects may reside in multiple systems.

A policy describes the legal framework including rules and regulations, the organizational and administrative framework, functionalities, claims and objectives, the principals involved, agreements, rights, duties, and penalties defined, as well as the technological solution implemented for collecting, recording, processing, and communicating data in information systems. For describing policies, methods such as policy templates or formal policy modeling might be deployed. For example, the Organization for the Advancement of Structured Information Standards (OASIS) Web Service (WS) Policy provides a general purpose model and syntax to describe and communicate the policies of a web service. It specifies a set of common message policy assertions within a policy and attachment mechanisms for using policy expressions with existing XML service technologies.

Regarding the flexibility in handling properties and policies, the domain is generic in nature. It may consist of sub-domains and building super-domains. Sub-domains will inherit policies from their parent domain. The smallest domain is the working place or sometimes even a specific component of a system (e.g., in the case of server machines). The domain will be extended by chaining sub-domains to super-domains forming a common domain of communication and co-operation, which is characterized by establishing an agreed security policy. Such transaction-concrete policy has to be negotiated between the communicating and co-operating principals, which is also called *policy bridging*.

Users may perceive a collection of objects from different information domains as a single object. This compound object is referred to as a multi-domain information object. Multi-domain information objects must be subject to a common security policy. The security policy must state the privileges that a user must have to view, print, create, delete, or transfer multi-domain information objects between information systems.

Different middleware enables different interoperability with direct invocation (middleware is restricted to communication services) or chained invocation (middleware services). The latter is characterized by different models of delegation.

The general purpose of communication is the provision of services to a client requesting these services. Most of the services have to be provided by the functionality of the healthcare information system often combined with human users' interactions. Such application services are end-system services, limited to communication services, and do not provide additional application functions. Therefore, application security services are restricted to the communicating principals' domain.

Middleware concepts are being introduced increasingly into the new(er) versions of healthcare information systems. In this model not only both principals, but also the middleware can provide requested functionality and application security services. Such an architecture can be represented by chains of different domains.

From the security point of view, a domain ensuring intra-domain communication according to its own policy is commonly considered with need of protection only at its boundary to external domains with their specific policies (or even the policy-free domain of the Internet). This is done by, for example, firewalls, proxy servers, etc. Regarding the external environment, a domain is therefore often considered closed. The internal domain is mistakenly assumed to be secure, often neglecting internal threats and attacks, which are the majority among all security attacks.

Regarding the specific requirements and conditions of health care, the underlying security model must consider the whole specter of security services and mechanisms, which can be accomplished by secure micro-domains.

6.2. Control Model

The control model illustrates how control is exerted over access to the sensitive object operation. There are four components in the model: the Claimant, the Verifier, the Target, and the Control policy. The Claimant has privilege attributes, contained in an attribute certificate. The Target has sensitivity attributes, which may be contained in a security label, attribute certificate, or in a local database. The techniques described here enable the Verifier, who may be the owner of the Target or an independent authority, to control access to the Target by the Claimant, in accordance with the Control policy and optionally taking other environmental variables or components (EnvironmentalVariables) into account (e.g., local time).

The Claimant's privileges are typically encapsulated in its attribute certificate/credential. This may be presented to the Verifier in the service request (push strategy), or it can be distributed by some other means, such as via a Directory (pull strategy). The Control policy must be protected for integrity and authenticity and, for this purpose, it may also be combined with the Claimant's privilege in its attribute certificate. Normally, it will be conveyed in a separate structure.

The Claimant may be an entity identified by a public key certificate, or an executable object identified by the digest.

6.3. Delegation Model

In addition to the control model, there is a need for a delegation model. There are three components of the delegation model: the Verifier, the Source of Authority, and the Claimant, as shown in Figure 11.3.

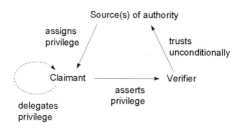

FIGURE 11.3. Delegation model.

The Verifier endows an entity known as the Source of Authority with unlimited privilege. The Source of Authority is a special type of Attribute Authority. It delegates privilege to Claimants by issuing attribute certificates. The Claimant asserts its delegated privilege by demonstrating its identity. This can be done by proving its knowledge of a private key whose public counterpart is contained in a public key certificate referenced by an attribute certificate that includes the claimed privilege. In the case of an executable object, it may alternatively done by demonstrating that the digest is the same as the owner value of an attribute certificate that includes the claimed privilege.

Optionally, the Claimant may delegate its privilege to another Claimant. The Verifier must confirm that all entities in the delegation path possess sufficient privilege to access the target requested by the direct Claimant.

The Source of Authority may also process a request from an entity to delegate its privilege by issuing an attribute certificate to another entity. However, this process is outside the scope of this standard.

The Claimant and the Verifier may be entities in different security domains. In such cases, the Source of Authority may be located in the Verifier's domain, and a continuous section of the delegation path, which includes the direct Claimant, shall be in the other security domain.

The delegation path is distinct from the certificate validation path used to validate the public key certificates of the entities involved in the delegation process. However, the quality of authenticity offered by the public key certificate validation process must be commensurate with the sensitivity of the Target being protected.

Specifying interoperability between distributed objects or components, respectively, the Object Management Group has defined an alternative Delegation Model within its CORBA Security Services Specification. In an object system, a client calls on an object to perform an operation, but this object will often not complete the operation itself, so will call on other objects to do so. This will usually result in a chain of calls on other objects, or *call chain.*

In privilege delegation, the initiating principal's access control information (i.e., its security attributes) may be delegated to further objects in the chain to give the recipient the rights to act on its behalf under specified circumstances.

Another authorization scheme is reference restriction where the rights to use an object under specified circumstances are passed as part of the object reference to the recipient. Reference restriction is not included in this specification.

The following terms are used in describing delegation options:

- Initiator: the first client in a call chain
- Final target: the final recipient in a call chain

- Intermediate: an object in a call chain that is neither the initiator nor the final target
- Immediate invoker: an object or client from which an object receives a call

Communication of health information is frequently connected with a supplier chain performing this activity (e.g., involvement of secretaries, clerks, service departments, but also any other principals). This delegation model must be used for any such chaining of services.

6.4. Document Model

Processes, entity roles, etc., must be documented and signed expressing the particular relations between entities and processes. The combination of processes and relations leads to multiple signatures (e.g., in the case of delegation).

Cryptographic message syntax supports multiple signatures on a document. Each signature is computed over the document content and, optionally, a set of signed attributes specific to the particular signature. These attributes may include timestamps, signature purpose, and other information.

6.5. Policy Model

A security policy is the complex of legal, ethical, social, organizational, psychological, functional, and technical implications for assuring trustworthiness of health information systems. A policy is the formulation of the concept of requirements and conditions for trustworthy creation, storage, processing, and use of sensitive information. A policy can be expressed in the following ways:

- Verbally unstructured
- Structured using schemata or templates
- Formally modeled

For interoperability reasons, a policy must be formulated and encoded in a way that enables its correct interpretation and practice. Therefore, policies have to be constrained regarding syntax, semantics, vocabulary, and operation of policy documents, also called policy statements or policy agreements (agreements between the partners involved).

6.5.1. XML Schema

Figure 11.4 presents a simple XML instance for a security policy statement. One common way to express constraints is the specification of user-defined XML schemata. This schema should be standardized for interoperability purposes mentioned above.

To reliably refer to a specific policy, the policy instance must be uniquely named and identified via a unique policy ID. The same is true for all the policy components such as domain, targets, operations, and their policies, which have to be named and uniquely identified as well. Like any other component, policy components can be composed or decomposed according to the generic component model. A policy is therefore characterized by a policy identifier, a policy name, a policy authority, a domain identifier, a domain name, a target list, target identifier, target name, Target object, operations allowed, and related policies.

6.5.2. Policy Baseclasses

The Policy class can be specialized as Basic Policy, Meta Policy, and Composite Policy classes (Damianou et al. 2000), as shown in Figure 11.5. The specializations of the

```
<policy>
      <policy_name/>
      <policy_identifier/>
      <policy_authority/>
      <domain_name/>
      <domain_identifier/>
      <target_list>
             <target_name/>
             <target_ID/>
             <target_object>
                   <operations/>
                   <policies/>
             </target_object>
      </target_list>
</policy>
```

FIGURE 11.4. Policy template example.

Composite Policy abstract class are interrelated in a complex way, which has been indicated in outlines as simple association.

6.5.3. Object Management Group Security Services

Another way for policy decomposition has been provided by the OMG's Security Services Specification. This distinguishes between the following policies:

- Invocation access policy implementing access control policy for objects
- Invocation audit policy controlling event type and criteria for audit
- Secure invocation policy specifying security policies associated with security associations and message protection

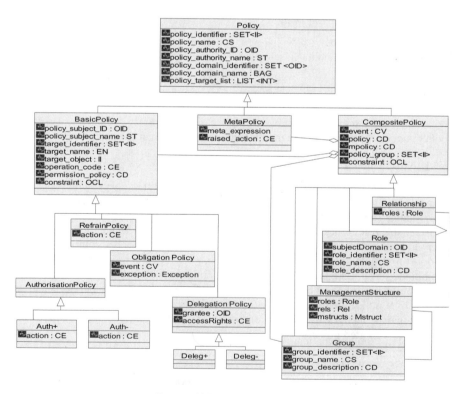

FIGURE 11.5. Policy base-classes.

It also addresses requirements for different object types:

- Invocation delegation policy
- Application access policy
- Application audit policy
- Non-repudiation policy

Health information systems such as the EHR should at minimum have a Patient Policy, an Enterprise Policy, policies defined by laws and regulations, and one policy per Structural Role as well as one policy per Functional Role.

Every creation, access, or modification to an EHR component must be covered by one or more policies. The reference model of the EHR Extract includes a Policy ID attribute within the Record Component class to permit references to such policies to be made at any level of granularity within the EHR hierarchy. The policies that apply specifically to an EHR may be included within the EHR Extract, eventually including any bridged policies.

6.6. Role Model

For managing relationships between the entities, organizational and functional roles can be defined. Roles may be assigned to any principal. Principals are the actors in health care. Therefore, roles are associated to actors and to acts.

6.6.1. Healthcare-Related Roles

In general, two types of roles can be distinguished: structural roles and functional roles. Structural roles reflect the structural aspects of relationships between entities. Structural roles describe prerequisites, feasibilities, or competences for acts. Functional roles reflect functional aspects of relationships between entities. Functional roles are bound to the realization/performance of acts.

Possible examples for structural roles of healthcare professionals are:

- Medical director
- Director of clinic
- Head of the department
- Senior physician
- Resident physician
- Physician
- Medical assistant
- Trainee
- Head nurse
- Nurse
- Medical student

Possible examples for functional roles of healthcare professionals are:

- Caring doctor (responsible doctor)
- Member of diagnostic team
- Member of therapeutic team
- Consulting doctor
- Admitting doctor
- Family doctor
- Function-specific nurse

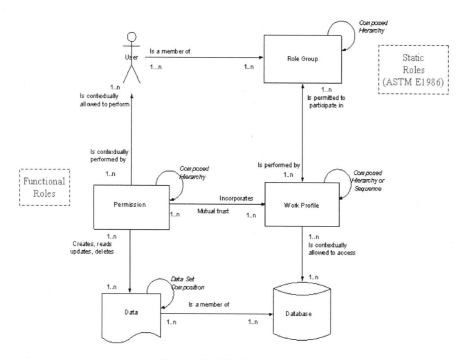

FIGURE 11.6. Role engineering.

Figure 11.6 illustrates the core unified service-oriented role viewpoint describing the relationship between static and functional roles based upon a role engineering approach.

Standard discussion regarding role-based access control treats roles from a functional role perspective. On the other hand, static[2] roles being defined in ASTM[3] and elsewhere can be used to provide connect authorizations to members of these work profiles prior to user activation of functional roles. Figure 11.6 places the function role into a context that includes static roles. The basic role can be considered to be a type of prerequisite role, that is, a role that a user must have activated before other roles can be activated. In this case, the static role is a prerequisite role that a user must have before additional roles may be activated in a user session.[4] Static (rarely changing) roles would be typically managed in identity certificates or directories.

On the right half of the figure, users granted static roles are permitted to participate in work profiles that contextually allow access to specific enterprise databases. In a client–server context, this amounts to an authorization to establish a session. In a distributed security service scenario, this access control decision is made at the network level. On the left-hand side of the figure, from the user point of view, s/he has been

---

[2] Basic roles are defined in Blobel B. 2002. Analysis, Design and Implementation of Secure and Interoperable Distributed Health Information Systems. Studies in Health Technology and Informatics 89. Amsterdam: IOS Press. These are alternatively called static roles or role groups by other sources.
[3] Formerly the American Society for Testing and Materials, now known as ASTM International.
[4] A basic role could also serve as a functional role, should the security policy permit.

granted the permissions (aggregated into Functional Roles according to the principle of least privilege) that allow performing operations (create, read, update, delete, and execute) on protected information objects associated with the work profile scenarios. By analyzing workflow and decomposing actions on objects, permissions and functional roles can be defined (Neumann and Strembeck 2002). Functional roles would be typically managed in attribute certificates or directories.

6.6.2. Functional Role Model

Functional roles consist of all the permissions on health information system objects needed to perform a task. Functional role names associate groups of permissions for convenience in assigning to users. A user may be assigned one or more functional roles, and thereby be assigned all of the permissions associated with a corresponding health-care workflow. Permissions will ultimately be used to set the system operations (create, read, update, delete, execute, etc.) for data and software applications. Functional roles may be found as entries in a user attribute certificate or stored in a distributed authorization directory.

Regarding the healthcare business process, functional roles can be defined in levels of authorizations and access right in the following generic way that reuses slightly changed definitions established in the Australian HealthNet Project and cross-referenced against other works:

- Subject of care (normally the patient)
- Subject of care agent (parent, guardian, caregiver, or other legal representative)
- Responsible (personal) healthcare professional (the healthcare professional with the closest relationship to the patient, often his general practitioner)
- Privileged healthcare professional
  — nominated by the subject of care
  — nominated by the healthcare facility of care (there is a nomination by regulation, practice, etc.)
- Healthcare professional (involved in providing direct care to the patient)
- Health-related professional (indirectly involved in patient care, teaching, research, etc.)
- Administrator (and any other parties supporting service provision to the patient)

This list fixes the set functional roles applied to manage the creation, access, processing, and communication of health information.

Additionally, functional roles can be grouped according to the relation to the information created, recorded, entered, processed, stored, and communicated:

- Composer
- Committer
- Certifier
- Authorizer
- Subject of information
- Information provider

Another approach for structuring functional roles related to information and its use has been introduced through the Information Distance Model, discussed below. This approach complies with the European Data Protection Directive and the related ISO CD 22857, Health Informatics: Guidelines on Data Protection to Facilitate

Trans-Border Flows of Personal Health Information (International Organization for Standardization 2004).

6.6.3. Structural (Static) Role Model

Static roles place people in the organizational hierarchy as belonging to categories of healthcare personnel warranting differing levels of access control. Similar to organizational roles, static roles allow users to participate in the organization's workflow (e.g., tasks) by job, title, or position but do not specify detailed permissions on specific information objects. Static roles allow a user to connect to a resource but do not grant functional authorizations. Some role group examples include physician, pharmacist, registered nurse supervisor, and ward clerk. Static roles may be found as non-critical certificate extensions entries to an X.509 certificate as specified in ASTM 2212-00.

An Entity–Entity relationship may concern a contracting act resulting in a contract between entities playing specific functional roles (see below). The contract could define the structural role of being, for example, a head physician. Another example may concern an Entity–Entity relationship for education resulting in a special qualification as well as a certificate certifying this qualification as a structural role.

These structural role constraints another Entity–Entity relationship influencing the functional role plaid by the entities involved in an activity. The establishment of a structural role is provided within an act between entities according to specific act-related functional roles. Figure 11.7 gives an example for the provision of a structural role certificate given from a certification authority to a client to be certified.

Considering both structural roles and functional roles in the same context, structural roles provide the prerequisites/competences for entities to perform interactions (an act) within their specific functional roles. Qualifications, skills, etc., are influencing both the assignment of the structural roles and the performance of activities according to their functional roles.

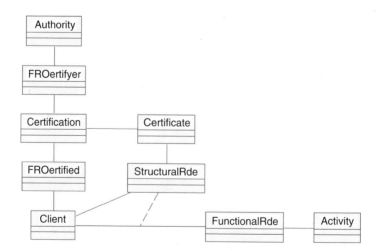

FIGURE 11.7. Establishment of a structural role within an act according the specific fiunctional roles.

6.6.4. Generic Role Specification

Roles may be generically described, including administrative constraints that may need to be enforced, using XML constructs. For example, separation of duties as an authorization constraint is widely used.

Health*e*People will manage the use of roles for access control through standards-based XML structures. The OASIS Security Assertion Markup Language (SAML) and eXtensible Access Control Markup Language (XACML) defines XML protocols and policy structures suitable for roles. For example, SAML supports the distributed service-oriented security architecture discussed earlier for federated and server–server exchanges.

6.7. Information Distance Model

Regarding the distance of persons to personal information, three types can be specified, each increasingly distant from the information:

- Originator of information (holder of data)
- Producer of information (interpreter of data)
- Administrator of information (user of information)

In a healthcare environment, the originator of information is normally the patient and the producer of information is the doctor. An example of an information user is a pharmacist.

Following the need-to-know principle, an increasing distance to information causes greater restrictions regarding privileges granted.

6.8. Authorization Model

6.8.1. Role and Privilege Assignment

Roles provide a means to indirectly assign privileges to individuals. Individuals are granted one or more roles defined by role attributes. Privileges are assigned to a role by role specification certificates, rather than to individuals. The indirect assignment enables the privileges assigned to a role to be updated without impacting the mechanisms that assign roles to individuals. Role credentials may be based upon attribute certificates, public-key certificates, or entries in a directory service.

The following scenarios are all possible:

- Any number of roles can be defined by any Attribute Authority (AA).
- The role itself and the members of a role can be defined and administered separately, by different AAs.
- Role membership, just as any other privilege, may be delegated.
- Roles and membership may be assigned any suitable lifetime.

For role assignment, the *role* attribute is contained in *attribute* components. A privilege asserter may present a role assignment certificate to the privilege verifier demonstrating only that the privilege asserter has a particular role (e.g., "manager" or "purchaser"). The privilege verifier may know a priori, or may have to discover by some other means, the privileges associated with the asserted role in order to accept/reject/modify a request. The role specification certificate can be used for this purpose.

A privilege verifier must have an understanding of the privileges specified for the role. The assignment of those privileges to the role may be made within the Privilege Management Infrastructure (PMI) by a role specification certificate or outside the PMI (e.g., locally configured).

Note that The use of roles within an authorization framework can increase the complexity of path processing, because such functionality essentially defines another delegation path which must be followed. The delegation path for the role assignment certificate may involve different AAs and may be independent of the AA that issued the role specification certificate.

The general privilege management model consists of three entities: the object, the privilege asserter, and the privilege verifier. Based on database access control models, Figure 11.8 shows a general privilege management model (Castano et al. 1995).

It should be mentioned that there are three principle decisions made in the privilege management context:

- Request authorized
- Request denied
- Request modified

Credentialing, privileging, and authorization are performed by connecting roles to policies.

6.9. Access Control Models

The role models specified above and advanced access control models such as the proposed NIST Standard Role-Based Access Control may be harmonized (Ferraiolo et al. 2001) in an adapted Role-Based Access Control Schema, as shown in Figure 11.9.

Each model component is defined by the subcomponents:

- A set of basic element sets
- A set of RBAC relations involving those element sets (containing subsets of Cartesian products denoting valid assignments)

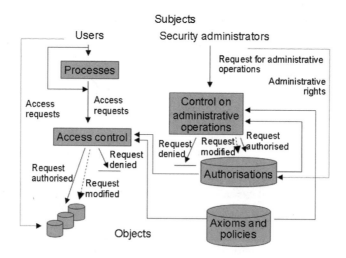

FIGURE 11.8. Privilege management and access control model (Castano et al. 1995, changed).

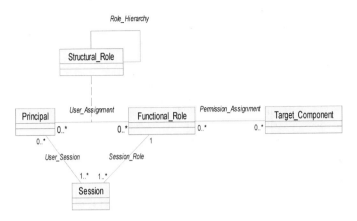

FIGURE 11.9. Role-based access control schema.

- A set of mapping functions that yield instances of members from one element set for a given instance from another element set

7. Conclusion

HealthePeople security meets the needs of law, custom, privacy, and patient care by providing security services through a practical service-capability infrastructure. It provides essential open, modular confidentiality, integrity, and availability services.

Uniform enterprise-wide fine-grain access control decisions are made without requiring time consuming and costly modification to individual application systems. This simplifies security management and enhances scalability. At the same time, information access mechanisms continue to operate locally.

Cost benefits accrue from HealthePeople's centralized authoritative information sources and enterprise cross-cutting security infrastructure. Here again, the security infrastructure allows sharing of security information in a way that decouples security mechanisms previously tightly integrated with specific applications. Users will be authenticated once and centrally, with centralized authorization and security management information bases supporting distributed access control decision function architectures. For managing relationships between the entities, organizational and functional roles can be defined. Based upon flexible access decision rules, user authorizations to multiple systems are managed, negotiated, and decided without the need to manually modify each individual system.

The HealthePeople environment for secure and reliable communication and co-operation requires participants to analyze and define their security needs and requirements. This is done in reference to well-defined security service models. Several practical models are presented that can help organizations to establish their own specific strategies.

HealthePeople security is a flexible infrastructure not a prescription. It will continue to evolve standards-based security architecture for health care promoting the interoperability and openness needs of HealthePeople participants.

References

CEN ENV 13608. 2000. Health informatics: Security for healthcare communication—Part 1: Concepts and terminology.

Damianou N, Dulay N, Lupu E, Sloman M. 2000. Ponder: a language for specifying security and management policies for distributed systems. The language specification, version 2.3. Imperial College Research Report DoC 2000/1. London: Imperial College.

Ferraiolo DF, Sandhu R, Gavrila S, Kuhn DR, Chandramouli R. 2001. Proposed NIST standard for role-based access control. ACM Trans Inform Sys Security 4(3):224–274.

International Organization for Standardization (ISO). 2004. ISO CD 22857 Health informatics: guidelines on data protection to facilitate trans-border flows of personal health information. Available from: http://www.medis.or.jp/iso/tc215wg4.html. Accessed 2003 January 10.

ISO 7498-2. 1989. International Standards Organization: Information processing systems, Open Systems Interconnection, Basic Reference Model—Part 2: Security Architecture. Note: ISO 7498-2 is superseded by ISO/IEC 10745 (ITU-T X.803), ISO/IEC 13594-IT-Lower layers security (ITU-T X.802) and ISO/IEC 10181-1 (ITU-T X.810).

Neumann G, Strembeck M. 2002. A scenario-driven role engineering process for functional RBAC roles. Available from: http://wi.wu-wien.ac.at/home/mark/publications/sacmat02.pdf. Accessed 2004 May 12.

12
Open Source Health Systems

DIPAK KALRA and DAVID FORSLUND

1. The Requirement for Health Software

Computers are now necessary for the delivery of contemporary health care in most countries. An obvious example of this includes digital imaging studies in which a computer is directing the investigation itself and processing the measurement values in order to make them capable of display to a human expert.

Today, however, computer systems play much wider and mission-critical roles in patient-centered clinical care:

- Parts of a patient's health record are captured in a range of diverse clinical applications in many different care settings, increasingly without a duplicate paper record being made of the encounter, test result, or prescription.
- The terminology systems and reference data that underpin manual coding activities and clinical applications are usually stored and accessed electronically.
- There are increasing numbers of alerts, electronic prompts, and guidelines incorporated within medical systems that direct clinical workflow, warn against out-of-range readings and potential hazards, or advise on care management.
- Demographic systems and regional or national registers are relied upon to ensure consistent patient identification across multiple enterprises, and to operate population health screening and recall programs.
- Computers are used to manage personnel registries and to enforce access control policies within single enterprises and across health regions.

These and other roles for computers will increase considerably across the whole of health care in the near future. A vast set of information systems and components need to collaborate efficiently and reliably in order to deliver a coherent set of such information services to the healthcare workforce. This is a significant challenge for the design of both large and small systems, requiring pre-planned approaches to interoperability across development teams within and between vendors.

Interoperability between systems is important to ensure:

- Reliable communication of patient records and other data to enable safe shared clinical care
- Consistent application functionality and workflow to support evidence-based clinical practice and efficient, joined-up, clinical services
- Access to common information services such as demographic, terminology, guideline, and security components

The challenge is greater still because the user requirements for health software are legitimately diverse across care settings, professions, and specialties, and they inevitably evolve as patterns of care delivery change and as a consequence of innovations in clinical practice. This places requirements on health systems and components to be highly configurable, adaptable, and, if necessary, easily upgraded or replaced.

It is recognized internationally that good (i.e., well-liked and well-used) clinical systems often arise through iterative cycles of development and clinical piloting in small-scale settings, and are often driven by locally recognized needs and championed both by the clinical and by the development teams. These departmental systems, of which any large hospital might have from 50 to 100, only occasionally evolve sufficiently to become suitable for widespread use. They are regarded as mixed blessings across the enterprise, for many well-understood reasons, but it cannot be denied that it is these kinds of innovations that have underpinned the global growth and acceptance of clinical computing and helped to shape the visions of larger-scale healthcare systems.

One of the major counter-challenges to adopting diverse and tailored clinical systems is the considerable training need within the clinical workforce in the use of computer applications. Almost universally, there are limited resources allocated to this activity on an ongoing basis, and efforts to build up well-trained teams are confounded by high staff turnover and the general mobility of clinical personnel. The commonly advocated solution to this is the use of identical systems across a health service, but in fact the major difficulty faced by staff using systems is not about knowing which button to click. Rather, it is about how to interface their routine clinical workflow and spontaneous information needs with the systems that are available. What we really need is not identical, but *intuitive* information systems.

2. Problems with the Current Marketplace

Although intuitive and interoperable clinical systems are what we need in health care, procurement decisions are rarely based on those values. In particular, the decision-making purchasers of health software are rarely also the intended downstream users of the systems. Thus, the purchasers typically underestimate the need for and the value of interoperability within their enterprise and for communications outside it, lack knowledge of the existence of relevant standards that might be leveraged to ensure that interoperability is built-in, and do not provide adequately for their future needs for adaptability and systems evolution.

Procurement decisions tend to focus on:

- The perceived attraction of meeting global enterprise information system requirements in a single shot
- The particular support of efficient workflow, the inclusion of (statutory) standard data sets and reporting functions to meet internal and external accountability requirements
- The initial cost of the system, although the gross total cost of ownership in the medium term is, surprisingly, not considered to be so critical
- The perceived scalability of the system and the range of support services offered by the vendor (but often not the projected cost of such support)
- The perceived reliability of the supplier as judged by the company size and turnover, but not particularly by that company's strategic direction within health care

- The perceived safety and respectability of the decision—following conventional practice and avoiding personal risk, not going out on a limb

A very clear and delightfully written paper on these and other factors was published by Bleich (1998); it remains a pertinent commentary on the procurement process as it is today.

A whole series of market forces and concerns about accountability promote a tendency toward electing a single vendor solution set within any one enterprise or health region. The recent approach adopted in the United Kingdom by the National Health Service is a massive-scale example of this. (For an overview, go to http://www.doh.gov.uk/ipu/whatnew/prognoun.htm.)

In general, this approach to procurement does not encourage the adoption of standards:

- Large vendors do not need them, but can instead use private interfaces internally and leverage their size and position to dictate the interfaces they choose to offer to others.
- Standards compliance is sometimes claimed but in practice often partial, and rarely verified by the purchaser; DICOM conformance has proved to be a good example of this problem internationally.
- There is no financial incentive for vendors to adopt standards because the customer requirements for interoperability within a procurement specification are usually quite weak and are not key determinants within the selection process.
- The whole financial model leans toward vendor ownership of the software, and of the strategic direction of its evolution; the private finance initiative (PFI) approach adopted by several countries is perhaps an extreme example.

Limitations in a new enterprise system are often identified some time after its arrival, and the need for additional modules or the inclusion of third-party components has therefore to be retrofitted to the original contract. The need to communicate with other enterprises and external systems seems often to extend beyond the scope originally anticipated. Such post-hoc interoperability is often achieved through expensive custom-made interfaces, which are also expensive to maintain as each system evolves. The cost of these interfaces is typically based on single customer cost recovery, the argument being that every custom-made interface is unique. Any customization or local tailoring of the systems at either end of the interface adds to the costs incurred, creating a pressure to avoid significant localization and thereby rather defeating the object of having adaptable systems.

Vendor lock-in with respect to data is a well-known problem that surprisingly does not seem to be disappearing yet.

The importance of standards in the healthcare arena has been discussed numerous times with clear emphasis on interoperable data standards. However, besides data standards, there is great need for functional standards so that systems can functionally work together rather than just sending data from one system to another, hoping that they can figure out what to do with it. This importance has been treated well in the paper by Forslund and Kilman (2000) as well as its impact on the global healthcare management infrastructure. The value of the health record as a way to collaborate on the treatment of a patient has also been discussed (Kilman 1997). Unfortunately, commercial pressures frequently work against this need for world-wide interoperable medical records.

As we discuss in the next section, open source has opened avenues of meeting the needs of interoperability and wide-scale integration by changing the way that one approaches the software in health care.

3. What Is Open Source?

Open source software is neither new nor radical, but offers a different approach to the provision of information systems that has the potential to harness the best features of the departmental systems described earlier, combining this with some of the perceived value of large-vendor systems.

The term *open source* may have different meanings for different people; for some, it is thought to be synonymous with public domain. However, open source actually has a formal definition, and software must meet a set of requirements and actually have a license of some type before it can properly be called open source. The motivation for open source is really quite simple. If the source of an application is readily accessible, many programmers can read it, evaluate it, and provide improvements so that the source code can evolve. Many people believe that, because of the large number of people reviewing such software, the quality of the software can be much better than is produced by the traditionally closed model.

The primary issues are the protection of intellectual property and the ability to make money in the process of developing and deploying the software. Contrary to popular views, the open source approach does not have to sacrifice either of these principles. In order to provide intellectual property protection, a formal license is normally required for open source. There are a wide variety of licenses that are used within the larger open source community, but they always involve these principles:

- Free Redistribution: There is no restriction on the distribution of the software in a royalty-free manner
- Source Code: The source code must be included in the distribution or readily made available in some form
- Derived Works: The license must allow for modifications and derived works to be distributed under the same terms as the original software
- Integrity of the Author's Source Code: There must be some provision to protect the integrity of the original authors' code

There are other important principles involved in open source licensing, not discussed here. For more information about the open source process, go to http://www.opensource.org.

There are many different licenses involved with open source, and they tend to fall into two primary camps. Perhaps the most well known is the General Public License (GPL) from GNU (a recursive acronym for GNU's Not Unix, pronounced "guh-noo"). The GPL probably provides the greatest protection of the various licenses, but also restricts the ability of a user to commercialize the software without making the derived works also freely available. Another well known license is the Apache Software license (and derivatives) which allows for commercial products to be derived from an open source base without requiring giving back that software to the community. In fact, the Apache Software Foundation is probably one of the most successful and prolific contributors today to the open source effort.

Some times open source software is spoken of as free software. However, there are two meanings to the term *free*, which sometimes confuse the situation. The first is *free*, as in no cost. The software is not charged for. This is normally a requirement as indicated above for open source. The more important term is the use of *free*, in the sense of liberty, that is, what can be done with the software, in terms of redistribution, modification, and so on. *Free* does not mean non-commercial. There may be very commercial implementations of *free* software. Apache's web server is one of the well-known examples. It is used heavily in commercial enterprises and commercial versions of the software can be purchased.

4. Advantages of Open Source Software

Open source software is frequently written initially within a small-scale and close working partnership of healthcare domain experts and systems developers. It is therefore very likely to be well tailored to the functional requirements of its specifying community. More importantly, because these are domain-specific specialized software components, they will have been developed on the assumption that they will in practice be used alongside other components that have not been developed by that group, and eventually in multiple and diverse settings. In contrast to the typical large-vendor approach, interoperability and standards compliance are therefore critical to the success of the open source software.

Open source software is usually not complemented by commercially available support services (from the development team or from anyone else) to customize and adapt the software for individual settings. The normal assumption is that user sites will be able to adapt the components themselves and be able to plug the component into any reasonably anticipated computing environment. Open source components are therefore more likely to interoperate with other standards-based components with minimal interface configuration. They are often (but not invariably) quite readily adapted to local contexts—at least, it is normally transparent to the local site how they can do it. The corollary, though, is that systems wanting turnkey solutions sometimes shy away from open source solutions because since they may require more customization. This could be viewed as an opportunity, however, for a system integrator.

Open source software is often a minority or niche player within its marketplace. Even Linux began that way. Functional excellence, innovation, and evolution have to be actively fostered within the development community to ensure that the component or system has credibility and remains useful in the medium and longer terms. Because open source teams rarely have a successor product they wish to market, built-in obsolescence is largely unknown. This is particularly true at the moment, when open source systems have to prove themselves to be better than their nearest commercial rivals in order to be treated as an equal to them.

While usually not seeking to provide a comprehensive solution set, open source teams often make use of other open source components, creating a standards-based and highly flexible and adaptable deployment environment. However, there are some very large open source projects. For example, the U.S. Veterans Administration has historically adopted an open source approach to the systems used throughout its U.S. hospitals and clinics.

As reflected by the definition of open source, there are two important characteristics of open source software that underpin the approach. First, the source code for the software is accessible:

- It is available for scrutiny, for peer review by the wider development community, providing a kind of quality assurance other than the black-box testing of software, which is the norm.
- It can be held by any user site as a form of protection against the original team folding: the user is empowered to take over the software's evolution or to commission this from another source.

- Vendor lock-in is practically impossible.
- Other component developers can understand in detail how they might best interface with it or incorporate it into other components and systems.

Second, the compiled, executable software is usually available at no cost or at a nominal cost:

- Potential user sites can pilot the software quite extensively before making a final decision on its adoption.
- It can be adopted for a lower capital cost and probably maintained at a lower ongoing cost of ownership.
- The costs are based on recurring services rather than on recovering the full development costs from each client.
- Because open source often makes use of and interoperates well with other open source software, the cost benefits of the approach tend to propagate across the overall enterprise information technology (IT) solutions.

Most importantly, the open source software is often nurtured within an active community of end users in a wide range of settings. Clearly, if the user community providing input on the requirements and feedback on the components is extensive, the component will evolve functional breadth and adaptability, and more comprehensive testing, making it suited to a diversity of settings.

The source code is often critiqued and contributed to by a number of voluntary teams and individuals, sometimes at an international level. An extensive and distributed development team can offer the benefits of a wider range of engineering experience, richer quality assurance and testing facilities, and the capacity to extend the development beyond the potential of the originating team. Very often, a site will elect to adapt a component in order to make it more suited to their environment, offering such adaptation back to the community as a functional enhancement or improvement. Other groups might develop interfaces to other components, new database bindings, extensions to a user interface, etc. It is by this means that the component or system can evolve in the directions that are needed by its user communities, thereby remaining relevant and usable over long periods of time.

The technical capacity of a distributed set of participants, working voluntarily and often with no dedicated budget for the collaboration, does not inherently guarantee anything better than could be achieved by a single vendor employing staff with equivalent expertise. It is the enthusiasm, energy, and the close, almost pioneering, collaboration of users and developers that creates an environment that is very difficult to reproduce commercially. Rapid iterative cycles of development and in vivo evaluation can replicate the best features of small-scale departmental systems but complement it with the technical rigor of source code peer review and the potentially rapid broadening of the community by making it freely available.

5. Adopting an Open Source Solution

It would be wrong to imply that the case for adopting open source software is overwhelming and without risk. There are a number of genuine concerns that healthcare services and organizations (or their IT departments) have about using such software. Some of these are common perceptions and misconceptions, but others reflect the weaknesses inherent in the open source approach as it is largely realized today.

Many open source projects have limited financial backing. The components might have been written by a team for their own enterprise; once they are completed to the extent required by that organization, the team might not be in a position to continue to evolve the software to incorporate requirements and contributions from other settings. Because of the initial small scale, the project might not have a well-documented architectural approach, but rather one created on-the-fly by the developers. The whole project might have arisen from a time-limited grant, such as funded research, with little assurance that the group will continue to exist after that project has finished. Because the work is largely fuelled by enthusiasm, there is always a chance that key members of the original team, or the team as a whole, will move on to new areas of interest. A rare but conceivable risk is that the group will decide to redirect their efforts in favor of a commercial successor to the open source software.

Vendors with a reasonably successful system and/or a positive branding image in the health sector will have sound business drivers to stay in the field, to recruit successor staff to maintain teams, to build against a well-defined architecture, and to ensure business continuity for their clients. Open source groups might have a moral commitment to this, but usually lack a business model that enables them to provide any long-term assurance of presence or dedication to the components they have developed. It would be wrong to imagine, however, that commerce is without equivalent risks: changes in market fortune, take-overs, or changes in high-level corporate strategy can lead to products being discontinued or to companies folding. Major players in the healthcare computing market have been known to abandon this sector altogether, leaving significant problems for their user base.

Both proprietary and open source paradigms share a common risk for the customer: the system provider might stop supporting or evolving software that has come to play an important role in the user's healthcare enterprise. Open source groups might appear at first sight to be flakier in this regard, as they are usually smaller teams with lower revenues deriving directly or indirectly from the developments. However, open source projects inherently offer some insurance against the disappearance of the originating team: the source code is available and there may be other groups already familiar with it and participating in its ongoing development. At worst, migration to a successor product can be informed and thereby made safer by having the source code. The relative risks of each approach are therefore more difficult to quantify and to evaluate formally. As a result, the case for open source is partly a subjective one.

Open source projects have a moral commitment to quality, but frequently lack the kind of accountability that is commonplace in commercial contracts for health software. Open source components usually carry disclaimers and limitations that would prevent litigation should the team prove to have been negligent or the software not fit for purpose. For this reason, commercial vendors are sometimes reluctant to invest the person-time needed to understand code within an open source component or to acquire the in-house expertise necessary to reduce the risk they might incur in using that component. Still, most consumer software also carries a disclaimer that is quite extensive.

Another area of concern more open to evaluation is the engineering quality of the components. In particular, there may be doubts about the application of quality assurance measures that ought to be used during software development and testing. There are often concerns about the diversity, quality, and coherence of contributions that may be arising from a distributed (and somewhat unregulated) pool of development volunteers. This is countered by the open source movement with the argument that the developers involved are often commercial grade (i.e., they also work or have worked for commercial software companies), and that the originating groups do regulate and eventually adjudicate the inclusion of code from other collaborators. The general experience of open source projects is that contributions are usually of very high quality and provide much-valued enhancement to the core component. Furthermore, the components are often tested quite widely in different settings soon after release— a kind of wide-area beta testing phase with full awareness of this role, while commercial customers sometimes find themselves hapless beta testers of software they thought was complete (i.e., an unintentional reference site). Basically, open source projects benefit from a broad, informal code review process. This code review may be far more comprehensive than is usually done even in the finest commercial software establishments. Although not formally certified as higher quality, this process can be very rigorous (although formal software engineering processes are by no means universal).

All of this presumes that the open source developments *are* being widely deployed, tested, or extended by collaborating teams across the globe. In the early stages, which might last for some years, there may be a significant dependence upon the original development team. There may be few external parties who can genuinely support and extend the code base because it is too complicated to understand without significant investment of time and skills, because it lacks good design documentation, or because in its early releases it may be too rudimentary for what is needed by most sites for anyone to invest in adopting the code and extending it to meet local functional requirements. There is a critical scale of interest and participation beyond which technical support will keep the component going, and ensure the benefits described earlier can be realized. Below this critical scale, the founding group may have to continue solo development at a pace they can afford and manage, even if a wider user community is impatient to see it develop more rapidly.

Limited overall resources for an open source activity may mean that there is a lack of advisory support for the software, and frequently paucity of trainers and of training materials. In their absence, however, such support as can be managed by the development teams and core user communities is usually freely given (e.g., through discussion lists) and of high quality. While such support services cannot be assured or specified in a service-level agreement, the authors are very familiar with the alternative: commercial suppliers providing expensive, contracted 24-hour helpline support that is delivered by poorly trained operatives and leaves its customers very frustrated.

Adopting an open source component does not necessarily imply that an enterprise has to go on to incorporate other open source components. However, in the present marketplace, vendor products and open source products do not always mix and match seamlessly. Polarized positions are more common to find than complementary ones. This means that few commercial health software systems directly interoperate with open source components. In fact, most commercial software only interacts with vendor-specified third-party components, or requires an expensive interface. Inevitably, for financial and perhaps evangelistic reasons, open source components tend to have been tested alongside other open source products. This clearly brings several benefits, including the ability to design a solution set that is entirely free of license costs. However, this may at times also mean that it is difficult to adopt a particular well-developed component because the complementary open source components necessary to build an overall solution might not be available or exist only at a lower level of maturity.

When weighing the various concerns discussed within this section, it is clear that the open source approach has some counter-arguments against its major perceived weaknesses. In the end, a somewhat subjective value judgment has to be made when attempting to evaluate the overall relative risks of adopting commercial versus open source software.

6. Considerations for the Principal Software Development Team

Thus far, we have focused on the strengths and weaknesses of the open source approach from the perspective of a potential user or adopter. Such views have generated the popular vision of open source software and projects. It is the kind of vision that will appeal to some development teams and not to others. Any team or organization needs to consider a range of factors when deciding if their activity should be made available as open source.

6.1. Is the Philosophy Appropriate?

The team has to be comfortable with code transparency: the source code will be open to peer review and feedback. The general approach to development should have been to adopt public domain interfaces, and to seek conformance to relevant standards. The component(s) will normally have free access, almost always not-for-profit (at least, not from the software itself).

The team needs to be prepared to host an open development process, using tools that enable collaborative software development, such as SourceForge. The responses and contributions will initially be bug fixes, modifications, and enhancements, but will progressively include suggestions for the strategic direction of the software as a whole. The originating team has to be ready and willing to progressively adopt democratic software development and project processes, in essence, to share autonomy.

6.2. Is the Software (Component) Suitable?

The team or organization needs to be satisfied that the component or system is fulfilling a role in an area that is not already well served by another open source component or good low-cost commercial products—in short, that it is really needed. It will also be more likely to generate interest if it is intended for use in an area of innovation or rapidly evolving requirements, which will probably be an area of healthcare computing that is less attractive to commercial developers. To stimulate a committed and contributing community (vital to realizing the benefits of open source development), the components should be relevant to a sufficient number of sites and settings, preferably in diverse settings and ideally at an international level.

On a technical level, it will be suitable for open source if it is appropriately componentized to fit within a range of different pre-existing software environments in different settings. Ideally, sufficient standards should exist (or be in the pipeline) to offer confidence about the interoperability interfaces that have been incorporated.

6.3. Could a Community Be Established?

The team needs to have a sense of the scale of community that might be generated around the open source project. At least a few other participating groups will eventually be needed to fulfill each of several different kinds of role:

- Interested users, to contribute ideas and requirements
- Active users to deploy and evaluate the software, and to enlarge the experience base
- Potential demonstrator sites, attracted by the prospect of active involvement in the development process (and perhaps by the low cost of participation)
- Developers offering a peer review of the code
- Developers interested in contributing new code for enhancements and extended functionality
- Other developers, particularly open source, wishing to integrate their components
- Other stakeholders, including research and teaching communities

6.4. Is the Code Suitable?

In order to be accessible to other online code reviewers, the source code, including historic versions, needs to be held in a formal repository. Concurrent Versions System (CVS) is the most common tool for configuration management in open source projects. It provides support for a moderately large team to work together on the development of an application with complete preservation of the changes made. (For more information, see http://www.cvshome.org.) The efforts of SourceForge.net, providing a home for open source development with rigorous support for full configuration management, are a major help to open source projects. SourceForge provides CVS support as well as mailing lists, announcements, documentation, and related tools for managing large projects. Not only is the open source code freely available on their web site at http://www.SourceForge.net, but the entire development process can be accessed by others in the community. This enables collaboration on a scale unprecedented in software engineering, and allows for people to see what ideas are being worked on by a wide community. In early 2004, SourceForge.net was hosting almost 70,000 open source applications and had over 700,000 registered users. The code, and the participatory framework offered to open source contributors, needs to be structured in a way that accommodates and organizes feedback responses and also change-manages any new code contributions.

6.5. Is the Team Ready?

The original authoring team has to recognize that niche software will be relevant and comprehensible to a small number of third parties, specifically, those who can actually picture what the intended functionality of such a component ought to be. There needs to be enough documentation for a code reviewer to navigate and understand it (at least to make some sense of it). Accompanying documents and/or slides are essential to enable clinical, or other kinds of end users, to understand why this component has been produced, how it might best be deployed and used, what requirements it aims to meet, and, importantly, what the group's immediate plans and intentions are. Installation instructions might also be nice!

Once a decision has been taken to "go open source," some months may be needed to prepare materials and to ready the team members themselves for the launch. Steps to migrate toward open source are detailed in Table 12.1.

The group must be ready and committed to foster an e-community (often using discussion lists) and to respond to inquiries about the project, the software, and the code. For registered open source projects, SourceForge.net hosts such capabilities. Most importantly, the team members must be ready for the code to move forward in new and exciting directions.

TABLE 12.1. Migrating toward open source: stepping stones.

Any team considering the open source approach to a project needs to take a number of steps:
- Reach agreement with the sponsoring agency that it is the right approach. This may be non-trivial because of the lack of understanding of how costs are recovered in an open source project.
- If the intent is to attract a number of people in addition to the local team, work to advertise the approach, plans, and vision for the project.
- Use a web site including some form of content management, to enable the discussion and review of ideas. We have used the plone system, itself an open source project, for this purpose. (Go to *http://plone.org* for additional information.)
- Consider how the participants will work together, particularly if it is a project that will have a number of contributors.
- Assess the licensing strategies that will protect the intelleotual property of the various contributors. Pick one of the many open source licenses that meets your needs, rather than writing one for yourself.
- If you need funding, pursue various organizations that might be interested in your project. In the United States, many research agencies are sympathetic to the idea of open source because it makes the results of federally funded projects available to a broader audience.
- If you have an existing, non–open source project you want to make open source, determine whether you are at risk of violating some implied license the software may already have. Ask for knowledgeable legal advice in this area.
- Establish a robust configuration management system and procedure for the software, so that its integrity can be properly managed. SourceForge.net is a good place to consider, but there are others as well.
- Understand that the more open you make your project, the more likely you are to get external participants in the development process.

7. Case Study: openEHR

7.1. *Deciding to Launch an Open Source Endeavor*

Two research teams, at the University College London (UCL) in the United Kingdom and Ocean Informatics in Australia, came together in an initiative to use the open source in electronic health record (EHR) development. Both teams had established strong pedigrees in the publication of requirements for EHR interoperability, the design of information architectures to meet these, and proof-of-concept implementations of EHR systems in small-scale demonstrator sites.

Members of the teams, which included one of the authors of this chapter, had worked together previously. In late 1999, we recognized that each team had achieved valuable new results with some degree of overlap and some complementary strengths, which might helpfully be combined.

Research on generic information models to represent and communicate EHRs has been active within Europe since the early 1990s. The European Union sponsored several multi-national projects, including the Good European Health Record (GEHR; Ingram 1995), Synapses (Grimson et al. 1998), and Synergy on the Extranet (SynEx; Sottile et al. 1999). In addition, the European Committee for Standardization (or CEN, for Comité Europeen de Normalisation) produced two generations of standards for Electronic Healthcare Record Architecture, ENV12265 (Hurlen 1995) and ENV13606 (Kay and Marley 1999). However, uptake of such specifications commercially has been limited for several reasons, including the perceived complexity of building robust and scalable systems underpinned by a generic hierarchical model and the apparent success of use-case-specific messages to communicate, for example, laboratory and billing information (using EDIFACT or Health Level Seven Version 2).

Our two groups felt that coming together would allow a synthesis of the best features of each approach, including a harmonization of the two archetype-like techniques that had been developed in Europe (Kalra 1996, 2003) and Australia (Beale 2000). A union of developmental efforts would enable more effective use of our scarce research grant resources. Promoting the need for generic and interoperable EHRs under a common banner, and with harmonized specifications, would make the efforts of each party more effective and better coordinated.

We all agreed that active engagement in implementation and clinical evaluation was essential to validate the integrity of the approach and to continue learning cycles to evolve the requirements and refine the specifications.

In particular, we all felt that, in the absence of readily available interoperable (standards-conformant) commercial EHR systems, a good quality open source reference implementation would:

- Have value as a highly visible proof that the generic information architecture approach is valid and scalable
- Offer a means of seeding new EHR demonstrators and user communities internationally, to promote the approach, to widen the requirements input base and to extend the field of empirical evaluation
- Engage a wider group of developers to complement and supplement the capacity of our small teams
- Provide a software exemplar of how the documented specifications can be implemented, which might be used as another kind of specification, namely, a kind of Implementation Technology Specification (ITS), to assist other developers making their own versions of an interoperable EHR.

7.2. Working Together

The joining together of our two groups entailed many threads of activity. We established a not-for-profit organization, which we agreed to call the openEHR Foundation, and defined its mission statement, vision, and objectives. We largely agreed on our intended approach on access to our future specifications, tools, components, and code, including if and how we want to distinguish non-commercial and commercial users. In principle, we were reluctant to propose any form of charged licensing for the eventual openEHR record server, but felt we might instead seek donations from national or other large-scale enterprises that elected to utilize it. We are still a long way from knowing whether this will prove to be a wise position to take.

The founding partners, UCL and Ocean, have each invested significantly in establishing openEHR. In 2002, we launched our new-look web site (http://www.openehr.org) and e-discussion forums. We continue working to extend the international community of interest through conferences and other meetings. In this regard, we have been very helpfully supported by the EuroRec Institute (http://www.eurorec.net) that has frequently promoted our work within its activities.

We worked with lawyers to draft a set of legal instruments, such as memoranda and articles of association, to establish and run the openEHR Foundation, which has been formally registered. To protect the name openEHR as we grow and become better known, we registered the name as a trademark in several parts of the world. We believe we need to establish a sensible license for our current and anticipated materials, to protect their integrity and to limit our liability, while facilitating their use within the openEHR community and by others. We have produced a copyright notice that is now included on all of our documentation, and a data protection policy for the web site and discussion lists. We are considering adopting the Mozilla triple license for our open source code, to permit the deployment of openEHR components within other open source or commercial software products.

We actively critiqued our two sets of information models in the light of the implementation and demonstration experience we have each gained, in order to design a new converged comprehensive reference model, an archetype specification, and related models and services. Published as evolving releases on our web site, these were widely downloaded, stimulating valuable feedback.

We began planning a program of implementation that can take advantage of the skills and existing tools of each site, taking account of the funding and capacity each team as it might vary over the coming years. We are also establishing change control systems to maintain integrity of the development process, in particular for when the contributing team expands beyond the founding pair of teams.

7.3. Ready for Take Off

If, in early 2000, you had asked us how long it would take to achieve much of the above and to begin writing code, we might have guessed up to two years. With no dedicated funded posts committed full-time to this challenge, progress has been a little slower, made in bursts whenever gaps arose in our day jobs and whenever our Australian colleagues were able to get time and funding to join us in London. Contrary to all the promises of e-working, we have always found that progress really accelerates when we are brainstorming together in the same room.

An active discussion community has been established with over 300 members, which has brought us some very rewarding positive feedback, and also lots of stimulating issues that have challenged us to extend and refine our scope. This has also brought us into contact with other health informatics communities, such as clinical guidelines, terminology, ontology, images, and security.

The process of developing appropriately worded licenses and disclaimers has taken us several iterations, despite good legal support. Trademarking the name openEHR is certainly quite an expensive affair.

Perhaps what has excited us the most has been the launch of important new standardization activities in Health Level Seven (HL7) and the European Committee for Standardization (Comité Européen de Normalisation, or CEN). In HL7, the Structured Documents Technical Committee, the EHR Special Interest Group (SIG), and the Templates SIG have all established rich interfaces with the openEHR work, and involved us as individuals. In Europe, there is currently a major revision of the CEN EHR Communications standard (ENV 13606), with significant input from members of our groups. Reciprocally, we have found that the participation in these has provided us with fresh ideas, and a rationale to harmonize the openEHR specifications with those activities— the main reason why we have delayed some of our specification releases during 2003.

We are now at the stage when stability is being reached in these standardization activities, and we have issued a formal release of the openEHR specifications as the basis for implementation. We have established an Architecture Review Board to oversee further revisions, through a formalized change control process. We are now ready to begin the exciting implementation path, and are actively seeking collaboration from industry and participation in national EHR demonstrator projects.

While we will inevitably begin in-house, we hope soon to be announcing access to some initial source code, and to begin enticing participation from our many international friends.

7.4. Case Study: VistA

Probably the most successful and widespread open source effort in health care began in the U.S. Department of Veterans Affairs (VA) as the Decentralized Hospital Computer System (DHCP) more than 20 years ago. To automate their widely distributed medical centers, VA chose the language MUMPS, from the American National Standards Institute (ANSI), as their implementation framework and created a suite of applications that still sets the standard for managing electronic health records.

Renamed the Veterans Health Information Systems and Technology Architecture (VistA), it remains at the forefront of open healthcare software today. Over the years, versions of it have been adopted by the Indian Health Service as well as the Department of Defense. The software is in the public domain today. More information about it is available at http://hardhats.org and at http://worldvista.org. Recently, this effort has benefited with the release of an open source MUMPS platform known as GT.M, available through http://www.sanchez-gtm.com.

Although not intimately familiar with the details of VistA, we recommend it as probably the most important open source case study in healthcare software. VistA contains probably the largest volume of clinical patient information and thus would be a rich resource to engage in the providing of a medical record directly to patients as envisioned in the HealthePeople effort.

7.5. Case Study: OpenEMed

OpenEMed has had a fairly long history. It started as an example of the National Information Infrastructure in the fall of 1993 as part of the internal Sunrise project at Los Alamos, to demonstrate a common infrastructure that would support the use and value of distributed applications to a number of disciplines. The TeleMed project developed out of this effort, with no initial intent to be open source. The project first succeeded in managing computerized tomography image sets for cases of multi-drug resistant tuberculosis, including queries for images that had the same features. After this work, done with the National Jewish Medical and Research Center in Denver, Colorado, the system evolved into a more general medical record system with the help of the Telemedicine and Advanced Technology Research Center (TATRC) at Fort Detrick, Maryland.

At that time, the system was completely rewritten in Java and participated in pioneering standards within the Object Management Group (OMG) for distributed medical records management set by its Healthcare Domain Taskforce. Java was chosen as the implementation language because it supported rapid prototyping and was an adequate object-oriented language to support the object-oriented approach of OpenEMed. The system was designed around services that were designed to be very flexible in the support of patient identification, terminology discovery, clinical observations, and distributed access control. The standards developed and implemented actually used the original GEHR model as one of its objectives and fully supports that model.

In doing so, we adopted and helped create an open architecture before we adopted the open source model. We wanted the system to be fully interoperable with any system that implemented the same standards. We contributed significantly to the standardization of these core services in the medical record. We had several companies show interest in licensing the software, but found that it really did not make sense for us to enter into a restrictive licensing agreement.

Because mostly public funds were used to develop the software, it made sense to make the software available freely to the public. Thus we adopted our current open source licensing procedure based on the open source license from Berkley Software Design (BSD). We changed the name from TeleMed to OpenEMed to avoid any possible trademark conflicts. We positioned our work as a type of reference implementation of the relevant OMG specifications, which we believe is crucial to ensuring that the standards are fully implementable, not just a paper standard. By following this strategy, we have attracted more funds than we could have obtained from licensing, and brought more people to contribute to the software base. We have been able to use OpenEMed far beyond its original medical domain and closer to the original vision we had for the Sunrise project as a whole. Through the open source mechanism we have invited others to participate with the Los Alamos team in developing the software. Most of that participation has occurred from partners in Europe, most notably from the University of Maastricht. The project continues to invite interested participants both from the commercial and research sectors to participate.

The licensing strategy we use enables us to utilize much of the very significant Apache software project funded as part of the Apache Foundation. Our open source license is compatible with this. It has enabled us to adopt some of the best new Java technology available and allows OpenEMed to continue to be a state-of-the-art development effort. We have demonstrated the ability to create a system that quickly adapts to changes in requirements and in the technology.

An important observation we have made over the development of a number of versions of the OpenEMed software is that open source provides a very solid foundation for our software. We try to have multiple implementations of various services we use (such as databases, object-relational mapping, security, etc.) so that we are not dependent on a single vendor for any of our technology. We have used commercial products in OpenEMed, but they are not needed for most of its functionality. We have found that the support for an actively supported open source project is light-years ahead of the support provided by a commercial vendor for a similar technology. We have found numerous times that bugs are fixed in as little as 30 minutes to about 24 hours, where bugs in commercial products (with support contracts) frequently are never fixed, even in the next major revision of the software! This is not true of all open source projects, but, because there are so many, it is not hard to find those that provide this kind of support, even if it is not from the original developers. Picking a mainstream programming language is a significant help in this area.

The OpenEMed software is primarily a framework rather than a turnkey system, although it has complete implementations of several important areas of health care including a full-blown medical surveillance system (Forslund 2004) and pilots of an immunization registry and a National Electronic Disease Surveillance System (NEDSS) Integrated Data Repository (IDR). The component approach we have adopted has gained interest within the U.S. federal sector as an example of the value of components in building complex systems. By reconfiguring our components, we are able to solve a number of problems without having to rewrite of substantial amount of code. The components we are using compose a service-oriented architecture that has gained in popularity in recent years. The whole concept of providing reusable medical services is what the entire project is about.

The architecture that was used in OpenEMed has been used in other projects, including the large federal Government Computerized Patient Record (GCPR) project that was seeking to integrate the Indian Health Service, the Department of Veteran Affairs, and the Department of Defense healthcare systems. In addition, it has been used in

Brazil and in the European project called Professionals and Citizens for Integrated Care (PICNIC; http://picnic.euspirit.org). The service-oriented approach used in OpenEMed is gaining wide acceptance today in the Web Services community and provides a significant data integration framework for many applications.

Currently, OpenEMed is the core architecture of the FIRST project at the City of Hope, which is seeking to create a distributed collaborative system for managing clinical protocols. It also is a core component in an effort to provide a comprehensive integration strategy for biosurveillance within the United States.

8. What Makes an Open Source Project a Success?

Open source has been proven in many areas to be the most robust and economical approach to software development and deployment. This is now widely accepted outside the domain of health care because of the broad success of the Linux operating system and tools like the Apache web server, which is the most commonly used web server in the world today.

We find open source to be a viable business model. For the developer, it can provide a broad base for the code development, substantially lowering the cost of developing of quality software. For the end user, it can provide economies by reducing vendor lock-in and enabling costs to be placed in the service area where they are incurred.

Contrary to the widespread notion that open source reduces the protection of intellectual property, open source can actually provide greater protection for intellectual property by enforcing the acknowledgement of who developed the code by placing the entire process under public scrutiny. However, some open source licenses, such as the GPL, provide more intellectual property protection than others.

In the domain of healthcare informatics, knowledge is spread around an enormous number of enterprises, and systems need to meet a diverse set of needs. Open source provides an excellent basis for meeting those needs. It enables a local organization to customize an open source solution to meet their needs rather than relying on specialized commercial solutions, which can be very expensive. The model of physicians sharing knowledge is very similar to the open source software model. The several examples we have provided for case studies also demonstrate this suitability.

End users have quite reasonable protection of their software investment, especially with the high volatility of software companies these days. With open source, they are able to ensure that the capability they have today will still be around tomorrow and not lost in some commercial buy-out, with the product removed from the marketplace. This does not totally protect from rising costs of maintenance, but does enable them to continue their business with reduced risk of code abandonment.

The community nature of open sources generally provides excellent support for upgrades and bug fixes to open source software. If individuals cannot solve a problem, they frequently can find a solution in the broader community. In essence, open source increases the effective size of their development team and support base, and they no longer have to rely on a single vendor for support and maintenance. The cost benefit of this is enormous and, for some projects, is the major motivator.

We clearly demonstrated the emphasis on the adoption of open architecture and open standards by open source efforts. This effort to support open standards is driven by the community approach of open source software and the desire to reduce the cost by adopting standards. The architecture typically is open and enables other applications to plug into an infrastructure, again, to reduce costs and risks of a particular software approach. The weakness of some open source efforts is in not adopting an over-arching architecture, but rather building it as needed over time. This can lead to difficulties in maintaining the code. This extreme programming (or XP) approach can be quite valuable, however, in enabling a software system to adapt to new requirements, as long as it is combined with a fairly rigorous software methodology.

In terms of making healthcare information available to the consumer and the person of primary interest, open source has a major role because it can enable the consumer to have the tools necessary to understand his healthcare information without being constrained by a vendor that may preclude his ability to track his own personal healthcare information. This should be a major motivator by all people involved in healthcare informatics.

References

Beale T. 2000. The GEHR archetype system. The Good Electronic Health Record Project, Australia. Available from: http://titanium.dstc.edu.au/gehr/req-design-documents/artchtypes_3.1B.pdf. Accessed 2004 Mar.

Bleich HL. 1998. Why good hospitals get bad computing. Medinfo 9(2):969–972.

Forslund DW, Kilman DG. 2000. The impact of the global, extensible electronic health record. In: Eder LB, editor. Managing healthcare information systems with web-enabled technologies. Hershey, PA: Idea Group Publishing.

Forslund DW, Joyce E, Burr T, Picard R, Wokoun D, Umland E, Brillman J, Froman P, Koster F. 2004. Setting standards for improved syndromic surveillance. IEEE Eng Med Biol 23(1):65–70.

Grimson J, Grimson W, Berry D, Stephens G, Felton E, Kalra D, Toussaint P, Weier OW. 1998. A CORBA-based integration of distributed electronic healthcare records using the synapses approach. IEEE Trans Inf Technol Biomed 2(3):124–138.

Hurlen P, editor. 1995. Project Team 1-011. ENV 12265: Electronic healthcare record architecture. Brussels: Comité Europeen de Normalisation.

Ingram D. 1995. The Good European Health Record Project. In: Laires MF, Laderia MJ, Christensen JP, editors. Health in the new communications age. Amsterdam: IOS Press. p 66–74.

Kalra D, editor. 1996. The Synapses User Requirements and Functional Specification (Part A). In: EU telematics application programme. Brussels; The Synapses Project.

Kalra D. 2003. Clinical foundations and information architecture for the implementation of a federated health record service. PhD Thesis. University of London.

Kay S, Marley T, editors. 1999. Project Team 1-026. ENV 13606: EHCR communications: Part 1 Electronic healthcare record architecture. Stockholm: Comité Europeen de Normalisation.

Kilman DG, Forslund DW. 1997. An international collaboratory based on virtual patient records. Commun ACM 40:110–117.

Sottile PA, Ferrara FM, Grimson W, Kalra D, Scherrer JR. 1999. The holistic healthcare information system. In: Brown P, editor. Proc. Toward an electronic health record Europe '99. CAEHR (centre for the Advancement of Electronic Health Records), 14–17 November 1999. London, UK. p 259–266.

13
Critical Standards Convergence

STEVEN WAGNER and J. MICHAEL FITZMAURICE

Good health is essential to enjoyment of life and human activities. A critical under-pinning of good health is delivery of appropriate health care. The efficiency and effec-tiveness with which health care is delivered have a major and direct impact on individuals, populations, and the providers and organizations engaged in its delivery. Timely access to accurate information is essential to delivering high-quality health care and achieving the goal of good health. Today, the amount of information pertinent to the care of individuals is quite large and often cannot be located when needed for care decisions. In the future, such information will be enormous and well beyond the ability of individual providers to effectively absorb and process it, even though access will more easily be accommodated. To make sense of this vast amount of information, providers and patients will want to apply their own filters or views to the information. Information technology applied to health care will be the vehicle for compiling, inter-preting, and delivering pertinent information to patients and providers in a timely and easy-to-understand manner.

Health data collection and repositories of patient care data, access to medical knowl-edge, and decision support systems that provide prompts, alerts, and reminders to healthcare decision makers are all essential tools. The most crucial substructure of this vision, the one that has the most potential at this time to advance the effort to achieve good health, is healthcare data standards.

The purpose of this chapter is to describe:

- A vision of health care in the future from both the patient and provider viewpoints
- The current state of healthcare standards activities and the standards organizations involved
- The major obstacles to achieving the vision and establishing the system of standards that is so essential for high-quality health care
- Approaches for getting from the present to the vision by reducing or eliminating the major obstacles

1. The Vision

The scenarios that follow describe a vision of health care in the future from two points of view—the patient's and the provider's (Veterans Health Administration 2001). Each perspective is followed by an examination of what is needed to achieve this vision.

1.1. The Patient's View

A cancer patient logs into his personal healthcare website from home and receives personalized electronic information about a new treatment. The information is automatically retrieved from credible sites, based on previously established criteria, including his age, gender, and medical condition.

After reviewing the information, the patient uses the interface to access insurance benefits and eligibility information and to schedule an appointment for next week at a community-based outpatient clinic close to his home.

At the visit, the patient shares the new treatment information with his physician and receives guidance and education regarding its relevance to his condition. An oncologist from a renowned specialty cancer center participates in the discussion via videoconference. Based on a mutual decision to pursue the potential treatment further, the patient takes several tests to determine if he is an appropriate candidate for the treatment.

Once the test results are ready, the patient is alerted that they have been automatically added to his health record. Using his web interface the patient reviews the results, authorizes consent to the remote clinician, and makes the results available to the remote care team so that treatment planning can begin.

1.1.1. Analysis

The Patient View scenario indicates how patients will be able not only to access their healthcare records, but also to control their health information and influence their health and treatment in general. Technology will increasingly allow patients to take a more active role in their own health care. Personalized access to online preventive and healthcare information will be provided to patients based on individual preferences and patient characteristics. Educational information will educate and empower patients. Ratings of preventive and healthcare knowledge sources will be employed to increase the use of credible information. Online preventive and healthcare information will be combined with a patient's own healthcare information including test results and treatment plans in a single record.

Patients or their designees will act as information stewards granting others access to their healthcare information based upon the receiving party's need to know. Security mechanisms will be present to ensure the privacy, availability, integrity, and confidentiality of patient healthcare information.

Patients will be able to enroll, schedule appointments, request prescription refills, and provide and receive health information with increased ease via the Internet, e-mail, or voice mail. Patients will have a greater ability to communicate (using wireless and other devices) with clinicians remotely, to participate in online discussions with support groups, and to participate in online health surveys.

Advances in telecommunications will enable the delivery of information and services to smaller, remote locations and enable remote monitoring, such as home monitoring through electronic devices and self-monitoring, and reporting to the physician's office. Around-the-clock surveillance of patients at remote facilities will allow staff to be alerted in seconds when needed.

The use of smart cards and advanced authentication methods such as biometrics (i.e., retinal scans or hand geometry) will become prevalent for focused applications such as patient and caregiver identification and authentication. Further, these smart cards will support patient identification and provide access to online information.

1.2. The Provider View

A primary care physician prepares for a routine healthcare visit with a new patient who is under his care. Using his online clinical system, he assembles the patient's history and physical exam results.

Replacing the need for the physician to delve into paper records and charts, clinical systems now offer interoperability across care facilities and organizations, not to mention across specialties, making a patient's health record available to the primary care physician within moments of the patient's authorization.

This longitudinal record offers a broad-view perspective on the patient. The key aspects of the patient's problems, a health summary, and interventions are available, as are references to points-of-care and timeframes in which these interventions occurred. Clinical decision support is available and its computational range extends across the full composite record.

The clinician notes the existence of a stress test, taken only three months earlier at a cardiology facility, that appears to be particularly relevant for understanding the patient's condition. With a few keystrokes, he is viewing both the progress notes and the electrocardiograms (EKGs) themselves, with all coded terms displayed in the local institution's normal vocabulary.

When the clinician prescribes medication for this patient, the decision support system double checks the known applicability of the drug for the patient's conditions, including allergies, verifies that the recent lab tests are consistent with his diagnosis of these conditions, and analyzes the dose relative to the patient's weight, age, and contraindications. It then presents suggestions and medical knowledge sources for the clinician to evaluate.

1.2.1. Analysis

In the future, physicians, nurses, and other clinical staff will access integrated longitudinal health records (care points, time, locations, and providers) across the healthcare system. The underlying, shared medical concepts in these records will be presented in terms that have meaning to the local clinician, based upon national vocabulary standards mapped to locally accepted terms.

On-line clinical images, including EKGs, magnetic resonance imaging, and CAT scans, will be available to clinicians and integrated with patient records to create a more complete patient view.

Clinical staff will also be empowered with decision support tools that are integrated with caregiver workflow and that act upon clinical data repositories and data warehouses to assist the provider's evidence-based diagnosis, predictions, and care recommendations. Physicians will be able to determine expected treatment outcomes and practice preventive medicine effectively, in addition to obtaining guidelines for clinical practice at the point-of-care and obtaining the credentials of other providers of care. Providers will have electronic capabilities to verify insurance and eligibility, order tests and receive results, submit insurance claims, and manage referrals. Physicians will also have the ability to offer remote teleconsultations to health management teams.

The use of pervasive devices (smart phones, personal digital assistants, and laptops) will provide clinicians with location independence and persistent, secure connectivity to a vast pool of knowledge resources. Clinicians will be able to receive drug alerts and laboratory test results on these devices. Electronic prescription and continuous speech recognition services will be offered as alternatives to data entry by hand, especially in clinical settings such as hospital emergency and radiology departments, significantly enhancing hands-free care and documentation.

Security will operate seamlessly in the background, verifying the integrity of information, protecting the confidentiality of sensitive patient information, and assuring the availability of information resources. Physician–patient relationships, patient safety, security, physician productivity, and quality of care will be strategically and significantly enhanced.

1.3. The Need for Standards Convergence

What does all this have to do with healthcare standards? Everything! Health care is provided by a large community of providers to an even larger community of patients. It is an inherently distributed environment. The only way to achieve the integration of information described in the scenarios above is through the development of a comprehensive, integrated set of healthcare standards—a set of model-based standards that seamlessly and efficiently join to support the exchange, representation, interpretation, security, and confidentiality of healthcare information.

This comprehensive, integrated set of standards must support the collection and retrieval of clinical information about patients that is accurate and uniformly defined. The systems must link to medical knowledge that is helpful in the care of the patient, such as clinical practice guidelines. And the systems that perform these functions must interoperate with each other without adversely affecting the provider and patient.

To move quickly in this direction, our healthcare system must identify the standards that are needed, spell out the specific requirements, produce the required standards, implement them, and update the standards as medical advances occur or as problems and gaps are found.

To guide the development of standards, there should be a healthcare information model and strong encouragement for interoperability of information systems that use these standards. The availability of the Health Level Seven (HL7) Reference Information Model and the Australian Information Model illustrate complexity on one hand and simplicity on the other.

The competitive marketplace currently rewards health information system vendors who obtain a customer base and hold on to it through use of proprietary standards. These standards are specific to the vendor's own software and account for the way health data are defined and coded and moved around in their own system's operations. Because these vendor-specific, proprietary standards are not made readily available by the vendor for widespread use by other vendor systems, the actual interoperability with other information systems is hampered. This can be good news for specific health system vendors who want to keep a customer dependent on the vendor's system and its standards. But it is bad news for hospitals and physician groups that want to choose among the systems (for example, laboratory, radiology, pharmacy systems) offered by different vendors and make them work together efficiently.

For efficiency and promotion of effective health care, healthcare standards must be developed with the goal of permitting interoperability among the health information systems that use them. Purchasers would like to pick the best laboratory information system for them and link it to the best pharmacy information system that meets their needs. The market finds it difficult to give purchasers what they want. Why is this?

First, purchasers know what functions they want but not how to specify how those functions should interoperate with the functions of a complementary system, for example, laboratory systems with pharmacy systems. There is a lack of knowledge regarding how to specify what they want to buy. Second, many consultants can link any two systems together but it takes significant effort related to translation of data and modeling. The translation process seems to take place in a black box where data from one system enters on one side and the data (transformed) requested by another system exits the other side. Data and modeling standardization could make this black box simpler, or unnecessary. Third, the market does not push vendors toward common ways of coding their data and modeling their exchange. The market rewards the vendor who waits till someone else does it—the waiting vendor gets a free ride. And if all vendors wait, there will be few common healthcare standards. All too frequently, the cost of developing a healthcare standard exceeds what any one vendor can capture in benefits from the market, even if the aggregate benefits exceed the costs of development.

The case for government standards development support and leadership can be made here because there is a common good (reduction in adverse health events and quality improvements that can be made available to all) that, when combined with the private good (added value derived from the sale of systems that interoperate with common healthcare standards and from additional services in support of patient care), exceeds the cost of developing and implementing healthcare standards that support interoperability of systems. Without government action, each health information system vendor will wait for someone else to do it while investing in its own proprietary standards for defining clinical data and how it is stored and transmitted.

On the other hand, without private sector leadership and collaborative action, government will not have the broad input necessary to properly determine which standards to support and which concepts to codify. Clearly, standards development and implementation is an area in which the public good requires both government and private sector leadership and support.

Individual studies have shown that benefits can be gained from systems that interoperate, such as drug and laboratory test ordering systems that interoperate with laboratory reporting systems (Tierney et al. 1993; Bates et al. 1998). These results, however, are usually found in a controlled study in an advanced teaching hospital and not spread widely among other hospitals for many reasons. One of these reasons is the lack of standards to link data exchanges and functions of hospital departments across department systems. Among the many other reasons is the fact that, at each hospital that is successful, there is often a driving, energetic physician pushing his or her peers to adapt information technology solutions to everyday tasks. The supply of such physicians to date has not been sufficient to populate the more than 5000 U.S. hospitals with at least one per hospital.

2. The Present

Health care is blessed with a number of healthcare standards–related and standards development organizations. A previous chapter on critical areas of standardization lists the major private sector organizations involved in the development of healthcare standards and their accomplishments. A graphical representation of these organizations and their relationships is provided in Table 13.1.

Of note is the Healthcare Informatics Standards Board (HISB) that provides a coordinating function across U.S. healthcare standards development organizations (SDOs) to avoid unnecessary duplication of effort and to identify gaps among existing standards. Within HISB, the SDOs are joined by vendor, government, professional association, and other members to learn and debate current standards issues. When gaps

TABLE 13.1. Standards-related organizations and their relationships.

Government		Private sector		
Standards setting	Healthcare providers/users	SDOs		Healthcare promoters
		ANSI HISB coordinated	Other	
CMS	AHRQ	ADA	DICOM	CFH
FDA	CDC	ASC X12N	JCAHO	eHealth Initiative
NLM	CHI	ASTM E31	WEDI	HIMSSNLM
	CMS	HL7	ISO	
		CAP	TC215	
	DoD	IEEE 1073	ISO	
	DVA	NCPDP	TC215	
	NCHS		US TAG	
	NCVHS			

are identified, members have an opportunity to present their standards needs and to supply subject matter experts and financial assistance to the standards development organizations (SDOs) to close the gaps.

In the government sphere, the National Committee on Vital and Health Statistics (NCVHS), composed of 18 private sector appointees, advises the Secretary of Health and Human Services on health data and information policy. In recent years, NCVHS has taken extensive testimony and provided recommendations to the Secretary in such areas as:

- Implementing the HIPAA Transactions and Code Set standards; national identifiers for providers, health plans, employers, and individuals; the HIPAA Privacy Rule; and the Security Rule
- Replacing ICD9-CM diagnosis and institutional procedure codes with ICD10 codes
- Building the national health information infrastructure
- Developing and adopting patient medical record information (PMRI) clinical message and vocabulary standards

Also in the government sphere, the Departments of Health and Human Services (HHS), Veterans Affairs (VA), and Defense (DoD) combined to form an eGovernment initiative called Consolidated Health Informatics (CHI). Using about 100 experienced government staff, CHI has undertaken a role to evaluate existing healthcare standards and determine which ones in each of 24 identified health domains are appropriate for use in federal programs that exchange health information.

In early 2003, the Secretary of HHS announced the adoption by HHS, VA, and DoD of four standards recommended by both NCVHS and CHI, plus one more recommended by CHI (U.S. Department of Health and Human Services 2003a). More recommendations are forthcoming from both groups. The intended result of this activity is greater use of these standards not only by the federal government, but also by those in the private sector who would choose to follow the lead of the federal government.

Also in 2003, the Secretary of HHS announced the purchase of a permanent national license to use a healthcare terminology known as SNOMED-CT (Systematized Nomenclature of Medicine-Clinical Terms) as a reference terminology (U.S. Department of Health and Human Services 2003b). This five-year contract permits free use for all United States users of SNOMED—both government and non-government.

3. The Obstacles

Most healthcare SDOs in the United States develop standards that address specific healthcare areas, for example, dental, pharmacy, medical devices, and business transactions. Some SDOs, such as HL7, American Society for Testing and Materials (ASTM), and others, have tried to tackle the broader needs of healthcare standards, including modeling, messaging, security, and identifiers.

In the early 1990s, as a result of early problems and issues around fragmentation of standards and territorial disputes that arose concerning the development of healthcare standards, the SDOs recognized the need for a forum to coordinate healthcare standards efforts. Ultimately, this led to the formation of the American National Standards Institute (ANSI) Health Informatics Standards Board (HISB). It is not teeth of enforcement but voluntary collaboration that accounts for the acceptance and success of HISB. However, as part of ANSI, HISB has only the authority to coordinate the activities of SDOs that are members of HISB itself. This limits the breadth and degree of coordination HISB can accomplish. The results of a survey conducted by HISB in the summer of 2003 identified significant agreement among survey respondents that the key to exchanging information between information systems is closer coordination and development of harmonized standards (American National Standards Institute 2003). Seventy-five percent of the survey respondents agreed that current standardization activities would benefit from enhanced coordination.

In a field as complex as health care, there are many obstacles to developing a comprehensive, integrated set of standards to support a seamless, interoperable healthcare system. The major obstacles are discussed below.

3.1. Obstacle: Lack of a Common Vision, Direction, and Roadmap for Healthcare Standards

Health care has always lacked a roadmap for healthcare standards development partially due to the decentralized and uncoordinated way in which healthcare SDOs were initially formed and standards were initially developed. A desirable roadmap would include a common vision, direction, and set of guiding principles, as well as an overall framework for healthcare standards development. The framework would include a comprehensive taxonomy of healthcare-related standards areas (preferably based on an information model) and assign responsibility for development of each type or category of standards to a specific SDO.

Some progress has been made in this area. American National Standards Institute (ANSI) HISB has adopted a basic set of principles and an overall strategy for the development of healthcare standards. However, a comprehensive roadmap does not yet exist. A broader effort is needed.

3.1.1. Approach

Produce a comprehensive roadmap (that includes a timeline, milestones and funding) for healthcare standards development to which all healthcare standards groups can agree. This effort will require broad coordination and collaboration. Government organizations can play a significant leadership role in this effort. For example, through CHI government organizations could develop a roadmap that meets government needs and share it with other healthcare standards organizations. This government roadmap could provide a starting point for discussions and lead to development of a more comprehensive roadmap to which all healthcare standards organizations and standards users could agree.

3.2. Obstacle: Lack of Well-Supported Coordination and Collaboration (Harmonization) of Standards among SDOs

Coordination and collaboration has always been a challenge for healthcare standards development. Over the years, a variety of coordination efforts have been attempted with limited success. Some effective improvements have been made in the area of standards coordination by ANSI HISB and by the Markle Foundation's program, Connecting for Health, which includes the eHealth Initiative. The latter program is particularly strong in pulling together the private sector users of health data standards. However, though successful in good part, these efforts are limited in scope. There have been successes in the area of collaboration and harmonization between SDOs, but often on a one-to-one basis. Health Level Seven has established a number of joint special interest groups with other SDOs that show signs of promise. Nevertheless, to conserve resources and produce a common infrastructure, a comprehensive standards coordination, collaboration, and harmonization process is needed that all standards-related organizations and users of standards can agree to follow.

3.2.1. Approach

Establish a comprehensive public–private process for coordination, collaboration and harmonization of the development of healthcare standards.

Several SDOs currently use processes internally to coordinate among SDO organizational elements. These processes can potentially be leveraged to develop a process that can be used across healthcare standards–related organizations. This is another area where government can play a significant leadership role. With CHI identifying critical standards gaps for the government, and an equivalent private sector organization doing the same for the private sector, federal funding could provide the resources to develop and refine the process to promote collaboration and produce coordinated and harmonized healthcare standards.

3.3. Obstacle: Lack of Consistent Information Models for Representing Healthcare Information

The use of modeling in health care has evolved to the point that modeling is now seen as an integral part of the process of developing healthcare standards. Health care is an information intensive field, and information modeling is critical to the future development of healthcare information systems and applications. Information models provide the basis for ensuring that the information in standards developed by different SDOs fits together into a comprehensive, integrated whole with minimal overlap and duplication. Healthcare SDOs have begun using modeling to support the development of standards, particularly the DICOM Committee, HL7, American Dental Association, and X12. Currently, information models are being developed separately by multiple healthcare SDOs. This leads to overlaps and inconsistencies among the models and requires that each separate model be mapped to the other models—a time-consuming process. At this time, there appear to be sufficient interest and expertise with modeling to develop a better approach.

3.3.1. Approach

Develop a comprehensive, integrated healthcare information model that all healthcare standards groups agree to adopt and use in their standards-related efforts. This effort would not have to be started from scratch. There are a number of existing models to draw upon for content. The HL7 Reference Information Model covers a significant amount of healthcare information. Several of the large healthcare providers (e.g., DoD, VA, Kaiser Permanente) are standards users that have much experience with information models and can help with both developing and validating the model that is produced. Again, what is needed is overall guidance, coordination, and resource support.

3.4. Obstacle: Lack of Common, Comprehensive Terminologies and Code Sets

This obstacle goes hand-in-hand with the lack of an information model. In addition to lacking a common information model, healthcare has always lacked common, comprehensive terminologies and code sets to describe the data elements that would be encompassed in the information model. Major improvements have been made in this area, including government licensing of the SNOMED-CT reference terminology. There is also significant ongoing work in this area, particularly by HL7. However, this work needs to be enhanced to provide a comprehensive framework for terminology and code set development. All healthcare-related standards groups and users must be included in the process of developing the terminologies and code sets.

3.4.1. Approach

Establish a comprehensive framework for terminology and code set development and an open process in which all standards-related groups can participate. Efforts are needed to develop a core terminology set that maps well to its components (an NCVHS recommendation in 2003) with an evaluation process that includes representatives from all pertinent health groups. The federal government can contribute to this effort by mapping key clinical terminologies using UMLS.

3.5. Obstacle: Lack of a Common Security Framework

American Society for Testing and Materials made early gains in security and, more recently, HL7 has begun addressing this area. The HIPAA Security Rule provides substantial guidance and is applicable to every area of health care. There is a need to develop policies and procedures that allow for multiple levels of implementation—scope and scale. Healthcare SDOs need to share a common security framework in order for different implementations of security standards to interoperate in a secure and consistent manner. The security framework must address both security services (authentication, authorization, accountability, confidentiality, etc.) and security mechanisms (access control lists, digital signature, audit trails, encryption, etc.) as well as where and how the security services and mechanisms will be supported.

3.5.1. Approach

Develop a single common security framework for health care. American Society for Testing and Materials has a reasonably good standard that can be used as a starting point to support this effort. A more complete standard needs to be developed and adopted by all healthcare standards groups. Government organizations have significant experience in this area and can play a significant leadership role in the task of developing a common security framework. This work could be accomplished within ASTM, but with broad participation from all healthcare standards–related organizations.

3.6. Obstacle: Lack of a Common Messaging Paradigm

At least four different messaging formats (from X12, HL7, DICOM, and NCPDP) have been developed to support the exchange of healthcare information. Health Level Seven is now developing a fifth messaging format based on eXtensible Markup Language (XML). Supporting multiple messaging formats adds significant costs for users when they implement healthcare standards. The existence of different messaging formats is an historical fact, but it does not have to continue into the future. Extensible Markup Language is a web-based standard that is rapidly becoming a widely adopted messaging format outside of health care. Within health care, it is receiving more and more attention. Extensible Markup Language has many advantages over existing messaging formats and appears to only have one significant disadvantage, namely, increased size of the messages that are created. The cost of this disadvantage has been reduced significantly due to improvements in the processing power of today's computer systems and the bandwidth of today's networks. Most healthcare SDOs are currently considering defining messaging standards using XML. The time appears right for all healthcare SDOs to begin moving toward a reduced number of messaging formats and possibly a single common messaging paradigm.

3.6.1. Approach

All healthcare standards–related groups need to adopt a single (or minimal number of) messaging standard(s) to support the exchange of healthcare information. Each healthcare group should look to existing messaging standards rather than inventing its own, and should coordinate with other healthcare groups. Extensible Markup Language is becoming a widely adopted standard and has the potential to support virtually all healthcare messaging needs. The HHS federal advisory committee, NCVHS, has recommended the early adoption of XML-based messages, specifically HL7 Version 3.0.

Achieving an integrated system for the secure exchange of health information is a driving force behind HHS' National Health Information Infrastructure. Ultimately though, the direction for standards development must come from the users of the standards—both the private sector and government. Leadership, financial support, and experts in specific business and clinical functional healthcare areas must come from standards users. While no single group or organization currently exists that is developing a common roadmap for healthcare standards and overseeing its coordination and financing, there is strong interest in the federal government and in the private sector in achieving these objectives.

The delivery of clinical care and the business of health care cannot be separated in the U.S. economy. The use of healthcare standards to achieve interoperability must be seen as good business and good clinical practice in the long run, not only from an overall perspective, but also from the viewpoint of individual providers of care. Private and public health incentives and financial incentives must be aligned. If, however, there is currently a natural gravitational pull toward convergence of healthcare standards to achieve seamless interoperability between health information systems, it is not yet of industrial strength.

4. The Solution

There are options for overcoming the obstacles and problems that confront health care and stand in the way of achieving the critical standards convergence needed to reach the goal of a comprehensive, integrated set of healthcare standards. Some of these options are:

- Government does it all
- A private organization does it all
- HISB and SDOs do it all
- A consortium of all of the above organizations

Given the distributed nature of health care, the abundance of SDOs and other standards-related organizations, and the level of coordination, collaboration, and harmonization required, it quickly becomes apparent that the best way to accomplish the goal is through a cooperative effort of government organizations (federal and state), SDOs, and private organizations—in short, standards developers and users.

We will call it a consortium. But what is really needed, more than a new organization, is a new cohesion or alliance of groups, organizations, and individuals. This consortium must bring together standards developers and users and provide a common vision. It must also provide the impetus for achieving information interoperability in the U.S. health system in support of healthcare delivery demands. Participation must be voluntary. In spite of self-interested motives, the obligation of the members of the consortium must be to promote the effectiveness and efficiency of healthcare delivery—for the common good. This consortium should develop, adopt, and comply with guiding principles. It should develop and adhere to a roadmap for healthcare standards, making mid-course modifications when needed and agreed upon. Members must agree to abide by the decisions of the consortium as a whole.

There must be incentives for organizations to participate in the consortium such as endorsement of standards developed in accordance with consortium principles and requirements, and low-cost use of these standards by member organizations. Leadership and governance of the consortium must be fair and balanced among government and private sector members, standards developers, and users. Likewise, membership on committees, working groups, and other organizational structures should also be representative. There must be an ongoing source of funding for the consortium. Given the focus of the consortium on the public good, the preferred source would be from government. Membership and meeting fees to cover some costs would be acceptable; however, the bulk of standards consortia expenses are typically borne today by those who support the travel and time of its members. Participation by healthcare experts in the business and clinical side of healthcare delivery, along with the technical experts in computing, communization, and standards, is essential for rapid progress. This expertise is found in major healthcare financing and delivery companies, healthcare consulting companies, and in professional societies, associations, and other organizations.

The role of the consortium would be to address major obstacles, such as those listed in the previous section. The consortium would leave development of standards to other existing government and SDO groups. The consortium would establish or reaffirm a common vision, direction, roadmap, and priorities for healthcare standards. It would establish desired outcomes for each major obstacle and, with sufficient resources, a process and time line for achieving each high priority goal/outcome.

Government agencies and private sector organizations can contribute significantly to establishing and maintaining the consortium as well as to keeping the cost of membership low. They can support the consortium by providing access to:

- Audio/video conferencing facilities
- Collaborative software and servers (e.g., Webex, Groove, etc.)
- Personnel to accomplish administrative tasks (e.g., prepare meeting minutes, schedule face-to-face or audio/video conference meetings, prepare documents, maintain a web site and document repository, etc.)
- Meeting room space for face-to-face meetings

The case has been made for collaborative action between government and the private sector for developing healthcare data standards and implementing them. There is a large risk of failure to any one implementation project and often a longer payoff period than suits the private sector's investment needs; government support is needed to handle these risks. In addition to shared risk-taking, standards development and implementation must be guided by the needs of the market place. The market usually responds faster than government to changes in technology and to opportunities to supply better services. Of course, government finances a great deal of healthcare activity in the market place—further rationale for collaborative action.

Currently, we see increases in government and private sector leadership, collaboration, and funding. Both sectors are straining to determine just which health data standards are most promising to develop, map, and adopt. As computers become faster, data storage becomes cheaper, and data transmission paths become broader, the ongoing collaboration and resulting accomplishments in healthcare standards can remove large barriers to widespread and secure access to electronic health information. Health research, medical science, and clinical practice will then have better tools to improve the quality of health care in the United States and the well being of all its population.

References

American National Standards Institute. 2003. Survey says . . . ANSI Reporter 36(4):14.

Bates DW, Leape LL, Cullen DJ, Laird N, Petersen LA, Teich JM, Burdick E, Hickey M, Klafield S, Shea B, et al. 1998. Effect of computerized physician order entry and a team intervention on prevention of serious medication errors. JAMA 280(15):1311–1316.

Tierney WM, Miller ME, Overhage JM, McDonald CJ. 1993. Physician inpatient order writing on microcomputer workstations. Effects on resource utilization. JAMA 296(3):379–383.

US Department of Health and Human Services. 2003a. Federal government announces first federal eGovernment health information exchange standards. Available from: http://www.hhs.gov/news/press/2003pres/20030321a.html. Accessed November 13, 2004.

US Department of Health and Human Services. 2003. HHS launches new efforts to promote paperless healthcare system. Available from: http://www.hhs.gov/news/press/2003pres/20030701.html. Accessed November 13, 2004.

Veterans Health Administration. 2001. Enterprise Architecture. Washington, DC: Department of Veterans Affairs.

Section 3
Being in the Future: Case Studies

14
A European Perspective on the Cultural and Political Context for Deploying the Electronic Health Record

ANGELO ROSSI MORI and GERARD FRERIKS

In this chapter, we propose a scheme to describe the processes that lead jurisdictions to reach the holy grail, that is, the universal solution for the electronic healthcare record (EHR). We place Italy, the Netherlands, and the European Community within this scheme of developments. To do so, we consider the following eras:

- Prototaxic era, centered on the healthcare providers and technically driven (almost all countries are in this stage of development)
- Modern era, centered on the patient and politically driven
- Utopian era, centered on the citizen, accomplishing a worldwide integration of solutions on health care and the other sectors

Each jurisdiction is moving from a fragmented situation in the prototaxic era to a comprehensive, cooperative deployment of EHR solutions in the modern era. Only an extraordinary evolution of the cultural and political context can enable a jurisdiction to move quickly and safely toward the modern era, passing through five preparatory phases (i.e., community, white paper, supporting actions, roadmap, acceleration programs). This scheme enables each jurisdiction to locate where it is on the road to the EHR. It allows building a methodology to decide what kind of actions each jurisdiction should plan and execute to advance the context to the next phase. To move forward in the deployment of advanced EHR solutions without the suitable progresses in the enabling context may lead to severe waste of time and resources.

1. Information and Communication Technology in Health Care

This is a story of houses and skyscrapers. The old scenario of information and communication technology (ICT) solutions in health care looks like a series of individual clay and brick houses. The cultural and economic context for deployment was fragmented, because it was related to local drivers: local needs, local vision, local decisions, local solutions (perhaps locally integrated), and local benefits.

But now we want to build city blocks with skyscrapers. New design principles are needed, new ways of financing, new ways to actually manufacture and assemble the building, new kinds of services in the running structure. Moreover, a new culture is needed for authorities, designers, workers, and users.

The mere injection of (earmarked) money and the juxtaposition of optimal components are not enough. As we explain in this chapter, if the cultural and political background is not sufficiently mature for the new challenge, severe difficulties may arise in

TABLE 14.1. The cultural and economic context for deployment.

Old fragmented context	New structuring context
Technical awareness	Political awareness
Isolated decisions	Global direction
Local drivers	Global drivers
• Local needs	• Collective needs
• Local vision	• Consultation on the vision
• Local decisions	• Consensus on the roadmap
• Local solutions	• Concertation on the solutions
• Local deployment	• Cooperation on deployment

the deployment and may bring to a waste of time and resources, as experienced in the past by the most advanced jurisdictions. The wide consensus by the stakeholders' community on a clear vision and on a shared roadmap seems to be an important prerequisite, together with the availability of an adequate number of innovators.

So far, the ICT solutions in health care have been driven by the administrative and organizational needs of individual points of care. In the future, solutions must be properly extended to the clinical perspective on the care processes (Raymond and Dold 2002) and must be centered on the satisfaction of the health needs of the citizen across all the points of care.

It is clear nowadays that further progress is possible only if solutions are embedded in a political context that facilitates a pervasive, structural coherence and are integrated along two dimensions: geographic, within jurisdictions of increasing size; and thematic, relating data, information and knowledge that are administrative, organizational, and clinical in nature.

In other words, this phenomenon provokes a dramatic revolution in the cultural and economic context at several levels for an effective deployment of ICT. As shown in Table 14.1, it will be managed according to global drivers that we characterize as five C's:

1. Collective needs
2. Consultation on the vision
3. Consensus on the roadmap
4. Concerted solutions
5. Cooperation on the deployment

The challenge is huge, and in large countries it involves large figures (i.e., a budget of several billion euros per year, a heavy role for thousands of innovative ICT professionals, and the training of some million healthcare professionals).

The diffusion of specific international standards for ICT applications in the health sector (e.g., DICOM[1], HL7[2], ISO[3], CEN[4]), with pragmatic approaches for their effective usage (e.g., IHE[5]), is a prerequisite to reach the required levels of integration, at

---

[1] DICOM: Digital Imaging and Communication in Medicine. National Electrical Manufacturers Association (NEMA) and American College of Radiology (ACR). http://medical.nema.org.
[2] HL7: Health Level Seven. American National Standards Institute (ANSI). See http://www.hl7.org.
[3] ISO: International Standards Organization. Technical Committee on Health Informatics (TC215). See http://secure.cihi.ca/en/infostand_ihisd_isowg1_e.html.
[4] CEN: Comité Européen de Normalisation. Also known as European Standard Committee. Technical Committee on Health Informatics (TC251). See http://www.cente251.org.
[5] IHE: Integrating the Healthcare Enterprise. See http://www.rsna.org/IHE (International Committee) or http://www.ihe-europe.org (European Committee).

least from a technical point of view. However, the process of change can no longer be managed through separate and independent decisions of individual healthcare facilities.

In fact, this integration step cannot be performed by individual facilities in isolation, but it should be properly managed simultaneously by all the facilities within a whole jurisdiction, gradually increasing the area involved, up to a national and international scale, as shown in Figure 14.1.

In sum, the next generation of ICT solutions in health care faces an unprecedented challenge, due to the amount of resources simultaneously involved, the geographical scale, and the need to integrate many heterogeneous information systems.

Up to now, deployment was mainly a technical issue. Today, balanced and accelerated deployment becomes a key political issue, through an appropriate, permanent, cooperative process of change management. The complexity involved is significant, as depicted in Figure 14.2. At the same time, at many levels, and in several sectors, many actions have to be executed by many responsible persons and organizations.

In many countries, there is an increasing awareness about the opportunities, benefits, and potential long-term solutions about the deployment of ICT. Still, there are many questions:

• How does each jurisdiction get there?
• Why is this challenge dramatically different from the previous ones?
• How can the proper process of change management be triggered at the regional and national level?
• Is it possible for less reactive jurisdictions to learn lessons from most reactive jurisdictions or organizations (e.g., England, Canada, Australia, or Kaiser Permanente) and produce generalized methodologies and criteria for change management?

Clearly, there is a significant gap between the unstructured cultural and economic context of the past decade and the simultaneous, coherent context needed for the next one. According to our analysis, the most reactive countries have demonstrated that the

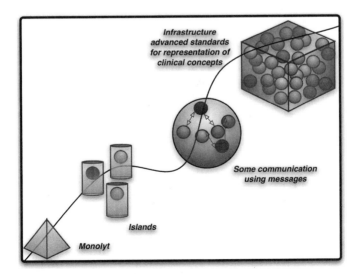

FIGURE 14.1. The evolution of ICT in health care.

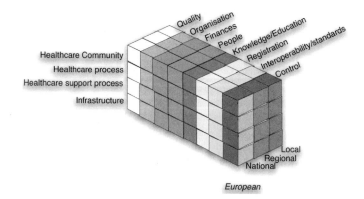

FIGURE 14.2. Complexity of the process.

necessary advancement of the context goes through five phases that eventually enable the movement toward a synchronized deployment across all hospitals and local trusts within a given jurisdiction.

In this chapter, we analyze these factors and apply them to our discussion of the current situation in the Netherlands and Italy and of ongoing efforts at rationalization at the European level. We believe that investing further in European cooperation offers opportunities and benefits that will allow us to face common challenges more effectively.

2. Three Eras of Evolution

The combined evolution of organizational models for healthcare delivery and of ICT solutions corresponds to a sequence of steps in health information systems, within and across organizations, up to a regional, national, and international scale. We represent this evolution conceptually as having three main eras and divide the first era into three periods. As shown in Figure 14.3, each step involves an optimal percentage of spending on ICT with respect to the healthcare budget.

The steps in this evolution determine the approaches to ICT standards, the focus of research and development efforts, and the selection of innovation transfer modalities.

2.1. Prototaxic Era

This was the era of the preliminary (proto-) organization (-taxon) of ICT solutions, when individual hospitals and local trusts were first bringing information technology (IT) into the healthcare sector. This era had three periods:

- In the ancient period of Health Information Technology (HIT), the paleoHITic period, a number of hospital wards and services autonomously decided to implement each single application.
- In the intermediate period, the mesoHITic period, communication between applications was pursued, by a first generation of international standards (e.g., HL7 and CEN). Decisions typically involved several units within a hospital.

- In the new period, the neoHITic period, platforms and common services were developed to integrate subsystems within the hospital or to harmonize views for continuity of care within networks for particular pathologies. The deployment of ICT was managed at the level of a whole hospital or a local community.

During the prototaxic era, the evolution across the periods was left to spontaneous local initiatives, with myriad decision makers following different priorities according to their local contexts. For that reason, many local situations at different evolutionary stages (or even in the pre-HITic period, i.e., paper and pencil) could co-exist within the same jurisdiction. Information systems in this first era were mostly *provider-centered*.

2.2. Modern Era

Several countries and regional authorities are realizing that nowadays the evolution should be suitably controlled, as described above. Therefore, they are now entering the modern era of e-health, which implies regional integration and strategic federal initiatives to synchronize, facilitate, and accelerate the local processes. Moreover, there is a need for specific resources and infrastructures deployed at the regional and national level. There will be the wide use of quality control measures and of Open Source Reference solutions based on open International Standards and an open International Reference Terminology.[6] Information systems should be *patient-centered*.

2.3. Utopian Era

If we go further in the future, we can ultimately envision a utopian era that brings the healthcare sector into the Information Society or, better yet, into the Knowledge Society. This would place us within a global systemic vision of ICT across all the eco-

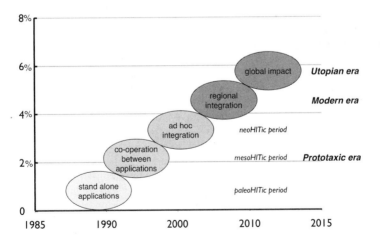

FIGURE 14.3. Eras and periods in the evolution of ICT solutions in health care.

---

[6] Among the candidates are EN 13606 on EHR communication (as co-operation between CEN/TC251, HL7, openEHR, and Standards Australia) and SNOMED-CT.

TABLE 14.2. Features of eras and periods for the deployment of information and communication technology (ICT) in health care.

Era	Timeline (period)	Status	Market description (euros per action)	Standards
Prehitic	<1980s	Pen and paper		
Prototaxic	1980s–1990s Paleohitic	Isolated applications	Isolated solutions, one provider (10–100 K)	
	1990s Mesohitic	Ad hoc communication	Communication as an art (0.1–1 million)	HL7 v2.x, EN/TC251, Edifact, DICOM
	1990s–2005 Neohitic	Ad hoc integration	System integrators (1–10 million)	OMG Middleware, HL7 CDA, CEN EHRcom, CEN Health Information Systems Architecture (HISA), IHE-USA, ISO/TC215, SNOMED-CT, Convergence HL7-CEN/TC251
Modern	2005–2015	eHealth regional and national impact	Infostructure, services, certification (1–10 billion)	HL7 v3, Archetypes, EbXML, Health Ontology
Utopian	>2010	Global impact	Global commodity (>10 billion)	Worldwide integration of sectorial solutions and harmonization of sectorial ontologies

Source: Adapted from Rossi Mori (2003).

nomic sectors, including social and health sectors and comprehensive e-government actions. In this era, health information systems will be fully *citizen-centered*.

Table 14.2 outlines the features of each era of ICT in health care.

3. Moving into the Modern Era

Before a region or country can enter the modern era, it must first cross the bridge between old context and new. The journey from the prototaxic era into the modern era is long and involves a series of steps that transform the cultural and economic context in which the actual deployment of innovative information systems will occur.

The experiences of various countries demonstrate that *technical awareness* alone is not adequate to face the level of the challenge. However, it seems to be a precondition that triggers the *political awareness* needed to embark upon an itinerary of interventions. Such interventions facilitate close cooperation among all the stakeholders, including national and regional authorities, standard development organizations, organizations responsible for quality aspects of the provision of health care and ICT, hospitals and health trusts, health maintenance organizations, health insurers, and other third party payers, ICT providers (software, services, telecom, security, hardware), and the communities of health professionals, health informatics professionals, and citizens.

Not only interventions at the level of ICT in health care must be the focus but changes in the way high-quality healthcare is provided, organized, and financed need to be taken into account. The healthcare ICT in only a facilitator of the healthcare reforms. This chapter will restrict itself to the ICT aspects.

Initially, ad hoc e-health alliances are created, to mediate the visions, monitor the process, and influence the political commitment.

In each country, the alliance may grow around one or more existing organizations, such as, for example, a PROREC Center, or an EHTEL-like organization, or the academic Medical Informatics association, or the national affiliate of HL7 or IHE, that is, the national expression of a European or international initiative.[7] The different weight of each of those initiatives in each national context depends on local historical reasons.

Next, political awareness progressively leads to action plans and the creation of permanent collaborative agencies at regional and national level.[8] These e-health agencies perform a set of structural tasks according to an explicit mission, that is, to support the community of ICT professionals and to rationalize what is already going on:

- Manage the task forces that produce strategic and technical material
- Organize meetings and portals to build consensus and disseminate know-how
- Produce surveys and to monitor the deployment of the strategies in regions and pilot sites
- Assist the establishment and the recognition of the community of health ICT professionals
- Set up basic services for ICT professionals, industry, and healthcare facilities

Successful initiatives in the most reactive countries demonstrate that increasing the speed of nation-wide infrastructures and creating synergy among different jurisdictions can help drive a balanced and accelerated process of change management. These countries have already completed their journey to the new context, and are now ready to enter the modern era.

---

[7] The National PROREC centres are a network supporting the EUROREC Institute for the promotion of the EHR, see http://www.eurorec.net/main.htm.
EHTEL, the European Health Telematics Association, is currently establishing a network of national EHTEL-like organizations, see http://www.ehtel.org.
EFMI, the European Federation of the Medical Informatics is grouping several national medical informatics associations, see http://www.efmi.org.
HL7, Health Level Seven, has about 30 national affiliates, including several affiliates in Europe, see http://www.hl7.org.
IHE: Integrating the Healthcare Enterprise. See http://www.rsna.org/IHE (International Committee) or http://www.ihe-europe.org (European Committee).
[8] Such plans or agencies include the following:
Canadian Advisory Council on Health Infostructure (ACHI). 2001. Tactical plan for a pan-Canadian Health Infostructure. Available from: http://www.hc-sc.gc.ca/ohih-bsi/pubs/2001_plan/plan_e.html.
Canadian Institute for Health Informatics (CIHI). 2002. Roadmap initiative: launching the process, year 3 in review. Available from: http://secure.cihi.ca/cihiweb/en/downloads/profile_roadmap_e_year3_review.pdf.
Fieschi M. 2003. Les données du patient partagées: la culture du partage et de la qualité des information pour améliorer la qualité des soins. Rapport au minister de la santé. Available from: http://www.sante.gouv.fr/htm/actu/fieschi/sommaire.htm.
U.K. NHS Information Authority. 2002. Strategic plan for 2002-2005. Available from: http://www.nhsia.nhs.uk/pdocs/board/Strategic_Plan_Summary_Final_Version.pdf.
Australian National Health Information Management Advisory Council. 2001. Health on line: a health information action plan for Australia, 2nd ed. Available from: http://www.health.gov.au/healthonline/docs/actplan2.pdf.
Australian National Health Information Management Advisory Council. 2003. La Junta ha invertido ya 160 milliones de euros para aplicar las nuevas tecnologias a la sanidad. Press release. Available from: http://www.andaluciajunta.es/SP/AJ/CDA/ModulosComunes/MaquestasDePaginas/AJ-vMagCanalNot-00/0,17657,214288_214389_39558,00.html.

We represent this transformation of the cultural and political context as a series of five phases, discussed in detail below.

3.1. Phase 1. Establishment and Recognition of the Community of ICT Professionals

In advanced countries, communities of ICT professionals in health care were established spontaneously in the 1970s and 1980s, usually growing out of academic medical faculties. Authoritative accreditation of those communities and their cohesion are crucial to create fertile ground for the successive steps and to assure the quality of consequent actions.

3.2. Phase 2. White Paper and Political Awareness

In several countries, the exchange of know-how and the comparison of ideas led to cultural growth in the 1990s—growth that brought all the stakeholders to an awareness of the opportunities and solutions offered by an innovative and pervasive usage of ICT in the modern era. The debate was moved up to the political level and formalized in white papers. This continuous evolutionary process of consultation and consensus is the only way to bring most stakeholders to a common vision, prerequisite for the accomplishment of the remaining three phases. Opportunities offered by the technology inspire the development of innovative organizational models and the political commitment.

3.3. Phase 3. Supporting Actions to Coordinate Independent Projects

In the most reactive countries, federal and regional authorities entrusted regional and inter-regional organizations (often new, ad hoc public agencies) with supporting actions costing up to tens of millions of euros a year as the 1990s ended. These supporting actions try to coordinate several ongoing independent projects; the intent is to gain knowledge of the lessons learned and to transfer the best practices. Such actions tend to create a technological and informative infrastructure and to provide basic services to the e-health community. After few years, however, it is evident that the mere coordination of projects cannot transform them into a systemic and comprehensive approach.

3.4. Phase 4. National and Regional Strategic Roadmap

In this phase, federal authorities set up a multi-year plan for e-health, with a stepwise roadmap involving synergistically several aspects: regulations, quality of health care and ICT, financing, incentives, education, organizational models, and specific research and development projects. Governments adopt international standards such as HL7 and DICOM, and support their development and promotion consistent with national profiles under the IHE approach. Crucial components of any action include consultation with the stakeholders and the involvement and consensus of the community of ICT professionals, who form the frontline for the deployment of the innovation.

3.5. Phase 5. Federal Acceleration Program

Recently a few countries and the largest health maintenance organization in the United States activated EHR acceleration programs, providing additional resources for deployment.[9] Mega-contracts that can exceed billions of euros per year are signed with system integrators, to deploy multi-vendor solutions under the control of the e-health community. In fact, the experience with the support actions (through the federal and regional agencies) and with the federal and regional roadmaps brings to the need for more coherence and timeliness. The transition to the citizen-centered integrated solutions should be balanced across jurisdictions and accelerated in order to anticipate the expected significant benefits.

3.6. A Slow Process

The ignition process, however, is very slow. For example, in England, the process took almost six years, from the National Health Service (NHS) Information Authority's Phase 2 White Paper to Phase 5 contracts for the Acceleration Program (National Health Service 1998, 2003). The actual deployment program will reach full maturity in 2010.

The Netherlands are now between Phases 3 and 4, while in Italy the health ICT community is just moving out of Phase 1. Italy and other less reactive countries have a strong need to understand the possible tactics to start the core process just described, for the proper advancement of the cultural and political context.

4. The Netherlands: Observations and Predictions

The Netherlands is a medium-sized country in Europe with a population of 16 million. Currently, it is focusing its healthcare policies on changing the way health care is funded, shifting to make Dutch healthcare providers operate in conformance with free market principles based on competition. Ultimately, the government will be the party responsible for setting the quality levels and control. For several intervening years, however, the government policy will be to leave healthcare IT developments to the healthcare and industry sectors.

4.1. Prototaxic Era

The policy for ICT in health care was to provide many small and medium-sized research and development subsidies; the motto was "Let many flowers bloom." Healthcare providers and the bodies representing them began to get used to ICT. Sectors that started to use ICT were general practitioners (GPs) and pharmacies. In the early years, GPs received an earmarked subsidy when they used certified systems. After a few years,

[9] Canada Health Infoway, Inc. 2002. Presentation of business plan. Available from: http://www.canadahealthinfoway.ca/pdf/CHI-Presentation-BussPlan.pdf.

U.S. National Committee on Vital Health Statistics. 2001. Information for health. National Health Information Infrastructure (NHII). Available from: http://ncvhs.hhs.gov/nhiilayo.pdf.

NHS. National Programme for IT in the NHS (NdfIT). Available from: http://www.doh.gov.uk/ipu/pgrogamme/index.htm.

Rundle RI. 2003. HMO Kaiser plans to put its medical records online. Available from: http://www.stdsys.com/kaiser_permanente.htm.

when this successful program ended, the immediate result was that no single ICT provider submitted new versions for certification.

This era lacked pervasive awareness of the final goal of full integration and of the need for a change management process. Evolution remained within the old fragmented context. It looked at optimizing the components, without first defining a shared vision and comprehensive solution.

4.2. Entering the Modern Era

Several years later, in 1999, at the request of the healthcare sector, the Ministry of Health started the ICT Platform Healthcare organization, known as IPZ. All actors in health care participated. The budget was a few million euros. At the same time, a national program was launched to introduce the health smart card and started the process to realize a healthcare information infrastructure. Its budget was 13 million euros. After the successful first phase, the health insurance sector brought the program to a halt. In 2002, the National ICT Institute in Healthcare (NICTIZ) was created with the aim of realizing the infrastructure and given a budget of 10 million euros per year for five years. All representative bodies in the healthcare sector were involved. (For more information on NICTIZ, visit http://www.nictiz.nl.)

In a separate initiative, the Ministry of Health is involved in the process of introducing Diagnosis Treatment Groups (DBCs), the Dutch extended version of Diagnosis Related Groups (DRGs). For the most part, the ICT implementations of this introduction are taking place outside of NICTIZ. It appears that NICTIZ is being run primarily as a project that has to deliver a medication list nationwide by 2006 with a minimal supporting infrastructure.

The NICTIZ project known as Aorta is focused on the infrastructure. Under the proposed architecture, all information that has to be shared (e.g., the medication list) is requested using an index mechanism that knows in what peripheral systems information is kept. The government is working to set up the public key infrastructure and unique identifiers for the healthcare sector to use. The law now in preparation on the use of the healthcare unique identifier will set minimal quality levels. All senders and receivers of healthcare information are required to use this identifier, but can do so only when the system they are using is secured according to a Dutch standard that has been developed for information security in health care.

Acceptance of this top-down approach has been mixed. Large ICT companies that operate worldwide take exception to the architecture proposed by NICTIZ. They have problems with the proposed solution for the national medication list. Although NICTIZ originally accepted HL7 Version 3 as the preferred standard to realize the infrastructure, it is likely the first medication lists will be realized using old Edifact messages. In addition, the Dutch organization of general practitioners decided not to take part in NICTIZ. Some healthcare insurers have started ICT services in competition with NICTIZ; some openly declare that they do not support the plans by NICTIZ.

So far NICTIZ does not participate actively in national or international organizations like Prorec,[10] IHE, or Eurorec.[10]

As it works to enter the modern era, the Netherlands is learning and struggling. So far the context for cooperative deployment has not proved sufficiently robust, and the

---

[10] The PROREC centres are a network supporting the EUROREC Institute for the promotion of the EHR, see http://www.eurorec.net/main.htm.

lack of a shared vision has hampered the transition. However, based on results from NICTIZ, the Netherlands is on its way to the next phase: a national acceleration program not for only one topic (the medication list) but for a complete healthcare information infrastructure.

There is still some concern that cultural and political context is perhaps not yet mature enough for this next step. Entering the modern era without fixing problems that arose in earlier phases entails an element of risk.

5. Italy: Observations and Predictions

Not all countries develop along the same lines and at the same speed. Clearly, Italy is a less reactive country, moving today from phase 1 to 2.

Although there are no precise figures, the average budget for ICT seems to be about 0.7% of the health budget, and the number of ICT professionals working in hospitals and local trusts may be between 1500 and 3000. These figures (which may in fact be optimistic) should be compared to 4% of the health budget that is considered appropriate in the most reactive countries, and with the 20,000 professionals in England, a country comparable to Italy for size and organization of health services.

Most hospitals and local trusts do not have a position responsible for ICT; if they have do, it is not at the level of the board of directors. There is no official documentation center to record experiences in the field and provide related technical documentation. Nor is there any attempt so far to facilitate comparison and synergy among projects and experiences. The delay of Italy with respect to the most reactive countries is estimated to be from five to seven years.

Figure 14.4 projects a theoretical federal acceleration program for 9.5 billion euros between 2005 and 2018. The simulated acceleration program should help the hospital and local trusts reach a consolidated budget for ICT amounting to some 5% of their total budget by 2018. The national and regional authorities should provide basic technical and information infrastructures and services, including research on e-health and an appropriate systematization of clinical information and knowledge for citizens and

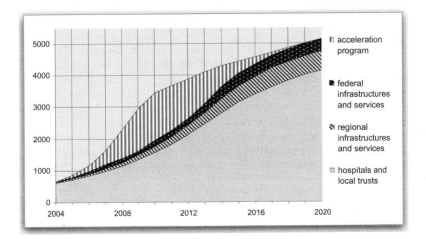

FIGURE 14.4. A simulation of a possible acceleration program in Italy.

healthcare professionals. A large amount of resources should be spent to increase the presence and the qualifications of ICT professionals and thereby support the optimization of care processes.

By 2012, the National Health Service should be able to take advantage of a net benefit of 2%. Moreover, government studies in the United States and Australia suggest that an appropriate ICT deployment of this magnitude could prevent many deaths due to medical errors. Extrapolating the parameters from these studies to Italy finds between 1350 and 3700 avoidable deaths every year, or from 4 to 10 deaths each day.

Most national and regional authorities, as well the managers of hospitals and local trusts, seem to have no real perception yet of the nature and the size of the challenge. There is no official document on the magnitude of the effort needed for the next few years by the hospitals and local trusts, no official document about the vision and the actions needed to assist them to deploy a effective solutions for the modern era of e-health. However, a recent announcement by the Ministers of Health and of Innovation states the intention to perform a feasibility study during 2005.

A steering committee comprised of representatives of federal and regional authorities is in charge of the management information system for surveillance and control of the set of regional health systems. The production of the strategic documents (few in number to date) is entrusted to a consortium of multinational consultant companies on behalf of the steering committee. There is no systematic involvement of the stakeholders, in particular with the ICT community that deals every day with the actual healthcare information systems that will feed the management information system.

What led to this situation? Circumstances over the last two decades prevented the ICT community in health from growing and being effective. Although there are many skilled professionals, they have been isolated until now, lacking the organizational support they needed to facilitate their cooperation. Bottom-up attempts failed, including efforts to establish a permanent liaison activity through national journals and scientific congresses.

5.1. Moving Forward

Today, the situation has changed. Finally, the nucleus of the community seems to have emerged, through the synergy of four organizations formally created during the last few years, including the association of those responsible for information systems in hospitals and local trusts (AISIS); PROREC Italia, for the promotion of the EHR (http://www.prorec.it/prorec-en.htm); HL7 Italia, the national affiliate of HL7 (http://www.hl7italia.it); and IHE Italia, the national mirror of IHE International (http://www.rad.unipd.it/ihe/).

Recently, the four organizations were involved in a Committee of the National and Regional Authorities on the deployment of EHR solutions. A report about the state-of-the-art in Italy and abroad, with a policy for collaborative developments in Italy, is due for December 2004. Moreover, the Federation of General Practitioners (FIMMG) is working with industry and experts in the field to develop a proof of concepts.

All the above organizations are de facto an informal but effective Alliance on e-Health, that plays the role of an EHTEL-like organization for Italy, initiated by CNR and FIASO, the other federation of hospitals and local trust through the OSIRIS project (see http://www.e-osiris.it).

Hopefully, this movement will raise political awareness and foster cooperative efforts to develop clinical information systems and to facilitate integration overall. According to our analysis, a long journey is still needed to prepare the context for the modern

TABLE 14.3. Some potential short-term actions to trigger a process of change management in a "less reactive" country.

1. Each hospital or local trust should recognize the crucial role of a proper deployment of information and communication technology (ICT). This implies the need for a Chief Information Officer (CIO) directly linked to the Chief Executive Officer and for an aggressive plan for the enrolment of a suitable number of ICT professionals, even in the presence of severe limitations on the total budget.
2. Each hospital or local trust should require, in the next contracts, the usage of open standards (e.g., DICOM, HL7) according to national implementation guidelines and profiles and thus the provision of tested applications (e.g., through IHE).
3. The e-health community should produce a white paper on the opportunities for ICT in health care, with an appropriate debate to reach consensus on a common vision across all potential stakeholders.
4. Each entity responsible for innovative experiences and projects should produce a structured description of approach, goals, expected results, and lessons learned, and make easily available the related promotion and technical documentation, in order to detect similarities with other activities and to begin to compare and merge the respective know-how.
5. Each jurisdiction should set up a permanent reference center, to transfer know-how to and from ICT professionals, support by a web-based virtual community and documentation center. Appropriate sources should be devoted to look for cooperation with reference centers in other jurisdictions.
6. The community of health professionals should begin to collect and compare the definitions of the structured content of the components of the electronic health record, in relation to specific tasks and contexts (e.g., including diagnostic reports, discharge letters, disease registries, etc.) in order to improve their coherence.

era, as shown in Table 14.3. A reference center with a permanent staff of full-time mediators should be set up in each jurisdiction, to select and transfer know-how among e-health professionals. Resources should be allocated to establish a national and international network among reference centers. Regions should gain knowledge of approaches to increase awareness, build the community of e-health professionals, and introduce the culture of standards. The most crucial investment must be in education. Within hospitals, the current role of technology manager should evolve into that a chief information officer, directly responsible to and on the level of the chief executive officer.

A large number of ICT professionals should be educated in the peculiarities of health care, and many new jobs for these e-health professionals should be created, especially in hospital and local trusts. In like manner, healthcare professionals should develop the skills needed for the innovative management of information with the support of ICT.

6. The European Level: Observations and Predictions

Here we present three aspects: the eEurope 2005 action plan, the e-health action plan,[11] and the European research program. In May 2004, e-health was the subject of a major official conference under the Irish Presidency.

6.1. The eEurope 2005 Action Plan

In the context of information technology and the EHR, the eEurope 2005 action plan was the most important policy document so far.

---

[11] Commission of the European Union. 2004. Communication on e-health—making healthcare better for European citizens: an action plan for a European e-Health Area, COM(2004)356. Available from: http://europa.eu.int/information_society/doc/qualif/health/com2004_356_ehealth.pdf.

The most relevant policy described in the eEurope 2005 action plan is the one on e-health. The plan emphasizes the benefits digital technologies offers health management, including the potential to reduce administrative costs while delivering healthcare services at a distance and providing medical information and preventative services. Notably, the eEurope 2005 action plan provides for:

- Presentation by the Commission, in the spring of 2003, of a proposal for the introduction of a pan-European health insurance card, to replace the paper forms currently needed to obtain care in another member state
- Establishment by the member states of health information networks between points of care (hospitals, laboratories, and homes)
- Provision of online health services to the general public (e.g., electronic medical records, teleconsultation, e-reimbursement)

This action plan is setting a political agenda—and doing so without substantial funding.

6.2. The e-Health Action Plan

In May 2003, the Health Ministers of EU Member States, Acceding and Associated countries, as well as EFTA countries signed a joint declaration,[12] where they expressed their commitment to the development of national and regional e-health implementation plans as an integral part of eEurope 2005. Ministers declared their willingness to work together toward best practices in the use of ICT as tools for enhancing health promotion and health protection, as well as quality, accessibility, and efficiency in all aspects of healthcare delivery.

In April 2004, a communication on e-health addresses the crucial role of new technologies and new ways of delivering health care in improving access to quality and effectiveness of care. The new e-health action plan takes a twin-track approach: making the most of new information and communication technologies in the health sector and better integrating a range of e-health policies and activities. In practice, this means making people and governments more aware of the benefits and opportunities of e-health; making a reality of interoperable health care information systems, online and digital patient records; new services such as teleconsultation and e-prescribing.

The action plan just adopted by the European Commission shows how information and communication technologies can be used to deliver better quality healthcare across Europe. The action plan covers everything from electronic prescriptions and computerized health records to using new systems and services to cut waiting times and reduce errors. The proposals will contribute to better care at the same or lower cost. The action plan sets out the objective of a European e-Health Area and identifies practical steps to get there through work on EHRs, patient identifiers and health cards, and the faster rollout of high-speed Internet access for health systems to allow the full potential of e-health to be delivered. To add momentum member states should develop national and regional e-health strategies and work needs to progress to allow measurement of the impact of e-health technologies on the quality and efficiency of services, as well as overall productivity. By the end of the decade, e-health will become commonplace for health professionals, patients, and citizens.

---

[12]EU Health Ministers. 2003. Ministerial declaration. Available from: http://europa.eu.int/ information_society/eeurope/ehealth/conference/2003/doc/min_dec_22_may_03.pdf.

Again, this ambitious action plan is setting a political agenda without any allocation of funds.

6.3. *European Research and Development Programs*

For over 20 years, European research and development programs have been in place. European research activities are structured around consecutive four-year programs, known as the Framework Programs.

The European Union's Sixth Framework Program sets out the priorities for research, technological development, and demonstration (RTD) activities for the period 2003–2006. For ICT, these priorities have been identified on the basis of a set of common criteria reflecting the major concerns of increasing industrial competitiveness and the quality of life for European citizens in a global information society. This is elaborated upon in the mission statement of the Information Society Directorate-General of the European Commission.

The Information Society Technologies (IST) program is the major source for project funding in Europe for ICT in health care. (For more information, visit its website, http://www.cordis.lu/ist/home.html.) While the First Framework Programs focused on pure research and development, the Sixth Framework is focusing on the patient and implementing lessons learned.

The Information Society Directorate-General is playing a key role in implementing the vision set by Europe's heads of state in Lisbon 2000: to make Europe the world's most competitive and dynamic economy, characterized by sustainable growth, more and better jobs, and greater social cohesion, by 2010. As set out in the eEurope action plan, this will require advanced and easily accessible IST to permeate throughout European business and society. The Directorate-General therefore:

- Stimulates research into information society technologies which can be integrated into the citizen's everyday environment, business, and administration
- Establishes and maintains a framework of regulation designed to generate competition and stimulate the development of applications and content
- Supports initiatives that encourage and enable all European citizens to benefit from, and participate in, the information society

The IST sponsors research activities consistent with its strategic objectives, by addressing major societal and economic challenges in the following areas:

- Toward a global dependability and security framework
  - Networked businesses and governments
  - eSafety for road and air transports
  - e-Health
  - Technology-enhanced learning and access to cultural heritage
  - Applications and services for the mobile user and worker
- Communication, computing, and software technologies
- Components and microsystems
- Knowledge and interface technologies
- Future and emerging technologies

(*Source*: http://www.cordis.lu/ist/activities/activities-d.htm)

The budget allocated to IST projects that address these priority areas is 3.625 billion euros for the duration of the Sixth Framework.

In particular, the e-health objective is to develop an intelligent environment that enables ubiquitous management of citizens' health status, and to assist health professionals in coping with some major challenges, risk management, and the integration into clinical practice of advances in health knowledge.

This strategic objective is managed by the e-health unit (shortcuts: e-health projects, e-health publications, e-health events, e-health who's who). The call for proposals on e-health that closed in April 2003 had a budget of 70 million euros; the next call will probably be issued in late 2004 or early 2005.

6.4. Assessment

The European policy is mediated by the governments of member states. The community of stakeholders is becoming proactive through two organizations: EHTEL, the European Health Telematics Association, and the EUROREC Institute for the promotion of EHR. However, the two organizations are so far not recognized and authoritative enough to be directly involved in the decision processes.

Action plans are worked out by the European Commission and spontaneously adopted by most national and regional authorities. Deployment is fragmented at the country level.

In these conditions, it is difficult to establish an effective synergy among the best practices across Europe and to set up common services for the whole community of ICT professionals.

In like manner, IST research and development have found it difficult to face the new challenge: they were looking at the houses, not at the skyscrapers. With few exceptions, research projects are focused on particular components, not on the global framework for the future deployment of EHR solutions. Research is not studying methodologies to manage the enabling phases needed to bring a country or a region into the new cultural and political context. It is not studying tactics to move from one phase to the next. In short, it is not developing a theory of the processes of change management.

Figure 14.5 depicts the readiness of the political and cultural context to afford in a synergic way the challenge of EHR deployment for different jurisdictions. The position of Europe as a whole is presented, together with the position of Italy, the Netherlands, and England.

7. Potential Areas for European Cooperation

Over the next few years, the challenge of moving into the modern era will be huge and will require the maximum of cooperation across jurisdictions (Rossi Mori 2003). Lizotte-MacPherson, president and chief executive officer of the Canadian Infoway, expresses both dimensions:

Our analysis shows that if jurisdictions were to implement EHR in isolation, the estimated one-time costs climb to $3.8 billion. However, with Infoway's collaborative approach, the cost is estimated at $2.2 billion—a potential saving of $1.6 billion.[13]

Each country in the European community faces the same questions. How can the process of bringing the whole country to the modern era be controlled, when multiple

---

[13]Quoted in Health Infostructure in Canada—Government Financial Investment at http://www.hc-sc.gc.ca/ohih-bsi/chics/finance_e.html.

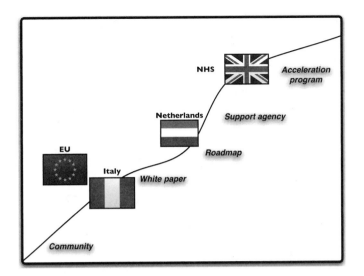

FIGURE 14.5. Status of the transition to the modern era in a few European countries.

heterogeneous local situations are still in the prototaxic era? How are organizational models changing the provision of health care to take advantage of the opportunities offered by ICT? What information infrastructure and logistic support should be provided by regional and national authorities?

The amount of work that must be completed in a timely fashion is titanic in scale, requiring billions of euros per year. European countries can certainly benefit from mutual support enabling them to share experiences on cost-benefit analysis and strategies, learn from best practices, and develop and maintain modules of the infostructure.

European cooperation is needed to develop advanced interoperability services and systemic regional applications: for example, regional master indexes of citizens and professionals (for secure access to the health network and for integration of patient data from different local systems), servers for clinical data (e.g., with extraction, storage, retrieval, transmission, and presentation of clinical summaries), data collection and analysis for data warehouses for governance and clinical support, and toolkits to build and maintain metadata registries. Open Source reference implementations based on open international standards could be critical to support regional networks, such as the Professionals and Citizens Network for Integrated Care (PICNIC) project and the openEHR initiative. (For more information about these projects, visit http://www.medcom.dk/picnic/ and http://www.openehr.org/.)

It is imperative to involve the people working in health ICT and canvass their opinions and solutions. Their input is critical to the field, defining new job profiles in the modern era and addressing how to educate thousands of decision makers, increase awareness in health professionals and citizens, and educate millions of health professionals.

Now is the time to develop and test effective methods to design interventions for change management that take local features into account. The goal is to create a European healthcare infostructure by fostering cooperation among national and regional activities across Europe and involving professional associations and local resources.

Creating a successful infostructure requires an enormous amount of effort of research and technology transfer (President's Information Technology Advisory Committee 2001). That infostructure needs careful control and appropriate methodologies and tools, including regulations, national and regional laws, directives, and guidelines; regional, national, and international observatories; open source and open content initiatives; pilot implementations and showrooms; and education about health information systems (Rossi Mori and Consorti 2002).

A cooperative EU effort should bring together the policy makers and the stakeholders to produce a feasible strategy to develop the infostructure within each country, according to the change management processes running in that country. Suitable studies should understand which parts of the infostructure could be common across EU, which parts need to be customized according to common principles, and which ones should be developed independently within each country.

7.1. Scale of Ambition and Critical Mass

The measures to promote the correct diffusion of health ICT in the European countries need to follow a precise methodology of change management. The scale of this kind of project is of an unusual size.

We can arrive at a rough idea as to the size of the potential European actions, based on the experience of a few countries with acceleration programs and the corresponding infostructure programs. The goal here is to demonstrate that it is worthwhile to perform a proper study to calculate the precise figures and refine the description of the opportunities.

The total expenditure for the European Union for health ICT (i.e., in the prototaxic era) is 11 billion euros per year, according to estimates based on costs for 15 countries in 2001 (European Commission 2003). According to the parameters of current experiences in reactive countries, if every member state would start its own acceleration program to enter the modern era of e-health, this total expenditure could double in a few years.

While the actual deployment of hardware and networks is intrinsically a local matter, the architectures, communication standards, and reference applications, data sets, and terminologies may benefit by joint developments and by sharing positive and negative experiences. More important, it is crucial to share the methods to set up the roadmaps and the criteria to monitor the change management programs.

Which benefits could arise from the cooperation among the 25 countries of the enlarged European Union? What amount could be devoted to common programs?

A set of national (federal) and regional agencies should provide logistic and organizational support to the working groups of experts developing the infostructure, and coordinate the distribution and promotion of their results. In large countries, this kind of agency seems to require several million euros annually.

Based on the cost of setting up the supporting agencies independently in each country, we calculate the order of magnitude of the expenditure across the whole European Union as more than 100 million euros a year. Most of the resources would be devoted to build expertise all over again in each country, to develop ontologies and innovative tools for cooperation, and to explore alternative measures. A joint European action facilitating the set up and the coordination of regional and national supporting agencies—of limited size, for example, between 10 and 20 million euros per year—could reduce the total cost, speed the process, increase the quality.

This action could build on the background prepared by the European Health Telematics Association, known as EHTEL (European Commission 2003) and the healthcare research projects known as WIDENET. (For more information on

WIDENET, see http://www.sadiel.es/Europa/widenet/acceso.htm and http://pi.ijs.si/ProjectIngelligence.Exe?Cm=Project&Project=WIDENET.) In particular, we cite the EHTEL-like organizations (i.e., the alliances of stakeholders on e-health), the national centers established as part of the PROmotion strategy for European electronic health RECords (PROREC), and the EUROREC Institute for the promotion of the electronic health record. For more information on the centers, see http://www.sadiel.es/europa/prorec/, http://www.sadiel.es/europa/prorec/Contenido_prorec_network.htm, or http://www.prorec.ro/; to learn more abut the Institute, visit http://www.eurorec.net/main.htm.

In the context of the OSIRIS project (http://www.e-osiris.it), the Italian National Research Council Institute of Biomedical Technology began collecting documents on national and regional strategies and made available a web-based inventory to collect clinical data dictionaries and data sets (Italian National Research Council 2003; Rossi Mori and Consorti, 2003).

8. A Common Vision and Robust Context for Europe

Reaching the holy grail of a European health record involves a complex developmental process in EU jurisdictions. Enabling phases make way for progress to a new cultural and political context, in which the deployment of a modern era of e-health can take place. Activities now underway in Italy, the Netherlands, and the European Union fit represent these different phases.

Information and communication technology (ICT) is ready to support the integrated management of clinical, organizational, and economic data. The eventual result will be dramatic improvements in the quality and appropriateness of care provision and in the effectiveness of clinical governance and managerial decision-making. These will be made possible by accurate and timely data coming from the actual care processes.

The effects on public health surveillance and control will propagate up to regional and national authorities. These authorities, each within its own scope, can facilitate harmonization of local subsystems and their integration by promoting the implementation of a technology infrastructure, an information infrastructure (infostructure), and basic common services.

Cooperation at the European level has the opportunity to create a common vision and robust context all over Europe, to serve healthcare organizations and encourage national and regional customization consistent with well established criteria and/or guidelines for the implementation of standards. Indirectly, the infostructure created will benefit industry, as the substrate to support the expansion of the European market. International convergence toward a common understanding of the framework and a robust methodology will in turn facilitate the development of new commercial services (indexes, registries, data warehouses, servers) and a proper diffusion of innovative commercial applications.

Today, we are entering the modern era, centered on the patient and politically driven. Tomorrow, the utopian era awaits, centered on the citizen and accomplishing a worldwide integration of solutions for health care and other sectors.

Acknowledgments. The ideas presented in this contribution were developed through discussions and meetings with many colleagues. Of particular relevance were the activities linked to the following projects and organizations: CEN, EHTEL, HL7, Mobidis,

Osiris, PROREC, and WIDENET. The collection and the analysis of the documents on
e-health strategies were performed in the context of the OSIRIS Project (http://www.e-
osiris.it), co-financed by the Italian Ministry of Health.

References

European Commission, Enterprise Directorate, General e-Business, ICT Industries and Services.
  2003. ICT and e-Business in the health and social services sector. The European e-Business
  Market Watch Newsletter 7.II.
Italian National Research Council, Institute of Biomedical Technology. 2003. A collection of doc-
  uments on national and regional strategies on e-health from several countries. Interim release.
  Available from: http://www.e-osiris.it/e-library/databaseOnStrategies.htm.
National Committee on Vital Health Statistics (NCVHS). 2001. Information for health: National
  Health Information Infrastructure (NHII). Available at http://ncvhs.hhs.gov/nhiilayo.pdf.
  Accessed November 17, 2004.
National Health Service (NHS) Information Authority. 1998. Information for health: an
  information strategy for the modern NHS. Available at http://www.nhsia.nhs.uk/def/
  pages/info4health/contents.asp. Accessed November 17, 2004.
National Health Service (NHS). 2003. National programme for IT announces suppliers short-list.
  Press release. Available from: http://www.publications.doh.gov.uk/ipu/programme/ICRS_short-
  list_release_approved_final_12-08-03.pdf. Accessed November 17, 2004.
President's Information Technology Advisory Committee. 2001. Transforming health care through
  information technology. Available from: http://www.itrd.gov/pubs/pitac-hc-9feb01.pdf. Accessed
  November 17, 2004.
Raymond B, Dold C. 2002. Clinical information systems: achieving the vision. Kaiser Permanente
  Institute for Health Policy. Available from: http://www.kpihp.org/publications/briefs/
  clinical_information.pdf. Accessed November 17, 2004.
Rossi Mori A. 2003. Cooperative development of the healthcare infostructure for Europe. In:
  Kevin Dean, editors. Connected health. Thought leaders. Essays from health innovators.
  London: Premium Publishing.
Rossi Mori A, Consorti F. 2002. A reference framework for the development of e-health: bringing
  the information systems into the health systems, bringing the health system into the informa-
  tion society. Available from: http://www.e-osiris.it/data/docs/it252_reference-framework-16.doc.
Rossi Mori A, Consorti F. 2003. The prototype for an inventory of clinical data sets. The description of the activity and the inventory are available at http://www.prorec.it/registry.htm.

15
Convergence Toward the Pan-Canadian Electronic Health Record

JULIE RICHARDS, SHARI DWORKIN, and NANCY GILL

New information and communications technologies strategically deployed in a pan-Canadian health information highway will provide Canadians with new opportunities to take greater responsibility for their own health and participate meaningfully in decisions about their health and their health system. This pan-Canadian health information highway, more commonly known as the Canada Health Infoway, will also improve the quality, accessibility, portability, and efficiency of health services across the entire spectrum of care.

The Canada Health Infoway refers not only to the use of information and communications technologies in health but also to the health information those technologies create, the policies and standards governing use of this information, and the people and organizations that create the information and use this infrastructure. It is not a single massive structure but will be built upon the existing and planned strategies and initiatives of all Canadian local, regional, provincial, territorial, and federal jurisdictions. While retaining their own identity and supporting their different legislations, it is the pan-Canadian vision which allows these diverse initiatives to complement each other in improving the health of all Canadians (Advisory Council on Health Infrastructure 1999).

Three key strategic directions will move Canada towards this vision:

- Health information for the public
- Integrated provider solutions
- The electronic health record (EHR)

All three directions are priorities, but the EHR is the critical gap requiring immediate attention. Thus, Canada's First Ministers[1] have agreed to invest Canadian $1.1 billion in the Canada Health Infoway to promote and facilitate the development of interoperable EHR and telehealth solutions. With this investment, along with investments by organizations, the provinces/territories, and previous federal initiatives, their goal is to have the basic elements of interoperable EHR solutions in place in half of all Canadian jurisdictions by 2010. This is a tall order, and gives rise to a series of questions: Can it be done? How will it be done? Why now? What is different from before? The answer is *convergence*.

---

[1] Canada's First Ministers are the jurisdictional leaders of Canada, including the Prime Minister of Canada, along with the Premiers of the 10 provinces and 3 territories.

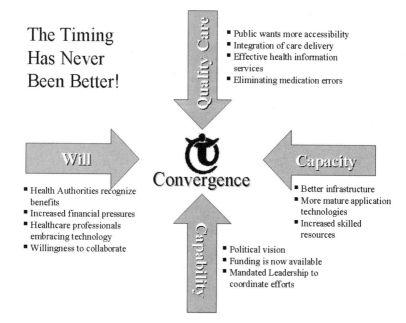

The Timing Has Never Been Better!

Quality Care
- Public wants more accessibility
- Integration of care delivery
- Effective health information services
- Eliminating medication errors

Will
- Health Authorities recognize benefits
- Increased financial pressures
- Healthcare professionals embracing technology
- Willingness to collaborate

Convergence

Capacity
- Better infrastructure
- More mature application technologies
- Increased skilled resources

Capability
- Political vision
- Funding is now available
- Mandated Leadership to coordinate efforts

FIGURE 15.1. Convergence.

1. The Timing Has Never Been Better

According to many Canadians, the timing for the realization of the pan-Canadian EHR vision has never been better. The drivers of quality care, will, capability, and capacity have converged, as shown in Figure 15.1.

1.1. Quality Care

The needs to integrate care delivery across sectors, respond to global epidemics, and ensure patient safety all fuel the urgency to improve the quality of care. Adding to this urgency, the public is demanding greater and timelier access to quality healthcare services and information. As a result, many regional care delivery organizations now encompass all of acute, ambulatory, emergency, home, community, and continuing care. Some regional organizations encompass mental and public health care as well. Even where such services are not integrated in a single entity, local community-based organizations increasingly collaborate on service delivery. The benefits of integration are never more apparent than in treating infectious diseases, such as SARS or the West Nile virus, or in eliminating medication errors. Effective exchange of health information using a pan-Canadian EHR is key to quality care delivery.

1.2. Will

Faced by growing financial pressures, many healthcare organizations recognize the need for EHRs. A general shift in attitude has made healthcare providers more willing to consider and actually use technology and to understand its potential benefits.

Federal, provincial, and territorial jurisdictions are increasingly willing to collaborate and to compromise to achieve greater (and potentially more interoperable) benefits at lower, shared cost. The First Ministers' agreement on health includes the commitment to work collaboratively to develop common data standards to ensure compatibility of health information networks (Office of Health and the Information Highway 2000). More than ever, Canadians have the will to take action.

1.3. Capacity

Better infrastructures are being deployed and are increasingly available. Networked application technologies are mature and proven. More Canadian universities and colleges are providing undergraduate, graduate, and post-graduate degrees in health informatics, increasing the availability and capacity of skilled resources.

1.4. Capability

Canada's Ministers of Health, in the role of the Advisory Council on Health Infostructure[2] (ACHI), believed that the values for the Canada Health Infoway vision should be the same ones that underpin Canadians' support for Canada's health care system. "First and foremost, the Canada Health Infoway should strengthen Medicare as a single-payer, publicly funded health care system guided by the five principles of the *Canada Health Act*—universality, accessibility, comprehensiveness, portability and public administration—within the framework of a strong federal, provincial and territorial partnership. The values of fairness and compassion underlie these principles and will help shape the evolution of the Canada Health Infoway" (Advisory Council on Health Infostructure 1999).

In September 2000, the Canadian federal government announced that it would invest Canadian $500 million in an independent corporation mandated to accelerate the development and adoption of modern systems of information technology, such as electronic health records, to help evolve the Canada Health Infoway. The corporation named after its mandate, Canada Health Infoway Inc., was announced in 2002 and is referred to as *Infoway*.[3] *Infoway* now has Canadian $1.1 billion in investment capital. Along with the initial Canadian $500 million in 2001, the federal government provided an additional Canadian $600 million based upon the 2003 First Ministers' Accord on Health Care Renewal (Canada Health Infoway 2003d).

Infoway has adopted a strategic investor approach to fulfilling its mandate. *Infoway*'s business is investing with partners to develop, replicate, and deploy robust, reusable interoperable EHR solutions faster, better, and more cost effectively than individual provinces or regions could do alone. Their strategic investment approach is intended to speed up implementation of the EHR across Canada while minimizing overall risk. *Infoway* focuses primarily on identifying investment opportunities with its partners. Once investment decisions are made, the partners lead the development, implementa-

---

[2] The term *health infostructure* refers to the development and adoption of modern systems of information and communications technologies (ICTs) in the Canadian health care system which would allow the people of Canada to communicate with each other and make informed decisions about their own health, the health of others, and Canada's health system (Office of Health and the Information Highway 2003b).
[3] In this chapter Canada Health Infoway is the vision of Canada's health information highway described by ACHI in 1999. *Infoway* is the corporation announced in 2002.

tion, and deployment of the EHR solutions with *Infoway* providing oversight and support (Canada Health Infoway 2003d).

All these drivers—a shared vision, mandated leadership, and funding; the need to improve the quality of care delivery; increased capacity in infrastructure and resources; and the willingness and motivation to collaborate—are moving toward and converging on *Infoway*, which is acting as the catalyst to make it happen.

2. Evolution from a Local Focus to a Pan-Canadian Focus

In Canada, 19 jurisdictions are responsible for providing healthcare services to Canadians. These include 10 provinces, 3 territories, and 6 groups whose public health care responsibilities fall under the federal order of government (First Nations and Inuit Branch, Royal Canadian Mounted Police, Department of National Defense, Correctional Services of Canada, Veterans Affairs Canada, Citizenship and Immigration Canada). Canada's multi-jurisdictional federation covers a vast geographic area. As a result, EHR implementations have developed and continue to develop to support a variety of local, regional, and provincial and territorial needs.

2.1. Local/Regional Initiatives

One local/regional initiative is the electronic Child Health Network (eCHN). Based in the Greater Toronto Area (GTA), eCHN is a partnership of hospital and community providers working together to build an accessible, family-centered, high-quality, regionalized health system for mothers, newborns, children, and youth. Network membership currently includes 10 community care access centers (CCACs) and 20 hospitals that provide maternal/newborn, acute pediatric, and rehabilitative services in the GTA. Within eCHN are three major components. The first is an Internet web site that provides health-related information to consumers. The second is a password-protected Internet web site that allows healthcare providers to access healthcare information generated by various individuals and contained on the network. The third component, a system that allows healthcare providers to access a health record spanning across many institutions, is critical to integrating a patient's EHR across various systems. Called HiNet, this system makes information such as laboratory results, x-rays, visit information, doctor's notes, and personal information available electronically to healthcare providers when needed (Electronic Child Health Network 2001).

The following scenario has been adapted from the electronic Child Health Network web site:

At the age of 10, Jason Pinney was diagnosed with epilepsy. About six months later, he was diagnosed with a rare form of cancer that required an immediate operation at The Toronto Hospital for Sick Children (HSC). Originally, Jason was a patient at Toronto's St. Joseph's Health Centre (SJHC), where he was under the care of Dr. Mark Feldman, the hospital's Pediatrician-in-Chief. Dr. Feldman referred Jason to the specialists at HSC. At that time, Jason's mother had to go to St. Joseph's Health Centre to pick up Jason's health records, including his diagnostic images and charts, and personally delivered them to HSC.

Now: Dr. Feldman explains that "Jason is a kid whom I follow at SJHC with regard to epilepsy and school problems and was followed at HSC for cancer. Epilepsy drugs and cancer drugs may interact—I knew exactly what he was on. If the parents had questions about his cancer treatments, I could answer some of them. If HSC had questions about his epilepsy treatment—they could get the info immediately. If he presented to either ER with symptoms related to his cancer or its treatment, his epilepsy or its treatment or unrelated problems requiring a treating MD to know his history in detail—HiNet made this possible."

Jason's mother, Ms. Gibson, explains that another reason she was happy to give consent to having Jason's health records included in HiNet is for future reference. "If he is ever taken to an Emergency Room, whether he is conscious or unconscious, I want somebody there to know what that big scar (53 stitches) is all about. I want them to know that his epilepsy is gone. I want them to be able to get on with trying to figure out what may be wrong with him at that time, rather than trying to figure out what his history might be. That part is known and it's all there for them to see." (Electronic Child Health Network 2004).

Today, HiNet makes health records for about 115,000 children available to healthcare providers at eight different healthcare organizations in Ontario (Electronic Child Health Network 2004).

2.2. Provincial/Territorial Initiatives

Many jurisdictions at the provincial and territorial level have their own EHR visions and strategies that they are aligning with the overall goal of a pan-Canadian EHR. Their different frameworks and blueprints share common elements such as privacy initiatives, EHR building blocks, and next steps to achieve the EHR.

British Columbia, for example, has an EHR framework that includes the key building blocks of systems or services required to fulfill the fully functional EHR and deliver value. That EHR framework, presented in Figure 15.2, with building blocks shown on the right, fits well with the *Infoway* Functional and Value Chain shown on the left and demonstrates how work done prior to *Infoway* has been effectively leveraged.

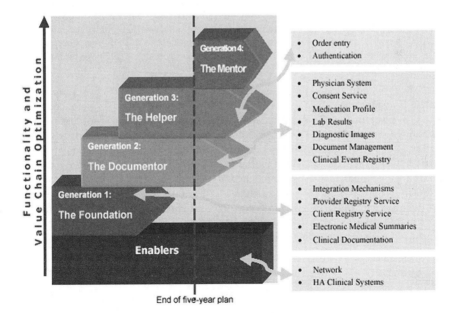

FIGURE 15.2. Example of aligning a provincial framework with the pan-Canadian model.

2.3. *Federal Initiatives*

Through the Office of Health and the Information Highway (OHIH), Health Canada established the Canada Health Infostructure Partnership Program (CHIPP) in January 2000. This two-year, Canadian $80 million funded cost-shared program was designed to advance the innovative use of information and communication technologies in the delivery of health care. In all, 29 inter-jurisdictional telehealth and electronic health record projects were selected for CHIPP funding (Office of Health and the Information Highway 2003a).

Current pan-Canadian initiatives are leveraging the work accomplished through CHIPP. One example of this is the development of a standards-based Provider Registry that will uniquely identify healthcare professionals within a pan-Canadian EHR system. Originally British Columbia led, this CHIPP initiative was undertaken by the four provinces and three territories that make up the Western Health Information Collaborative (WHIC). The registry is now being deployed in the neighboring provinces of Alberta, Saskatchewan, and Manitoba (Office of Health and the Information Highway 2002).

Many more EHR initiatives are underway at national, provincial/territorial, and local levels. It is now realized that, while each initiative is based on a distinct strategy, they must collectively contribute to the pan-Canadian vision of the EHR.

3. Pan-Canadian versus National Approach

3.1. *Pan-Canadian versus National*

At the Canada E-Health 2000 Conference, Dr. Tom Noseworthy described why a pan-Canadian approach is essential:

Many Canadians worry about the idea of having their personal health records stored on a single mainframe in a central location. It is equally untenable to accept an expensive, uncoordinated, piecemeal swirl of activity that will produce a sea of non-interoperability in health information systems. A pan-Canadian approach is essential for success, and the collective will to proceed will be a fundamental determinant of whether success is ultimately realized. (Office of Health and the Information Highway 2000)

While most Canadians inherently understand what pan-Canadian means and how it differs from a national approach, a formal definition of pan-Canadian is not commonly found in literature or dictionaries. The Cambridge and MSN Encarta (2004) dictionaries define national as "relating or belonging to, or representing a nation, especially a nation as a whole rather than any particular part of it or section of its territory; and owned, maintained, or controlled by the federal government" (Cambridge Advanced Learner's Dictionary 2004). The same dictionaries define pan- as "including or relating to all the places or people in a particular group" and "involving all collectively or in cooperation with one another." Both dictionaries define Canadian as "belonging to or relating to Canada", "or its people or culture." Therefore, pan-Canadian projects can be characterized as including or involving all places, people or culture in Canada collectively or in cooperation with one another.

A national EHR implies that there is only one solution to be implemented in the country that includes one large repository of an individual's information, one architecture deployed in all jurisdictions, and one set of standards, which is controlled by one government. Although there are many benefits to implementing one standard, this approach implies that one standard fits all. In Canada's case, it would fail to consider the differing business requirements, healthcare delivery models, and privacy legislations in its different jurisdictions. Such an approach is often unattainable in a large multi-jurisdictional country. At best, it takes an unacceptable length of time to implement.

3.2. Pan-Canadian Approach

The needed approach establishes pan-Canadian common infostructure standards for the EHR that simultaneously allow

- The exchange of information across jurisdictions, care settings, and disciplines
- The retention of local standards in operational systems that may or may not interact with the pan-Canadian EHR

One pan-Canadian infrastructure exchange requirement is to enable laboratory information, particularly test results, to be shared across jurisdictions. Work on this requirement was initiated at a workshop hosted by WHIC with participants from other provinces and several regions, as well as Health Canada and the Canadian Institute for Health Information (CIHI). This effort is demonstrative of the challenges involved in establishing the pan-Canadian infostructure (Western Health Information Collaborative 2002).

Currently, clinical laboratories in Canada use different data standards for the ordering, analyzing, and reporting of tests. This makes it difficult for an EHR to integrate orders and results from multiple laboratories either episodically or longitudinally over the lifetime of an individual. Similarly, although most laboratories have well-established interfaces (messaging system), these interfaces tend to be specific to the type of laboratory analyzer and the vendor application they use.

As illustrated in Figures 15.3 and 15.4, the strategy would use a pan-Canadian standard outside the laboratory and maintain the status quo inside the laboratory, facilitating the exchange of laboratory information in the health community or across jurisdictions. Laboratories that are upgrading or implementing new laboratory information systems would be encouraged to use common messaging and nomenclature where possible. This strategy would allow a physician to order one or more laboratory tests from a common test nomenclature without having to know multiple nomenclatures used in the various laboratories. The laboratory could perform the test and report the tests and results to the health community by mapping back to a common nomenclature. The physician reviewing a patient's EHR could view cumulative orders and results over time, regardless of which laboratory performed the analysis (Western Health Information Collaborative 2002).

This strategy of using common standards during the information exchange to enable integration and interoperability is not a reality today but is a fundamental component of the *Infoway* pan-Canadian Electronic Health Record Solution (EHRS). Within the EHRS, the services required to support mapping between the local and pan-Canadian standards are provided by the Health Information Access Layer (HIAL), which handles the receiving and sending of messages between any two systems.

4. The Pan-Canadian Electronic Health Record and the Health Level Seven Draft Standard

The preceding scenario assumes that the EHR supporting systems are interoperable from the point of view of both information exchange and of information management (entry, collection and accumulation, storing, normalization, etc.). Although the pan-Canadian EHR addresses interoperability largely at the information level, a fully

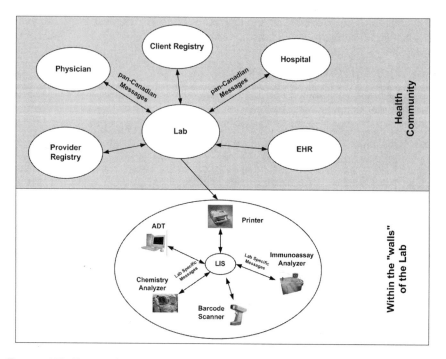

FIGURE 15.3. Strategy for pan-Canadian messaging standards. *Source*: Modified from Western Health Information Collaborative (2002).

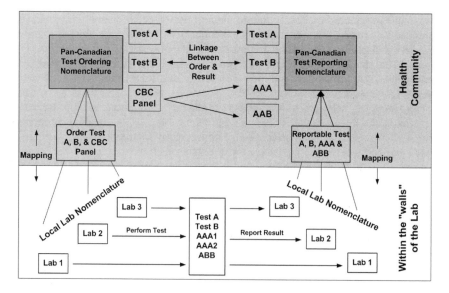

FIGURE 15.4. Strategy for pan-Canadian data standards.

functional EHR, capable of supporting integrated care delivery and quality and safety needs, is essential to efforts to accelerate the EHR's implementation and adoption.

Exactly what a fully functional EHR involves has yet to be determined. Canada has been actively involved in the development of the Health Level Seven (HL7) EHR Functional Specification. The hope is that participation in this international standards work will provide opportunities to reduce costs by reducing vendor customization and improving compatible access to the technology of global vendors. More importantly, adoption of international standards will result in interoperability with Canada's neighboring country in the future.

More immediately, there are specific pan-Canadian needs, limited federal investments of Canadian $1.1 billion, and the commitment to have basic EHR solutions in place in half of Canadian jurisdictions by 2010. Thus, work on a pan-Canadian EHR is proceeding while international participation continues. The approach is to develop the pan-Canadian EHR based on a common information model and then leverage the international initiative of the functional specification.

The drivers behind the pan-Canadian EHR and the HL7 EHR Functional Draft Standard for Trial Use (DSTU) are illustrated in Figure 15.5. The pan-Canadian EHR is foremost healthcare driven, based upon the desire to improve the quality of health of Canadians. The catalyst for acceleration of the HL7 EHR DSTU was a request by the Center for Medicare and Medicaid Services (CMS) in the United States to improve clinical information. The Center for Medicare and Medicaid Services believes that use of an EHR system has the potential to improve the quality of care, lower costs, and provide better clinical data upon which to base future policy and research. The Center for Medicare and Medicaid Services plans to offer incentives for physician participation by tying fee payments to the implementation of an EHR that meets specific functional specifications, thereby improving the quality of reportable clinical information.

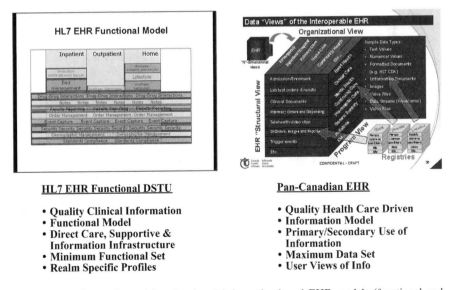

HL7 EHR Functional Model

Data "Views" of the Interoperable EHR

HL7 EHR Functional DSTU

• Quality Clinical Information
• Functional Model
• Direct Care, Supportive & Information Infrastructure
• Minimum Functional Set
• Realm Specific Profiles

Pan-Canadian EHR

• Quality Health Care Driven
• Information Model
• Primary/Secondary Use of Information
• Maximum Data Set
• User Views of Info

FIGURE 15.5. Comparison of functional and information-based EHR models (functional and information-based).

The pan-Canadian EHR is based upon an information model with a goal to provide the right information, to the right people, at the right time while respecting privacy. The HL7 DSTU is a general model of an EHR's functions, which can be applied to various care settings and realms.

The direct healthcare functions in the HL7 EHR DSTU are used for providing direct health care to, or direct self-care for, one or more persons. The supportive functions use existing EHR data in the management of healthcare services and organizations and the conduct of population health and research activities. This division of focus between the individual and the health system is similar to the difference between primary and secondary use of information in the pan-Canadian EHR:

Primary Use of the EHR refers to usage of the EHR data to directly contribute to the provision of care for a patient/person for a given encounter or episode. In most provinces today, primary uses are conducted under some form of implied consent with or without notification.
and
Secondary Use of the EHR refers to usage of the EHR data for activities that are not directly related to the care of a specific patient/person for a given encounter or episode. In most provinces today, secondary uses of the data are done via anonymized data and require some form of consent. Secondary uses may also be pertain to identifiable data and in that case always require explicit consent from the patient/person. (Canada Health Infoway 2003b)

The HL7 EHR DSTU is essentially a minimum functional set. The functional outline has an extensive list of functions, each of which is evaluated as essential now, essential in the future, optional, or not applicable. Grouped under direct care, supportive, or information infrastructure, these functions are applied to realm specific profiles such as various care settings, providers, or organizations. The goal of the pan-Canadian EHR is to have available all the necessary information to provide care to an individual. This maximum data set of information would be filtered as views of information specific to the needs of the provider regardless of the care setting or organization where the information originated.

These two models are not mutually exclusive. At the Fall 2003 Conference of the Partnership for Health Information Standards,[4] participants were asked: With regards to the HL7 EHR Functional Specification, how can a functional model and an information model fit together? Their response was that the information model encompasses more than just data; it is an object-based model that uses modern object-oriented techniques, resulting in more easily adaptable systems. Adaptability is key, because changes to traditional EHR models are expensive and difficult to implement. Thus, participants suggested overlaying the two models. The information model needs to accurately reflect the functional model, and vice versa. The information model needs to cover all necessary data for every decision that might be made in the functional model. Each new element (information or function) in one model must be validated against the other. Elements from the two models can be mapped using a matrix structure, making the two models somewhat self-validating. As one model changes, so does the other.

---

[4] In 1996, the Canadian Institute for Health Information (CIHI) formed the Partnership for Health Information Standards initiative to respond to the need for standards in health information systems in Canada. The Partnership brings together key players from the public and private sectors to discuss and promote universal and efficient standards for managing and exchanging health data and information. The Partnership provides the forum for the standards community to learn about, influence, and build consensus on pan-Canadian standards for health information.

5. The Canadian Conceptual Health Data Model

Canada's approach includes a focus on populating the information model with data commonly defined and understood across organizations and jurisdictions. In 1997, members of the Partnership for Health Information Standards developed the Canadian Conceptual Health Data Model (CHDM) to manage the capture of common health information and facilitate interoperability. The CHDM covers major healthcare entities and their relationships (people, governance, events, resources, and roles), creating a comprehensive picture of the Canadian health system. Use of the CHDM enables stakeholders to ensure common definitions are used across an organization and/or jurisdiction in collecting and exchanging data. Through the creation of common meaning, the CHDM supports the production of consistent and reliable information that can be used to populate the pan-Canadian EHR (Canadian Institute for Health Information 2001a).

Modeling of the CHDM began with the HL7 Reference Information Model (RIM). Starting with the RIM, chosen because it is considered a de facto, internationally recognized standard, and enhancing it with Canadian content produced a validated CHDM that represents the information requirements for the health system in Canada, including the pan-Canadian EHR (Canadian Institute for Health Information 2001a).

Success of the pan-Canadian EHR depends on capturing common data definitions to populate the EHR Information Model. *Infoway* plans to leverage the CHDM as it continues to work on the conceptual models for the EHR. Specifically, *Infoway* is recommending a model that will

- Allow integration of concepts and data models from *Infoway's* domain-centric program investments
- Allow integration of external information and data models into the interoperable EHR, particularly integrating constructs and patterns from the CIHI/Partnership Canadian Conceptual Health Data Model, and from the HL7 reference information model
- Provide the basis for the logical data model specification for the interoperable EHR (Canada Health Infoway 2003c)

6. The Pan-Canadian Electronic Health Record

The EHRS Blueprint: An Interoperable EHR Framework describes the Electronic Health Record (EHR), the Electronic Health Record Solution (EHRS), and the EHR Infostructure (EHRi) that supports the EHRS. The section that follows is excerpted, with permission, from this document (Canada Health Infoway 2003b).

6.1. Pan-Canadian Electronic Health Record

Infoway defines the concept of the pan-Canadian EHR as follows:

An electronic health record provides each individual in Canada with a secure and private lifetime record of their key health history and care within the health care system. Today, health records are largely paper-based and often not easily accessible to the right healthcare professional at the right time. An EHR would be available electronically to authorized healthcare providers and the individual anywhere, anytime in support of high-quality care. (Canada Health Infoway 2003b)

6.2. Electronic Health Record Solution

Infoway defines the electronic health record solution (EHRS) as "a combination of people, organizational entities, business processes, systems, technology and standards that interact and exchange clinical data to provide high quality and effective healthcare." It includes:

- Mechanisms to find and uniquely identify people, providers, and locations
- Patient-centric EHR
- Presentation solutions and intelligent agents
- Common services and standards to enable integration and interoperability
- Workflow and case management
- Decision support services
- Services to support health surveillance and research
- Services to ensure privacy and security
- Physical infrastructure to support reliable and highly available electronic communications across Canada

6.3. Electronic Health Record Infostructure

As illustrated in Figure 15.6, the EHR Infostructure (EHRi) is a collection of common and reusable components that support a diverse set of health information management applications. Consisting of software solutions, data definitions, and messaging standards for the EHR, the EHRi includes the following:

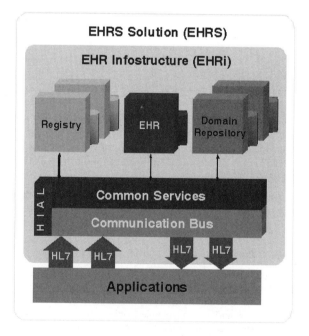

FIGURE 15.6. Key EHR system architecture components.

- Registry systems to manage and provide peripheral information required to uniquely identify the actors in the EHR. Specifically, these are the patient/person, the provider of care, and the location of care. Registries that hold patient/person consent information are also part of the EHRi.
- Domain repositories that manage and persist subsets of clinical data that pertain to the EHR domain. A picture archiving and communications system (PACS) is an example of a domain repository.
- An EHR system to manage and persist person-centric clinical information.
- Standardized common services and communication services to sustain the interoperability of the different components within the infostructure, as well as to sustain the interoperability between infostructures and with feeder or application systems.
- Standardized information and message structures as well as business transactions to support the storage and exchange of information in and out of the EHR.

6.4. Health Information Access Layer

The Health Information Access Layer (HIAL) is an interface specification for the EHR Infostructure (OSI Layer 7) that defines service components, service roles, information models, and messaging standards required for the exchange of EHR data and the execution of interoperability profiles between EHR services. The HIAL is broken down into two layers of services: the common services and the communication bus services. The common services layer is an aggregation of services that accomplish generic functions potentially reusable for any registry, domain repository, or EHR system available in a given EHRi. The communication bus services layer is an aggregation of services that pertain specifically to enabling communication capabilities in a peer-to peer, highly distributed network of EHRi systems. This layer handles the receiving and sending of messages between any two systems in an EHRS.

Figure 15.6 depicts the previously defined key concepts and illustrates how they assemble into the *Infoway* architecture for an EHRS. The information stored in the EHR and in domain repositories is patient/person-centric and longitudinal. Logically, this information forms a womb-to-tomb health history for the patient/person. Together, these systems and their associated databases form the complete EHR for a patient/person.

As depicted in Figure 15.7, an individual has one EHR with a network of EHRs across Canada. Because of the way health care is delivered, there must be flexibility in the solution architecture as to the location of a person's physical EHR data. For example, all of an individual's EHR data may be in the province where she resides or the province where she receives care, often but not always one and the same. Thus, the clinical data for any given encounter are in only one EHR. From the perspective of the system and its users, the person's data are located logically in one EHR.

Finally, *Infoway* defines interoperability as the capability of computer and software systems to communicate seamlessly with each other. As such, it is central both to making clinical data available across the continuum of care and across health delivery organizations and regions, and to promoting reusable and replicable solutions that can be aligned with jurisdictional priorities and deployed across the country more cost efficiently. Without the creation and acceptance of a common framework and sets of standards, EHR systems across Canada will continue to be a patchwork of incompatible systems and technologies (Canada Health Infoway 2003b).

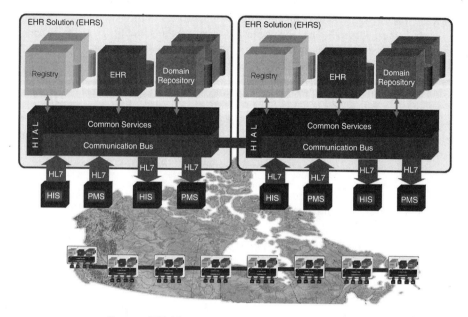

FIGURE 15.7. Network of EHR systems across Canada.

7. Standards

The case is clear: Without implemented pan-Canadian standards, there will be no meaningful exchange of health information. While there are many health infostructure standards, very few of those critical to the interoperable EHR have been implemented or can be considered pan-Canadian standards. So critical are standards to achieving the interoperable EHR that *Infoway* is investing a fourth of the Canadian $1.1 billion in infostructure, including standards. The intent is to leverage the work from previous and current standards initiatives and organizations.

Coordinating and promoting the development and maintenance of national health information standards is a core function of the CIHI. An independent, pan-Canadian, not-for-profit organization, CIHI is working to improve the health of Canadians and the healthcare system by providing quality, reliable, and timely health information. At a pan-Canadian level, CIHI has lead efforts to develop and/or adopt data and information standards for coding of diagnosis and interventions, minimum data sets, and health data messaging. Implementation of the International Statistical Classification of Diseases and Related Health Problems—Tenth Revision, Canada, (ICD10-CA), Canadian Classification of Health Interventions (CCI) and the Client Registry HL7 Message standards has demonstrated that pan-Canadian collaboration can result in the adoption of significant new standards. So too does the National E-Claims Standard Initiative (NeCST). In working toward the goal of a national electronic claims messaging standard, NeCST has demonstrated that the public sector, private entities, and provider associations can collaborate to develop and implement HL7 Version 3 messaging standards at a pan-Canadian level.

Canada's participation in international standards development is bi-directional: a top-down approach of adopting globally and implementing locally, and a bottom-up approach of working to influence development, as illustrated in Figure 15.8. Canada's National Standards System is overseen by the Standards Council of Canada (SCC), which also accredits standards development organizations in Canada. Another group, the Canadian Advisory Committee/Technical Committee (CAC/TC), was formed to present Canadian positions on health informatics standards to the International Standards Organization Technical Committee 215 (ISO TC215) and ultimately to serve the domestic need for standards through adoption and adaptation of the ISO standards. The CAC/TC is jointly administered by CIHI and the Canadian Standards Association (CSA). Canadian delegates play active roles and leadership roles on ISO Working Groups.

The Canadian Institute for Health Information also sponsors HL7 Canada, an international affiliate of HL7 Inc., as a forum to review and adopt HL7 standards for use globally and in Canada. It is through this affiliate that the HL7 Canada membership, including *Infoway*, contributed to the HL7 EHR DSTU.

In addition, CIHI is the Canadian liaison to the World Health Organization (WHO) and the North American Collaborating Center (NACC) for classification standards, as well as the domestic liaison to the joint American College of Radiology/National Electrical Manufacturers Association (ACR/NMEA) on imaging standards. The Canadian Institute for Health Information's Partnership for Health Information Standards brings together public and private sector experts to influence and develop consensus on health information standards that serve pan-Canadian needs. The goal of the Partnership is to leverage provincial, national, and international activities to contribute to the adoption and tailoring of existing standards for the Canadian health system. The Canadian

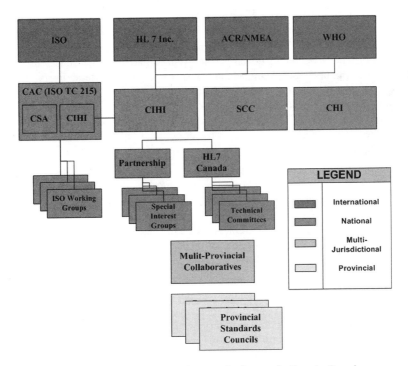

FIGURE 15.8. Health information standards organizations in Canada.

Conceptual Health Data Model (CHDM), discussed earlier, is an example of a Partnership initiative.

In May 2003, *Infoway* and CIHI announced a memorandum of understanding that formalized their relationship for the development and maintenance of standards required in support of EHR data definitions and standards. Under the agreement, *Infoway* is the catalyst for the development of EHR solution standards and the overall program manager for EHR standards-related work, while CIHI acts as Preferred Partner in the development of these standards. This partnership allows both organizations to take advantage of their collective expertise, ensuring a cost-effective and consistent approach to standards development. The organizational objectives of *Infoway* and CIHI are mutually beneficial, and their relationship furthers the goal of interoperable EHR solutions.

There is no pan-Canadian mechanism to mandate the use of health information standards. Constitutionally, the responsibility for the delivery of health lies at the provincial level, but even there the mandating of standards alone is not sufficient. Standards are effective only when their uptake is mandated or supported locally and when conformance and compliance are measured. Accordingly, a number of provinces have or are now establishing standards committees and councils. These councils oversee the development, coordination, adoption, and dissemination of health information and technology standards in their respective jurisdictions. To facilitate the interoperability, consistency, and comparability of health information and systems across Canada, the councils collaborate to share experiences, resolve common issues, and contribute to the pan-Canadian uptake of standards.

8. Standards Gaps and Priorities

The Canadian Institute for Health Information, the provinces, and other standards organizations have begun to develop some pan-Canadian EHR standards, such as methods of uniquely identifying clients, providers, and service delivery locations. Nonetheless, significant gaps remain. With convergence comes the opportunity to establish implementable and sustainable standards for the EHR. The key term is *establish*. This involves the use of existing standards, whether local, national, or international in origin, whenever possible. The strategy is to adopt first, adapt second, and develop when no other options exist. In short, we use the term *standards development*, but we mean:

- *Adoption* of existing standards (the preferred method for standards implementation)
- *Adaptation* of existing standards, preferably where the standard provides for localization to meet varied business requirements, or where the standard has a solid foundation but must be modified to suit Canadian requirements
- *Development* of standards, preferably through active participation in established Canadian and international standards development organizations and processes (Canada Health Infoway 2004)

In 2002, to address gaps in standards, *Infoway* initiated the Electronic Health Records Data Definitions and Standards Project. The goal was to define the strategy for key initiatives to develop and implement the interoperable EHR. A collaboration with CIHI, the project consulted standards experts and the stakeholder community through structured focus group workshops across Canada. Thus, the project identified key issues, priorities, and gaps in the establishment of EHR health information standards in Canada, and set out principles for collaborating with stakeholders in the selec-

TABLE 15.1. Principles identified by stakeholders in the Electronic Health Records Data Definitions and Standards Project.

1. Development of standards is driven primarily by the business of health care and must meet a clearly defined business need.
2. Standards development will be project based, with standards tested, refined, and evaluated as integral components of projects. This ensures a vital connection between the business need and the imperative to standardize, and facilitates re-use in successive projects.
3. The development, implementation, and maintenance of standards must be coordinated at a pan-Canadian level, and success will demand strong leadership coupled with broad support from all stakeholders.
4. Adoption and use of standards will succeed only if promoted by compelling incentives.
5. Efforts to develop and implement standards must focus on those standards that can be best sustained over the long term.
6. Two key components for successful standards implementation are management of change and the transition from current state to desired state. Tools and processes must accompany implementation, so as to minimize any negative impact while maximizing every opportunity for success.
7. Existing work will be leveraged wherever possible and practical. The process must always first encourage adoption, or adaptation, of existing standards, before development of new standards is considered. Additionally, development of new standards will be done through participation with and sponsorship of existing standards development organizations.
8. Standardized methodologies and tools will be a key consideration for any standards development model or process.
9. Vendors will be actively involved throughout the establishment of standards.
10. Provincial standards councils must play an integral coordination and communication role between various jurisdictions and pan-Canadian standards processes.
11. A commitment to building capability and capacity for standards work must be a key consideration in any standards development model or process. Stakeholders will need constant and ongoing education about standards initiatives and how they should be engaged.
12. Jurisdictions must be prepared to provide the leadership and resources needed to establish and implement standards.
13. Canada should increase its commitment to playing a leadership role in international standards. While developing pan-Canadian EHR standards represents an ambitious goal, it is also necessary to ensure that standards are harmonized with similar initiatives internationally. Canada's participation in international development activities will directly enhance efforts to adopt national standards. At a minimum we will be aware of international standards initiatives and participate and influence those that are relevant to Canada's needs.
14. Electronic health record standards development must be coordinated on a pan-Canadian basis. A clear stakeholder engagement strategy will be needed to foster appropriate representation in every aspect of development.
15. Alignment with standards, and with standards-development initiatives, will be key considerations in guiding *Infoway's* investment decisions for new projects. Project development lifecycles and standards lifecycles should be specifically coordinated.
16. Incentives will be available to existing projects to encourage alignment with standards or standards-development initiatives. In some instances, current projects will be mandated (and funded) to comply with the emerging standards vision.
17. Where applicable, *Infoway* projects will incorporate a standards component and will contribute to the evolution of a robust set of pan-Canadian standards for the EHR.
18. A mechanism must be established to encourage and engage non-*Infoway* projects to contribute to and align with the emerging standards vision.

Source: Canada Health Infoway (2004).

tion and implementation of standards on a pan-Canadian basis. Those principles, shown in Table 15.1, form the basis for the proposed strategy for EHR health information standards.

Findings from the project inform how *Infoway* invests in its programs and standards and resulted in a number of recommendations to address the gaps and priorities identified by Canadian stakeholders. These initiatives are listed in Table 15.2.

TABLE 15.2. Recommendations of the Electronic Health Records Data Definitions and Standards Project.

1. Methods for uniquely identifying clients, providers, and service locations on a pan-Canadian, cross-jurisdictional basis
2. Pan-Canadian vocabulary standards for diagnostics and interventions
3. Pan-Canadian messaging standards, including those for operational systems, registries, and those specific to the EHRS/EHR
4. Definitions for encounters, episodes of care, and health service delivery programs in Canada
5. Catalog of publicly available EHR Information/Data Models proposed or in use globally
6. Catalog of information use-cases for the interoperable EHR
7. Development of the EHR conceptual and logical data model
8. Development of EHR metadata and evaluation of data normalization services
9. Evaluation of HL7's CDA standard for semi-structured data
10. Development of a methodology or measurement system for applying standards criteria to determine if an existing standard is appropriate for adoption, an existing standard requires adaptation, or a new standard should be developed
11. Online catalog of standards implemented across various jurisdictions
12. Strategy for licensing standards in Canada
13. Tools to support the implementation and maintenance of standards in both official languages
14. Strategy to easily facilitate the transition of standards from implementation to maintenance
15. Establishing a mechanism in Canada that ensures quality and demonstrates conformance and compliance of EHR standards
16. Supporting participation in international standards development processes and organizations
17. Building of standards capability and capacity in Canada through knowledge management of standards
18. The need for a structured change management and transition processes as a critical component of data definitions and standards initiatives moving forward.

Source: Canada Health Infoway (2004).

Privacy protection is one of the four strategic goals and a key design feature for the Canada Health Infoway. For an EHR to be acceptable to the public, the privacy of patients and the physicians' duty of confidentiality must be adequately safeguarded. Fortunately, technologies like public key infrastructure and encryption offer the potential for a higher level of privacy protection in a well-developed EHR environment than in the paper-based world.

For an EHR to be effectively deployed in a pan-Canadian context, there must be a level of consistency in the privacy principles and policies on which the EHR is based. To this end, the Canadian Standards Association (CSA) Model Code is used extensively to formulate privacy legislation in Canada at the provincial and federal levels. Recognized as a Canadian national standard in 1996, the CSA code was modeled after the *Guidelines on the Protection of Privacy and Transborder Flows of Personal Data* developed by the Organization for Economic Cooperation and Development in 1980 and was developed by Canadian businesses, consumer groups, and governments (Canadian Institute for Health Information 2001b).

The CSA Code is comprised of 10 principles:

- Accountability
- Consent
- Limiting Use, Disclosure, and Retention
- Safeguards
- Openness
- Identifying Purposes
- Limiting Collection

- Accuracy
- Individual Access
- Challenging Compliance (Canadian Institute for Health Information 2001b)

By design, a successful pan-Canadian EHR will contain information that can be, when required, shared across organizations and jurisdictions in a controlled manner. Because of differing provincial legislation, however, there is no uniform process across the country to support the sharing of electronic health record data. "The issues that revolve around privacy and security do not pertain to the technologies and processes required to implement them, they pertain to the absence or lack of normalization of policies, laws, rules and regulations around privacy and security" (Canada Health Infoway 2003b). Efforts are underway to promote harmonization of policies and procedures specific to health information privacy across Canada.

9. Next Steps

The development of electronic health records in Canada has evolved from local individual independent systems to the current vision of a pan-Canadian interoperable EHR solution. The Canada Health Infoway vision is not a single massive national structure, but will be built by involving all people, places, and jurisdictions in Canada collectively in cooperation with one another. Convergence is the answer. As the drivers of quality care, will, capability, and capacity converge, *Infoway* will play the role of catalyst and strategic investor in the components that will make up the pan-Canadian EHR.

Consistent with Canada's goals, *Infoway* intends to have the basic components of EHR solutions in place in half of Canadian jurisdictions by 2010. To accomplish this, *Infoway* defined a three-year plan for investment in EHR component programs, as shown in Table 15.3.

TABLE 15.3. *Infoway* investment plans, 2003–2006: Targeted EHR components.

Program	Actions
Infostructure	• Infostructure components and services available in 50% of country • Further development of EHRS Blueprint, e.g., messaging standards, integration tools, etc.
Registries	• Provider Registry Application releases • Client Registry releases • Plans to deploy • Install country-wide
Drug information systems	• Interoperable system(s) implemented in one jurisdiction • Replicate system in second jurisdiction • Plans to deploy elsewhere • National messaging standards for dispensed drugs
Diagnostic imaging (DI) systems	• Regional DI operation to provide shared PACS and storage to 12 hospitals • Partnership and a regional DI operation to 8 hospitals • Replication of solution in 4 jurisdictions • Plans to develop Canada-wide
Laboratory information systems	• Approved investment strategy • Initial investment in one jurisdiction
Telehealth	• Approved investment strategy • Initial committed investment in three projects

Source: Canada Health Infoway (2004).

In 2003, 22 projects were underway or completed Canada-wide. These projects focused on developing solutions, and on the standards and architecture required to deploy these solutions quickly and comprehensively.

According to Francis (2004), "Within just a few short years, *Infoway* [and its project partners at the local, regional, provincial and pan-Canadian levels] will have developed the tools that provide Canada's health care community with more timely and accurate patient information so necessary for improved diagnosis, treatment, and health outcomes."

With those tools, Canada will be well on its way to achieving its vision of the pan-Canadian EHR.

Acknowledgments. On behalf of the Canadian Institute for Health Information, the authors wish to thank all those who contributed to this chapter. Special thanks go out to Brenda Shestowsky (Health Canada), Don Newsham (Sierra Systems), Grant Gillis (Canadian Institute for Health Information), Joan Roch (Canadian Institute for Health Information), Pat Jeselon (Pat Jeselon & Associates Consulting Inc), and Ron Parker (Canada Health Infoway), who reviewed and provided invaluable input into this chapter.

References

Advisory Council on Health Infostructure. 1999. Canada Health Infoway: paths to better health Final Report of the Advisory Council on Health Infostructure. Available from: http://www.hc-sc.gc.ca/ohih-bsi/pubs/1999_pathsvoies/fin-rpt_e.pdf . Accessed 2004 Feb 20.

Cambridge Advanced Learner's Dictionary, 2004. Available from: http://dictionary.cambridge. org. Accessed 2004 Feb 18.

Canada Health Infoway. 2003a. Infoway Pan-Canadian EHR Survey Phase 1 results and analysis. Available from: http://www.canadahealthinfoway.ca/pdf/EHR-Survey-PhaseI.pdf. Accessed 2004 Apr 30.

Canada Health Infoway. 2003b. EHRS Blueprint an interoperable EHR framework Version 1.0. Available from: http://knowledge.infoway-inforoute.ca/ehr_blueprint/en/printable/Printable.pdf. Accessed 2004 Apr 30.

Canada Health Infoway. 2003c. EHR Data Definitions and Standards Project. Available from: http://secure.cihi.ca/cihiweb/en/downloads/event_partner_may03_questions_e.pdf. Accessed 2004 Apr 28.

Canada Health Infoway. 2003d. Building momentum 2003/04 business plan. Available from: http://www.canadahealthinfoway.ca/pdf/2003_CHI_BusinessPlan.pdf. Accessed 2004 Feb 18.

Canada Health Infoway. 2004. Electronic health record (EHR) standards needs analysis. Available from: http://www.canadahealthinfoway.ca/pdf/EHR-StandardsAnalysis.pdf. Accessed 2004 Apr 27.

Canadian Institute for Health Information. 2001a. Conceptual Health Data Model v2.3. Available from: http://secure.cihi.ca/cihiweb/en/downloads/infostand_chdm_e_CHDMv2_31.pdf. Accessed 2004 Apr 28.

Canadian Institute for Health Information. 2001b. Report on the Recipient Identifiers and Registries Workshop. Available from: http://secure.cihi.ca/cihiweb/en/downloads/infostand_client_e_RIDWorkshopReport.pdf. Accessed 2004 Feb 11.

Canadian Institute for Health Information. 2003. Julie Richards. Canadian participation in HL7 EHR SIG. Available from: http://secure.cihi.ca/cihiweb/en/downloads/event_partner_oct03_participation_e.pdf. Accessed 2004 Apr 28.

Electronic Child Health Network. 2001. eCHN annual report 2000/2001.

Electronic Child Health Network. 2004. http://www.childhealthnetwork.com/chn/pdfs/Annual%20Report%20-%202000-2001.pdf. Accessed 2004 Feb 13. About the electronic Child Health Network (eCHN). Available from: http://www.echn.ca/hsc/chn-echn.nsf/pages/Pinney-Testivnaniel. Accessed 2004 Feb 13.

Encarta World English Dictionary (North American Edition). 2004. Available from: http://encarta.msn.com/encnet/features/dictionary/dictionaryhome.aspx. Accessed 2004 Feb 18.

Francis M. 2004. 2004 will demonstrate on-the-ground benefits of electronic health records for Canada. Healthcare Information Management & Communications Canada 17:21. Available from: http://hcccinc.qualitygroup.com/hcccinc2/pdf/Vol_XVII_No_5/Vol_XVII_No_5_5.pdf. Accessed 2004 Feb 13.

Government of British Columbia. 2003. Framework for an electronic health record for British Columbians. Available from: http://healthnet.hnet.bc.ca/pub_reports/ehr_framework.pdf. Accessed 2004 Feb 15.

Merriam-Webster OnLine. 2004. Available from: http://www.m-w.com/. Accessed 2004 Feb 16.

Office of Health and the Information Highway, Health Canada. 2000. Report on Canada E-Health 2000: from vision to action. Available from: http://www.hc-sc.gc.ca/ohih-bsi/pubs/2000_econf/report_rapport_e.pdf. Accessed 2004 Feb 14.

Office of Health and the Information Highway, Health Canada. 2002. Canada Health Infostructure Partnerships Program Project: Healthnet/BC Provider Registry. Available from: http://www.hc-sc.gc.ca/ohih-bsi/about_apropos/chipp-ppics/proj/healthnet_e.html.   Accessed 2004 Feb 12.

Office of Health and the Information Highway, Health Canada. 2003a. CHIPP Standards & Interoperability Report Part 1. Canada: Health Canada. In print.

Office of Health and the Information Highway, Health Canada. 2003b. Health infostructure in Canada. Available from: http://www.hc-sc.gc.ca/ohih-bsi/chics/hist_e.html. Accessed 2004 Feb 13.

Western Health Information Collaborative. 2002. Laboratory information strategies and standards. Available from: http://www.whic.org/public/whatsnew/WHIC_Lab_white_paper_v4.0.doc. Accessed 2004 Feb 11.

16
Health*Connect*: A Health Information Network for All Australians

David Rowlands

Like the majority of the health industry worldwide, the Australian healthcare system currently relies largely on paper-based records. However, experience has shown that such records can be difficult, time consuming, and expensive to access across the spectrum of health service providers. These problems in turn lead to gaps in the information needed for clinical care.

Health*Connect* is a proposed national electronic health information network that aims to improve individuals' access to their health information through the safe and secure collection, storage, and exchange of summary records. Subject to strict privacy safeguards, healthcare providers and consumers will have access to the records held on the network to ensure that all available information can be used to make informed health decisions.

Using leading-edge information and communications technologies to record health information for consumers, Health*Connect* will help authorized users draw together pieces of the health puzzle and provide safer, more holistic, and better coordinated care. Participation in Health*Connect* will be voluntary for both consumers and providers. Over the long term, the benefit for Australians will be a safer, better quality, and more sustainable health system.

This chapter provides an overview of Health*Connect*. It briefly describes the Australian health system and the state of health informatics in Australia as the contextual setting for Health*Connect* before outlining the major elements of the initiative.

1. The Contextual Setting

1.1. Australia's Health

Australia is an island continent nearly the size of the United States (Population Reference Bureau 2002) but with a population of only 20 million people. The majority of the population lives on the coastal fringes, with the vast interior being relatively sparsely populated.

Australia's population generally enjoys good health status. Average life expectancy is 77 years for men and 82 years for women, compared to 74 years for men and 80 for women in the United States (Population Reference Bureau 2002). Eighty-two percent of Australians aged 15 or over rate their health as excellent, very good, or good (Australian Bureau of Statistics 2003a). In terms of healthy life expectancy (HALE), Australia ranks eighth (after Japan, San Marino, Sweden, Switzerland, Monaco, Iceland, and Italy) out of 192 countries (World Health Organization 2003).

Australia has three levels of government: the Australian Government; six state and two territory governments; and around 700 local governments.

The Australian Government funds rather than provides health services. It subsidizes access to medical providers and pharmaceuticals; funds residential care for the aged; jointly funds public hospitals and community care with the states and territories; subsidizes private health insurance and regulates the industry; funds, promotes, and regulates public health and safety (with states, territories, and local government); and plays a major role in regulating the supply of the health workforce.

The states and territories fund and provide a broad range of health services. They administer public hospitals, mental health services, and community health services; regulate health workers; license and regulate private hospitals; and play a major role in public health activities.

Local governments engage in environmental health protection, are responsible for some public health services and public health surveillance, and are involved in disease prevention programs, such as immunization and child health screening.

Australia has substantial private sector involvement in health care. The main players are:

- Medical practitioners, the majority of whom are self employed and remunerated on a fee-for-service basis.
- Private hospitals. Forty-three percent of Australian hospitals are privately owned, accounting for 35% of the nation's hospital beds (Australian Institute of Health and Welfare 2003a); 39% of these hospitals operate on a not-for-profit basis and 61% are for-profit (Australian Bureau of Statistics 2003b).
- Diagnostic services.
- Private health insurers. There are currently 44 registered health benefit organizations covering approximately 43% (Private Health Insurance Administration Council 2003) of the Australian population. Private health insurance funds approximately 11% of total national healthcare spending.

Non-government religious and charitable organizations play a significant role in health services, public health, and health insurance.

Australia's health system is underpinned by the Medicare Benefits Scheme (MBS), a tax-funded health insurance scheme to provide universal access to health care. The MBS rebates 85% of scheduled fees for private medical services provided in the community, and 75% of scheduled fees for private hospital medical services. Public hospital services are provided free of charge. Under agreements between the Australian, state, and territory governments, consumers are guaranteed choice in accessing public or private providers.

Australia currently spends approximately 9.1% (Australian Institute of Health and Welfare 2003b) of Gross Domestic Product (GDP) on health services, which is about the average for member countries in the Organization for Economic Co-operation and Development (OECD). Figure 16.1 provides some international comparisons.

Key challenges for the Australian health system include:

- The aging of the population will put increasing pressures on costs. The proportion of the Australian population aged 65 years or more is forecast to rise from 12.5% in 2001 to 18% in 2021 (Australian Bureau of Statistics 2003a), accompanied by greater incidence of chronic illness. Health expenditure on older people is nearly four times that of people aged under 65 years (Australian Bureau of Statistics 1999).

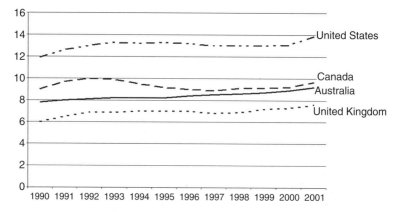

FIGURE 16.1. Total health services expenditures as a percentage of Gross Domestic Product, Australia and selected OECD countries, 1990–2001.

- The increasing cost of new medicines, treatments, and technologies is also placing greater pressure on the purchasing power of the healthcare dollar.
- Good health is not enjoyed by all. For example, the life expectancy of Indigenous Australians is significantly lower than for other Australians.
- Health workforce shortages are a problem.
- Rural and remote areas in particular are finding it difficult to attract or maintain equivalent services as urban centers.
- As in other comparable countries, consumer expectations of health care are rising, including expectations of safer, better quality, and more coordinated care.

1.2. Health Informatics in Australia

Australians tend to be relatively rapid adopters of information and communication technologies. However, Australia's large size and relatively low population densities provide significant challenges for the roll-out of infrastructure. The vast geographic distribution of regional, rural, and remote communities is resulting in considerable investment by the Australian government in broadband infrastructure to enhance the delivery of health and education. With the uptake of broadband being cost prohibitive to end users in less populated areas, the Australian government is seeking to achieve service quality, reliability, and performance in bandwidth through initiatives that enable demand aggregation, accelerate the roll-out of broadband to regional Australia, and enable regional Australians to access broadband services at prices comparable to those in metropolitan areas. Previous experience with the roll-out of TeleHealth activities in Australia indicates that the economic returns should be significant, including a reduction in costs associated with patient and clinician travel, improved access to specialist services, and optimization of health outcomes.

Approximately 90% of Australian general practices use computers on their desks. The Australian government's General Practice Computing Strategy has supported this strong uptake. Around 80% of general practitioners prescribe electronically, but only 40% currently use computers for other clinical purposes, such as recording patient notes or accessing decision support tools.

State and territory government health service providers, the private hospitals, and diagnostic service providers generally have sound computing platforms for patient management, financial transactions, and performance reporting. Significant investment in point-of-care clinical systems is now underway or planned in many of these jurisdictions, and most of the states and territories are also investing in supporting (infostructure) applications such as patient master indexes and provider directories to provide the capacity to link patient records as required.

The Australian health software industry comprises a few major international companies and a large number of smaller to medium enterprises that meet the Australian demand for specialized software solutions (for example, billing and claims, general practice, allied health, and primary care management). The majority of larger, hospital-based systems are imported, although they may be integrated with a range of locally developed best-of-breed applications. System integration is a major issue; larger organizations, including the states and territories, have made substantial investments in this area over the last decade particularly.

There is strong recognition that Australia's health information system needs greater capacity for connection as and when required. National health information management governance structures and mechanisms have recently been strengthened with the introduction of two groups: the Australian Health Information Council to advise on strategic directions, and the National Health Information Group to coordinate the development of national health information management capacity.

2. A Health Information Network for All Australians

Health*Connect* proposes to generate longitudinal, summarized, electronic health records (EHRs) to complement the records held by individual healthcare providers and consumers by filling in the gaps. Health-related information about individuals will consist of standardized event summaries containing information such as referrals, pathology results, medications prescribed, and diagnoses. The concept of event summaries essentially means selecting specific pieces of information, generated during a health-related event or episode, which are likely to be most pertinent to ongoing health care. The event summaries will be collected, with the individual's consent, in a standard electronic format at the point of care by providers such as hospitals and general practitioners and be available to health providers subject to the individual's consent, as well as to individuals themselves, at any location to assist with ongoing care.

As stated by the National Electronic Health Records Taskforce (2000), the specific objectives of Health*Connect* include:

Improved delivery of health care and better quality of care, consumer safety and health outcomes for all Australians while enhancing the privacy and respecting the dignity of health consumers by:

— empowering consumers to be able to take a greater responsibility for their own health care and be better informed about the choices available to them in respect of their health care;
— ensuring better decision making which is shared by both consumers and health providers at the point of care;
— providing a flexible, seamless and integrated process of care through the sharing and better exchange of information;
— providing better access to health care, particularly in rural and remote areas;

— building a best-practice, evidence based health system;

— encouraging better, more targeted health initiatives; and

— informing research, learning and training through developing a nationally coordinated and distributed system of electronic health records, which is based on the greater use of online technologies. (p xvi)

The Heath*Connect* project commenced in 2001 following unanimous endorsement by Australian, state, and territory health ministers of a report from a specially convened National Electronic Health Records Taskforce, available for viewing at http://www.health.gov.au. The health ministers collectively committed resources to a nationally collaborative project. While the task force had presented a compelling case, the first phase of activity, spanning 2001–2003, comprised testing the potential of Health*Connect* as a national system.

2.1. The HealthConnect Project[1]

To date, the major streams of activity in the Health*Connect* project have included:

1. Research and evaluation. This involves defining critical research questions, establishing the research framework, shaping and managing the various studies and inquiries designed to answer these questions, and compiling a research report at the end of the process. The critical questions are essentially:
    a. Can Health*Connect* prove its value?
    b. Is Health*Connect* technically feasible?
    c. Is there a preferred implementation model?
    d. What role should the private sector play?
    e. What will be necessary to manage privacy?
    f. How should Health*Connect* be governed?
    g. What would Health*Connect* cost and is it sustainable?

2. Governance and relationship management. What models of organization and what supporting processes and organizational infrastructure will be needed to manage Health*Connect*? In the interim, the project itself requires specific governance and relationship management arrangements to enable work to proceed in an accountable way and to draw in key stakeholders.

3. Design work. This is necessary to answer questions about a preferred implementation model and to help answer questions about costs and sustainability.

4. Common services. This involves the development of key components of Health-*Connect* for use in developmental trials. These include:
    a. Privacy and consent management
    b. Storage, messaging, and interfacing architectures and methodologies
    c. Standardized data capture and viewing protocols
    d. Security
    e. Approaches for reliable and accurate identification of key parties and entities

5. Health*Connect* trials. The trials have been developed to answer questions about whether Health*Connect* is technically feasible and whether it is useful in practice.

---

[1] The description of the Health*Connect* project and its findings to date is substantially cited from the Health*Connect* Interim Research Report, available at http://www.healthconnect.gov.au.

6. e-Health building blocks. This includes standards development for the broader e-health arena in which Health*Connect* will need to operate, including privacy, security, and identifiers.

7. New policy. This component of work aims to draw together learnings from the project and formulating the policy directions and frameworks for future phases of work.

2.1.1. Medi*Connect*

In addition, the high priority medications component of Health*Connect* has been progressed via the Medi*Connect* stream of activity. Medi*Connect* was originally envisaged as a secure electronic system that draws together personal medication records now held by different doctors, pharmacies, and hospitals. This would provide access to more complete information about consumers' medicines and improve quality and safety in prescribing, dispensing, and managing medicines. Medi*Connect* has now been incorporated as the medication record component of Health*Connect*. This component will help ensure that consumers are not prescribed medicines to which they are allergic or have had a previous adverse reaction, a major problem in the Australian healthcare system.

2.2. *What Will HealthConnect Look Like?*

Three key operating paradigms are central to the Health*Connect* business model:

- *The event summary paradigm.* Health*Connect* is intended to store event summaries rather than the complete health records of an individual. Health service providers would retain the responsibility to maintain complete health records relating to the services they provide. It is envisioned that health providers and consumers will use the Health*Connect* summary records to inform themselves of relevant external factors, such as treatments and diagnoses that have been provided by other providers. Health providers may choose to retain a copy of the Health*Connect* summary records as part of their clinical health records.
- *The push paradigm.* It is not intended that Health*Connect* pull data from operational systems, but rather that data will be pushed from the operational systems at the discretion of the consumer and the health provider.
- *The federation paradigm.* Health*Connect* is envisioned as a federation containing a number of independent nodes. Under this model, each node would maintain a subset of the total data repository either based on state, regional, or organizational boundaries. To maintain the efficiency of data retrieval, an individual's electronic health record would be wholly located within one node and the number of nodes would be small (less than 10). Each system, while geographically dispersed, would be linked to enable retrieval of any EHR from any user location subject to access and consent constraints.

Health*Connect* is therefore likely to comprise a national network of Health*Connect* records systems that would inter-operate with existing health information systems to establish, maintain, and provide access to a consolidated EHR for participating consumers.

2.3. Conceptual Model

The Health*Connect* service is conceptually similar to a library service or, more specifically, a national network of libraries with users adding, searching, and retrieving records from the libraries subject to a common set of access rules. In this case, the contents of the libraries will be consumer EHRs comprising many individual event summaries. Access to the libraries will be via users existing systems (as far as possible) or a general purpose computer interface (web browser). Health*Connect* will provide the capability to store, retrieve, and search the records; perform enforcement of the access rules; and provide standard interfaces to end user systems. Health*Connect* will interface with the information technology systems that support each user group. It will draw on external systems as information sources where these exist. Examples include provider directories as a source of provider registration information and data dictionaries as a source of EHR format definitions.

The Health*Connect* conceptual model is illustrated in Figure 16.2.

Accordingly, the draft systems architecture to date proposes that Health*Connect* organizationally consists of three layers, as shown in Figure 16.3.

- The coordination layer, representing the infrastructure, metadata, and services needed to integrate Health*Connect* into a common national network of Health-*Connect* records systems.
- A federated Health*Connect* records systems layer that comprises between 1 to 10 nodes each of which is an independent Health*Connect* records system servicing a defined user population.
- The user layer, which comprises the consumers' and providers' local information systems that they will use to access the Health*Connect*, services.

2.3.1. Coordination Layer

The coordination layer ties the Health*Connect* nodes into a common network of Health*Connect* Records Systems. It is at this level that any national governance func-

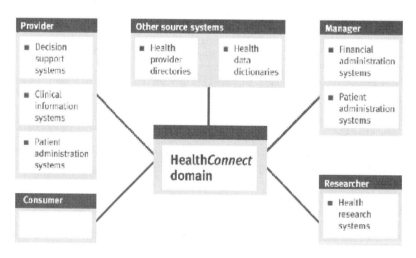

FIGURE 16.2. Health*Connect* conceptual model.

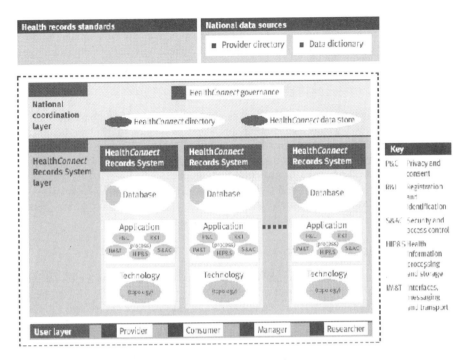

FIGURE 16.3. Health*Connect* conceptual systems structure.

tion would operate. The coordination layer would also include a directory spanning all of the Health*Connect* Records Systems nodes used to hold Health*Connect* data in the Health*Connect* Records Systems, and may also integrate all Health*Connect* data as a back up archival system. A by-product of this archival service would be the ability to tightly control the use of Health*Connect* data for secondary uses.

2.3.2. Health*Connect* Records Systems Layer

The federated Health*Connect* records systems layer would comprise Health*Connect* records systems operating as peer-to-peer Health*Connect* nodes. Each Health*Connect* records system would be an information technology system owned by an organization that specifically supports the management, storage, and exchange of a consumer's EHR.

Each Health*Connect* records system would provide the EHR function for a particular subset of the population, determined on a state, territory, regional, or organizational basis. To maintain the feasibility of retrieving records with high performance, it is proposed that an individual consumer would be affiliated with a single Health*Connect* Records System and that his or her entire EHR be wholly stored within that Health*Connect* records system. The alternative strategy of distributing parts of a consumer's EHR across multiple nodes introduces considerable complexity for the retrieval process, which may adversely impact on performance and scalability.

Providers and provider organizations would also be expected to affiliate with a single Health*Connect* records system. As far as possible, practical providers would share the same Health*Connect* records system as the consumers that they service. This would minimize the amount of inter-nodal communication necessary to locate the consumer's EHR. In line with the regional nature of healthcare delivery, the recommendation is for state, territory, or regional nodes to increase the likelihood that providers and their consumers would share the same node.

2.3.3. User Layer

The user layer would contain individual healthcare providers and consumers, all of whom, it is assumed, would have a computer available to them during the healthcare consultation. Their computers would connect to Health*Connect* using their provider organization's network connection. The provider organization would be entities such as hospitals, general practices, or physiotherapy practices.

Consumers would access Health*Connect* primarily through their preferred provider but would also have access through other means such as the Internet or perhaps booths in government shop fronts or via government agencies.

2.4. HealthConnect Trials

The Health*Connect* trial sites are the primary means of answering the action research questions. Essentially, the purpose of the trials is to test the feasibility of the health information network in a live setting and inform what might be the preferred model should Health*Connect* be implemented nationally. The trials are also expected to provide an understanding of the value of Health*Connect* to consumers and healthcare providers, including (in the long term) the impact on healthcare outcomes.

Fast-track trials in the Northern Territory and Tasmania were established to provide a live environment to test the Health*Connect* concept.

Results from the fast-track trials are being used to refine the models for testing in the longer-term trial sites in New South Wales, Victoria, Queensland, and possibly other States. The mainstream trials in New South Wales, Queensland, and Victoria are expected to be operational from late 2004 and will align with the Health*Connect* Business and Systems Architectures, which are expected to be more fully developed at this time. Figure 16.4 illustrates the locations of these trials.

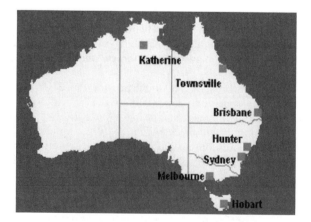

FIGURE 16.4. Location of Health*Connect* trials.

2.4.1. Tasmanian Trial

The Tasmanian Health*Connect* trial is focusing on adults (over age 18 years) with Type 1 or Type 2 diabetes mellitus in a local area of the capital city, Hobart. The major users are the Royal Hobart Hospital (including inpatient, emergency department and diabetes clinics, pathology, and pharmacy), consumers, and general practitioners located in the area.

2.4.2. Northern Territory Trial

The Northern Territory fast-track trial is testing Health*Connect* in a remote region, where a range of providers delivers healthcare services to a community of approximately 4500 people. The population has a very high representation of Indigenous Australians and healthcare providers recognize the importance of delivering culturally appropriate health care in close consultation with local communities. The population is also very mobile, meaning that individuals often seek health care from different providers in the region.

2.4.3. New South Wales Trials

The planned New South Wales trials are based on two separate target populations: the Child Health Information Network (CHIN) project at the Children's Hospital at Westmead in Western Sydney and the Chronic Disease Management System (CDMS) in the Hunter region in the Central Coast of New South Wales.

The CHIN will provide authorized access to the personal clinical information supplied by hospitals, child health centers, pediatricians, general practitioners, and private pathology. The information will be used to support the care of children with acute and chronic healthcare needs.

The target population for the CDMS will consist of approximately 2000 patients who are over 55 and have a diagnosis of one or more of the following: congestive heart failure (CHF); diabetes; chronic obstructive pulmonary disease (COPD); and other respiratory diseases (including asthma, emphysema, bronchiectasis, cystic fibrosis, pulmonary fibrosis, and other non-classified respiratory diseases).

2.4.4. Queensland Trials

Two Health*Connect* implementation trials are also being conducted in Queensland. These are (1) diabetes care, based on an extension of work already underway on the sharing of information and care plans by general practitioners in suburban Brisbane; and (2) an extension of research into electronic pre-operative assessment for elective surgery based around Townsville, a provincial city.

The Brisbane based trial will be based on *open*EHR, an open architecture and standard format for EHRs. *Open*EHR has evolved from the Good European Health Record (GEHR), which was conceived during the early 1990s.

2.4.5. Victoria

The Victorian trial aims to improve the information exchange between the acute and community sectors within a suburban area of Melbourne.

2.5. National InfoStructure Development

In the Australian context, infostructure has been defined as information infrastructure that provides shared resources and standards for healthcare agents/parties that enable information to flow in appropriately structured, identifiable (unambiguous), and secure ways.[2]

A sound national health infostructure is a prerequisite for the introduction of Health*Connect* on a national scale. The success of any future arrangements will require development and widespread adoption of the core resources and standards required to electronically support healthcare delivery and data processing nationally. Infostructure development activity sponsored by Health*Connect* includes:

- Development of a platform of EHR standards that emphasize consistency and interoperability at the semantic or knowledge level
- A nationally integrated health privacy framework
- Health sector identifier arrangements
- Standards development for a range of areas including messaging, coding and classification, data definitions, access, and consent
- An event summary classification framework together with instances of specific event summaries

Key achievements to date in these areas have included:

- Development of a draft national health privacy code via a widely consultative program. This code addresses disparities in the privacy regimes adopted by Australian, state and territory governments, and between the public and private sectors. (For more information, visit http://www.health.gov.au/pubs/nhpcode.htm.) While harmonization of these regimes is a very substantial task, sound but workable privacy protection is seen as a threshold issue for e-health initiatives.
- The definition of specific data requirements for Health*Connect*, including the specification of a national template for hospital discharge information. (These are expected to be available on the Health*Connect* website, http://www.healthconnect. gov.au, in the near future.)
- The development of a comprehensive program of EHR standards development, in conjunction and collaboration with key international standards organizations such as CEN, HL7,[3] and ISO.[4] This collaboration is seen as essential for two reasons:
  1. EHR development is as yet in its relatively early days, with limited numbers of experienced practitioners worldwide and a relatively narrow experience base of large-scale, integrated, longitudinal EHRs to draw upon. However, EHR standards promoting wide interoperability, very high data quality and clinically safe computer-based processing, including electronic decision support, will require robust standards. Accordingly, Standards Australia and the Health*Connect* Project have sought to leverage heavily from the pool of both Australian and international expertise. Australian contributions to these international standards processes have been significant.
  2. There are significant healthcare delivery and economic advantages in the compatibility of international standards promoting EHR interoperability, especially for a country such as Australia that imports many of its core elements of health information infrastructure.

---

[2] The definition of *infostructure* is paraphrased from the European Committee for Standardisation, Comité Européen de Normalisation, or CEN.

[3] Health Level Seven, originally U.S. based but increasingly international.

[4] International Standards Organization, in particular Technical Committee (TC) 215 on Health Informatics.

EHR standards development activity is scheduled to culminate in the publication of up to six Australian EHR standards over the next 18 months.
- Acceleration of a range of standards development activities, including the production of Australian Standards for Health Care Client and Provider Identification. (Standards Australia International 2002, 2004).

2.6. Infostructure Development Issues

The development and implementation of nation and sector wide capacity to locate and identify relevant and authorized parties to health service transactions; and to represent clinical information and knowledge in ways that can be reliably and unambiguously interpreted by both human and machine recipients present considerable challenges. These challenges range from technical to socio-political, and in many cases impinge directly on established clinical practice norms and health service workflow management processes.

2.6.1. Reliable and Unambiguous Identification of Health Service Transactors

The positive and unique identification of healthcare clients is a critical event in health service delivery, with direct implications for the safety and quality of health care.

Although Australian families are issued with a Medicare Card to enable claiming against the universal health insurance scheme, this card does not carry a unique identification number and its use is legislatively restricted to defined administrative purposes. Australia therefore currently has no national health identification scheme. Most states and territories are engaged in the development of master indexes of public sector health service clients to support the flow of clinical information within their jurisdictions. However, such indexes do not identify private health service clients.

Health*Connect*'s capacity to register, identify, and authenticate its clients is directly related to its proposed opt-in nature. Enrollment with Health*Connect* will be voluntary, and it is envisaged that registration will be accompanied by the provision of informed consent for the capture and use of personal information. Health*Connect* will therefore maintain its own client registry. However, the capacity to correlate and/or link Health*Connect* data with data holdings in other health services, under controlled conditions, remains dependent on the capacity to reliably identify and authenticate clients across the health sector more broadly. Accordingly, analysis of business and societal requirements for national healthcare client identification is still underway.

At a base level, however, an Australian Standard on Health Care Client Identification has been published with the aim of standardizing the capture and storage of information used to match individuals with the data that service providers hold about them (Standards Australia International 2002). The Standard provides a framework for improving the confidence of health service providers and clients alike that the data being associated with any given individual, and upon which clinical decisions are made, is appropriately associated.

Similarly, the reliable and unambiguous identification of health service providers is critical to ensuring that clinical information flows to them on a timely basis, and only to them. As for healthcare clients, most states and territories are currently implementing provider directories designed for specific purposes (e.g., professional registration, mailing lists, and service location) and unlinked. In some cases, the onerous requirements of maintaining such directories affect the quality and currency of their data holdings.

Health*Connect* has therefore initiated an assessment of the feasibility of establishing a national master index of healthcare providers that would preserve investment in existing fit-for-purpose directories but underpin them with a core of high-quality, up-to-date information required for unambiguous identification. The data elements required have been articulated in the Australian Standard on Health Care Provider Identification (Standards Australia International 2004).

2.6.2. Health Concept Representation

If it is to bridge existing gaps and address miscommunication within health service delivery processes, Health*Connect* will require the storage and interchange of information at levels of specification that not only assist human readability but also enable automatic processing of data by other EHR and decision support systems across different clinical settings. That is, Health*Connect* will require semantic interoperability of clinical data as described by the United States National Committee on Vital and Health Statistics (2000), that is, providing common interpretability, in that information within data fields can be used intelligently.

Accordingly, the Australian government has invested significantly in promoting international collaboration and debate concerning methodologies promoting the semantic interoperability of health information and knowledge, including *open*EHR archetypes and HL7's Clinical Document Architecture (CDA) and templates. As described above, the Brisbane based Health*Connect* Trial will utilize *open*EHR's archetypes to further test their potential.

The selection and representation of clinical data requirements has generated substantial interest and debate during consultation processes to date. This is in no small part reflective of the selection of clinical data elements being intrinsically linked to clinical practice. Standardized data are being developed in many cases in an environment of substantial variations in clinical practice and workflow. For this reason, consultation processes supporting development of the content of Event Summaries has sought to engender clinical ownership and governance of the agenda.

In addition, substantial information management infrastructure will be required to continue the longer term development and maintenance of clinical metadata, to ensure its lifelong relevance and version compatibility. Australia has a national Knowledgebase, maintained by the Australian Institute for Health and Welfare at its website, which provides a metadata repository. (To view the Knowledgebase, visit http://www.aihw.gov.au/knowledgebase/index.html.) This Knowledgebase is currently being redeveloped to upgrade its capacity and user-friendliness and to ensure its compliance with new ISO metadata management standards. Clinical metadata management requirements are being incorporated in this redevelopment.

Systematic approaches to enhancing and maintaining clinical data quality will also be required. Experience in some Australian clinical information systems projects to date has highlighted deficiencies in the quality of clinical data captured and stored, limiting the utility of such data for downstream care provision. Clinicians have also expressed concern about the professional and medico-legal implications of delivering care on the basis of potentially incomplete EHR data, for example, where clients may have chosen to withhold specific data or where not all of the providers associated with a given client have elected to supply information to Health*Connect*. While information gaps are not new in healthcare provision, there are concerns that EHRs may give the illusion of more complete recording than may actually be the case. All of these issues are closely associated with professional practices and norms, and require further investigation.

Another substantial issue is the use of standardized clinical terminologies or vocabularies. A Classifications and Terminologies Working Group has been established to determine the need for and implications of national standards for clinical terminologies, to assess candidates and to develop a comprehensive program of activities to progress toward these if required. (To read more about this group, see http://www.aihw.gov.au/committees/ctwg/index.html.) This is also an extremely complex area, with major ramifications for the vast array of legacy systems in place across the sector and for ensuring long-term compatibility between any nationally standard terminologies and the Australian Family of Classifications that provide a basis for the compilation of health data (Australian Institute of Health and Welfare 2003).

2.7. Key Findings to Date

Findings to date demonstrate that the Health*Connect* concept can work, and can be of value to and integrated into the day-to-day practices of healthcare providers.

Preliminary reports from the trials indicate that both consumers and providers perceive the information collected through Health*Connect* as being of value in providing clinical care, particularly in the area of improved information flow between providers. This feedback is further supported by the high take up of Health*Connect* by consumers and providers in the fast-track trials, and their support for continuing these trials beyond their original completion dates. These findings align with assessments of comparable initiatives internationally.

The capacity of Health*Connect* to lead to consumers being better informed and empowered is already evident from the Tasmanian trial. Consumers are able to manage their own health information by controlling who has access to it and which parts of it can be accessed. When enrolling in the trial, consumers consented to appropriate staff accessing demographic and personal information about their diabetic condition in Health*Connect*. They also had the right to consent selectively to their background information being loaded onto the Health*Connect* repository. When visiting their general practitioner, a small number of participants elected not to share information held in an event summary with the Health*Connect* repository. The option to choose which group of providers information can be withheld from will be introduced as the trials develop.

However, trial evaluations also revealed that neither consumers nor providers were fully aware of their consent rights and obligations. It is clear that both consumers and providers need to be fully informed about sensitive consent arrangements before they agree to participate in electronic health systems.

Interim findings from the Health*Connect* trial sites also show that using the system results in improved communication between healthcare providers, leading to the provision of higher quality health services. Half of the participating general practitioners at the Tasmanian site found that using Health*Connect* improved the flow of information and strengthened partnerships with hospital and pathology services and diabetes educators.

Evidence from the trials also indicates that Health*Connect* can provide substantial time savings for consumers and providers alike—a feature of the proposed network that is very important to these groups. The potential benefits of increased efficiency and improved workflow are very significant. It has been estimated that 25% of Australian doctors' and nurses' time is spent collecting data and information (Australian Audit Commission 1995).

Initial cost estimates for Health*Connect* have been developed, and are thought to be compatible with the scale of health information technology investments already underway in Australia. Work is still underway to assess the scope of the likely benefits. Notwithstanding this, initial cost–benefit analyses have suggested the potential for significant national savings in the costs of healthcare delivery, or at least offsets to potential healthcare cost increases.

However, while cost–benefit analysis is important, the future of Health*Connect* is likely to be determined more by demand and perceived usefulness. The world of electronic financial and business transactions is a good comparison. The costs and savings of establishing, maintaining, and operating these systems Australia-wide and worldwide are not entirely transparent. Although front office costs have been reduced by automatic teller machines, capital and back office costs have gone up substantially. Notwithstanding these considerable costs, consumers are happy to use these systems, and banks and financial institutions to provide them, because of their convenience and a dramatic escalation in access to financial services. If Health*Connect* is implemented nationally, it should be convenient and as seamless as the financial services industry. More importantly, Health*Connect* can also dramatically widen access to high-quality care, save lives, and mitigate suffering.

A big-bang approach to nationally implementing Health*Connect* is not recommended due to the likely funding requirements and significant risks associated with such an approach. Rather, the implementation model is an incremental approach that will integrate Health*Connect* with systems and infrastructure already in place or planned for development in the Australian healthcare system.

Accordingly, the implementation strategy is based on:

- Supplementation of existing infrastructure (including Health*Connect* trials) rather than replacement.
- Construction of a fully operational Health*Connect* as reference sites in two states (South Australia and Tasmania) within two to three years. These statewide reference implementations will be based upon the recently developed Health*Connect* architecture and used as the basis upon which future phased implementations could be introduced into other areas across Australia.
- Continued acceleration of infostructure development to underpin critical components of the Health*Connect* model. For Health*Connect* to be operational in a reference site within two to three years, policy work in the areas of provider and consumer identification, terminologies, legislation, governance, event summary and view definition, consent, security and messaging will need to reach maturity within 12 months of commencement of the implementation project.
- Completion of a comprehensive organizational change study across Australia in the first year of implementation activity. This project will investigate provider and vendor work flows and operation with the aim of improving work processes and delivery mechanisms through the introduction of Health*Connect* enabled processes.
- Completion of full implementation of Health*Connect* across Australia within 5 to 10 years.

2.8. Related Projects

Health*Connect* is a proposed EHR system for Australia that aims to provide core information infrastructure for healthcare service delivery. As such, it has much in common with other international EHR activities including Health*e*People in the United States and the Integrated Care Record Service in the United Kingdom's National Health Service.

Although forming a centerpiece for health service delivery, Health*Connect* is only one of a series of projects aimed at delivering a virtual health system in Australia. Other important projects include:

- TeleHealth—due to the sparse population distribution in regional, rural, and remote Australia, TeleHealth initiatives began in the 1980s, positioning Australia as a world leader in this technology adoption. While it is recognized that TeleHealth is an enabler to equitable healthcare delivery in non-metropolitan areas, the applications of TeleHealth in all settings is advantageous. A national approach covering all facets of TeleHealth planning and implementation has been established (National Health Information Management Advisory Council 2001).
- Electronic Decision Support Systems (EDSS)—a national approach to the development and implementation of EDSS has also commenced and is likely to scale up in the future akin to the Health*Connect* Project (National Electronic Decision Support System Task Force 2002).
- Several state and territory health department and private hospitals are currently deploying large-scale point of care clinical information systems. In many cases, these will form critical source and destination systems for Health*Connect*.
- Electronic prescribing has been successfully deployed for the majority of general practitioners, and several projects are underway to develop components of a comprehensive electronic medication management cycle.
- Electronic claiming and reimbursement and simplified billing initiatives have been deployed, and substantial and innovative approaches to hospital supply chain management and e-business in health care are being introduced.
- In terms of infrastructure, substantial programs have been operating for several years to widen and enhance access to telecommunications networks, particularly in rural and remote areas. A rural broadband initiative is currently underway, funded by the Australian Government. Public Key Infrastructure (PKI) componentry is also being made available nationally.

3. Better Information, Better Outcomes

Health*Connect* represents a response to both the deficiencies inherent in current arrangements regarding health information, and to new opportunities emerging from technological developments. While further research and development are required, the Australian Government is committed to implementing Health*Connect* in at least two states over the next two to three years.

The intent of Health*Connect* is to ensure that the health sector become better able to exploit information opportunities at the individual, clinical, institutional, planning, and research levels. This it will do by facilitating access to critical health information when it is needed, where it is needed, and in the form it is needed.

Health*Connect* promises other related improvements as well, including the availability, integration, and quality of other information holdings and flows, and the adoption of new skills by those using e-health infrastructure. Together, these are expected to lead to improved knowledge creation and use, more informed and appropriate decision making, more empowered users, and more effective targeting of healthcare delivery and resources.

In turn, these effects will contribute to higher-order goals such as improved health outcomes, more effective healthcare delivery, and increased satisfaction with the health system.

For further information about Health*Connect*, access the Health*Connect* website at http://www.healthconnect.gov.au.

References

Australian Audit Commission. 1995. For your information. Canberra, Australia: Australian Audit Commission.

Australian Bureau of Statistics. 1999. Australian social trends (4102.0). Canberra, Australia: Australian Bureau of Statistics. p 57.

Australian Bureau of Statistics. 2003a. 2003 Year Book Australia (1301.0). Canberra, Australia: Australian Bureau of Statistics. p 256.

Australian Bureau of Statistics. 2003b. Private Hospitals Australia (4390.0) 2001–2002. Canberra, Australia: Australian Bureau of Statistics.

Australian Institute of Health and Welfare. 2003. Australian Family of Health and Related Classifications. Available from: http://www.aihw.gov.au/committees/ctwg/public_resources/princ_australia_300802.doc. Accessed 2004 Nov 17.

Australian Institute of Health and Welfare. 2003a. Australian Hospital Statistics 2001–2002. Canberra, Australia: Australian Institute of Health and Welfare.

Australian Institute of Health and Welfare. 2003b. Health Expenditure Australia 2001–02, Health and Welfare Expenditure Series Number 17. Canberra, Australia: Australian Institute of Health and Welfare.

National Committee on Vital and Health Statistics. 2000. Uniform data standards for patient medical record information. Washington, DC: National Committee on Vital and Health Statistics. p 22.

National Electronic Decision Support Task force. 2002. Electronic decision support for Australia's health sector. Canberra, Australia: Australian Government Department of Health and Ageing.

National Electronic Health Records Taskforce. 2000. A health information network for Australia. Canberra, Australia: Australian Government Department of Health and Ageing.

National Health Information Management Advisory Council. 2001. *HealthOnline*: a health information action plan for Australia. 2nd ed. Canberra, Australia: Australian Government Department of Health and Ageing.

Population Reference Bureau. 2002. World Population Data Sheet 2002. Washington DC: Population Reference Bureau.

Private Health Insurance Administration Council. 2003. Operations of the Registered Health Benefits Organizations Annual Report 2002–03. Canberra, Australia: Private Health Insurance Administration Council.

Standards Australia International. 2002. AS5017-2002, Health Care Client Identification. Available from: http://www.standards.com.au. Accessed 2004 Nov 18.

Standards Australia International. 2004. AS4846-2004, Health Care Provider Identification. Available from: http://www.standards.com.au. Accessed 2004 Nov 18.

World Health Organization. 2003. The World Health Report 2003—Table 4 Healthy Life Expectancy (HALE) in All Member States, Estimates for 2002. Geneva: WHO.

17
The Veterans Health Administration: Quality, Value, Accountability, and Information as Transforming Strategies

JONATHAN B. PERLIN and ROBERT M. KOLODNER

The Health*e*People initiative builds upon earlier efforts within the largest integrated health system in the United States, the Veterans Health Administration (VA). Suffering, deservedly or not, during the 1980s and early 1990s from a tarnished reputation of bureaucracy, inefficiency, and mediocre care, VA sought to reinvent itself as a model system characterized by patient-centered, quality care of high value. This reinvention mandated structural and organizational changes, rationalization of resource allocation, measurement and active management of quality and value (and clear accountability for quality and value), and an information infrastructure that would increasingly support the needs of patients, clinicians, and administrators.

While predating the recent recommendations by the Institute of Medicine (Institute of Medicine 2001) for a more ideal health system, VA's improvement using remarkably similar strategies provides increasing evidence of the utility of those recommendations for closing the quality chasm. These strategies have allowed VA to emerge as an increasingly recognized leader in healthcare quality and value. Table 17.1 maps VA's value domains to the aims identified by the IOM.

1. Origins of the Veterans Health Administration

Although health and social support for aged or disabled soldiers has existed in the United States since colonial times, national programs for American veterans were consolidated with the establishment of the Veterans Administration in 1930. Resources for social services expanded rapidly following World War II with the Servicemen's Readjustment Act of 1944 (better known as the GI Bill of Rights), and a hospital system that specialized in meeting the rehabilitative needs of returning soldiers who had experienced physical and emotional trauma evolved. The Veterans Administration was elevated to Cabinet status and became the Department of Veterans Affairs in 1988, with financial support programs such as pensions administered under the aegis of the Veterans Benefits Administration and health services consolidated in the Veterans Health Administration. The Secretary of Veterans Affairs directs the activities of the Department, and the Under Secretary for Health serves as the Chief Executive Officer of the Veterans Health Administration.

TABLE 17.1. Mapping of VA value domains to ideal health system aims.

VA domains	Quality chasm Aims
Quality	Effective, safe
Access	Timely
Satisfaction	Patient centered
Function	Patient centered
Community health	Equitable
Cost effectiveness	Efficient

2. Structural and Organizational Transformation of the 1990s

Through the mid-1990s, VA operated largely as a hospital system providing general medical and surgical services, specialized care in mental health and spinal cord injury, and long-term care though directly operated or indirectly supported facilities. Medical centers and other facilities operated relatively independently of each other, even competitively reduplicating services. Anachronistic laws required that virtually all healthcare services were provided in hospitals, counter to the movement of care into the ambulatory environment. In 1996, the Veterans Equitable Resource Allocation Act (VERA) corrected this anachronism in support of restructuring from a hospital system to a healthcare system, as directed by then Under Secretary for Health, Kenneth W. Kizer. The structural changes were predicated on the assumption that the most effective, efficient care required coordination among facilities and synergy of resources, including the availability of care in the most appropriate environments.

The structural transformation was characterized by creation of 22 geographically defined Veterans Integrated Service Networks (VISNs). In addition to redirecting resource allocations to follow the geographically shifting veteran population, VERA allocated resources to each network, rather than each facility. Within VISNs, this created financial incentives for coordination of care and resources among previously competing facilities. While the portfolio of medical centers still exists today, medical centers are distributed among 21 VISNs (two VISNs were recently merged), as are community-based outpatient clinics (CBOCs), which increased from fewer than 200 in 1996 to over 700 today, and more that 300 other long-term care facilities, domiciliaries, and home-care programs. This structural transformation has shifted care from the hospital to ambulatory care and home environment, allowing a reduction of hospital and long-term care beds from approximately 92,000 to 58,000 with a concomitant decrease in hospitalizations and increase in ambulatory care visits and home care services. The trend is depicted in Figure 17.1.

It should be noted that during the period extending from 1996 to 2003, the number of veterans treated annually increased from approximately 2.8 to 4.9 million. The appropriated budget remained flat at $19 billion from 1995 to 1999; it increased to approximately $25 billion for fiscal year 2003, or about 32% cumulatively over six years.

3. Accountability for Quality and Value: A New Strategy

Because of its public nature, VA is perhaps the most scrutinized health system in the United States. In the late 1980s and early 1990s, VA was beset by increasing public anxiety about the quality of care. A movie entitled *Article 99* (Orion Studios 1992) parodied VA as a hapless and dangerous bureaucracy, and the challenging U.S. economy at the close of the 1980s and opening of the next decade raised concern about the economic viability of the system. The broader American healthcare context saw the increasing emergence of managed care, offering the hope of improved quality and the promise of a mechanism for controlling healthcare cost inflation. At the extremes, a tension between the desire to maintain a system dedicated to veterans' health needs and vouchering out (contracting for) care for presumably greater quality and efficiency emerged. It was increasingly apparent that if VA were to persist, it would need to prove its value to Congress and its quality to veterans themselves.

Two documents, *Vision for Change* and *Prescription for Change*, outlined the challenges facing VA and served as the template for organizational restructuring and a new strategy for systematizing quality and value (Kizer 1995, 1996).

The Department of Veterans Affairs sought to operationalize value in terms of the relationship of outputs to inputs in contrast to more simplistic, prevalent, and less meaningful concept of unit cost. Expanding from the concept of value as the relationship of quality to cost (Nelson et al. 1996), VA objectified quality as a constellation of outcomes of interest to veterans and stakeholders. These outcomes were known as the value domains shown in Figure 17.2.

The objectification of quality and value serves as the basis for internal performance improvement efforts and both internal and external accountability. Measures are determined in each of the value domains. In the arena of quality, performance measures largely derive from rates of provision of evidence-based healthcare services (processes and intermediate outcomes) in the areas of preventive health, disease treatment, and palliation. Novel composite measures, known as the Prevention Index (as shown in Figure 17.5), Chronic Disease Index, and Palliative Care Index, serve to focus provider attention on the respective areas and summarize performance. Representative measures in each domain are shown in Table 17.2.

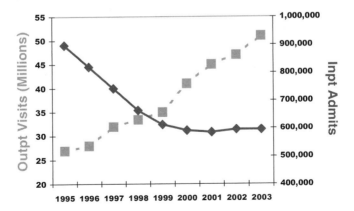

FIGURE 17.1. Decrease in hospital admissions (solid line) and increase in outpatient visits (dashed line) in VA from 1995 to 2003.

$$Value = \frac{Quality}{Cost}$$ Objectifying "Quality," this becomes: $$Quality = \frac{Outcomes}{Cost}$$

Value Domains:
- Quality   (Technical Quality in Prevention, Treatment, Palliation)
- Access   (Distance, Timeliness, Special Care Needs, Information)
- Satisfaction   (Patient Experiences, Perceived Quality)
- Function   (Health Related Quality-of-Life)
- Cost-Effectiveness (Efficiency)
- Community Health (Added 1999 - Teaching, Research, Contingency Disaster System)

Today, the "Value Equation" is re-expressed to clearly articulate the relationship of inputs to outputs:

$$Value = \frac{Quality + Access + Satisfaction + Function + CommunityHealth}{Cost}$$

FIGURE 17.2. Value domains and the value equation.

4. Accountability: The Performance Contract

VA operates with both formal external and internal accountability for performance. As part of the Government Performance and Results Act (GPRA), major federal agencies now engage in a performance agreement with the White House, administered through the Office of Management and Budget (OMB). Internally, since 1995, an annual performance contract has been in place between the Under Secretary for Health and senior network (VISN) leaders. The content of this performance contract has been constructed around the value domains, now known as the strategic goal areas.

Measures are developed using an evidence-based approach that extends beyond evidence-based medicine to embrace the concept of evidence-based quality management. Thus, the accountability and improvement system is both rigorous and data intensive. Operating in parallel with the Performance Measurement Program is the National Advisory Council for Clinical Practice Guidelines. In the clinical arena, VA has the strategic advantage of affiliation with 107 academic health systems, and in conjunction with its own directly employed professional work force, the expertise in specific clini-

TABLE 17.2. Representative measures in VA's value domains.

Value domain	Representative measures
Quality	Prevention Index (immunization, cancer & substance use screening)
	Chronic Disease Index (heart, lung, endocrine diseases, e.g., heart failure, COPD, diabetes)
	Palliative Care Index (pain screening & management)
Access	Wait times for new primary care appointments
	Wait times for specialty care appointments
	Percentage patients seen within 20 minutes of scheduled appointment
Satisfaction	Perception of quality as very good or excellent
	Performance on picker-based satisfaction survey*
Function	Percentage of spinal cord injury patients discharged to independent living
	Percentage of homeless patients discharged to independent living
Community health	Researcher satisfaction
	Learner perception survey
Cost-effectiveness	Days in accounts receivable & other fiscal measures
	Value equation

* Derived from Picker Surveys of Inpatient and Outpatient Care, Picker Institute, Boston, MA.

cal disciplines and evidence synthesis is robust. Many professionals are involved in VA Health Services Research and Development as well as VA's eight Quality Enhancement Research Initiatives (or QUERI programs), which focus on highly prevalent diseases such as diabetes or heart failure or conditions conferring unique vulnerability such as mental illness and spinal cord injury. The collective efforts serve to systematically translate the best evidence into recommendations for best practice.

Clinical performance measures evolve as the interrogative of the evidence-based clinical recommendations in preventive medicine, disease treatment, and palliative care. In the remaining domains of satisfaction, access, function, community health, and cost effectiveness, experts similarly reconcile data to identify and support areas for improvement. The guiding principle for selection into the performance contract is that the particular measures are ambitious and transformative, moving VA and its care of veterans meaningfully forward.

The performance contract is created as a collaborative process involving central management and field leaders. In fact, the Performance Measurement Work Group is both co-chaired by and comprised of central and field leaders, and it includes both clinicians and administrators. The group serves as a mechanism for vetting and prioritizing measures for inclusion in a performance contract recommended to the Under Secretary for Health. Thus, the ultimate contract between the Under Secretary and VISN leaders— the contents of which are cascaded formally or informally to clinicians and managers throughout the system—is a collaborative product, reducing the traditional us–them tension between central and field leadership or administrators and clinicians.

Results of the performance contract form the basis for quarterly management reviews. While extremely modest management incentives exist, the performance results are broadly distributed within VA and are known to key stakeholders such as Congress, veteran advocacy groups, and the OMB. Resulting performance data are published in hard-copy quarterly and annually, and are increasingly available as they accrue in real-time on internal intranet sites.

5. Supporting Systems

Effective information systems are the prerequisite for both the effective delivery of services that maximize value in each of the domains as well as the operation of the Performance Management Program. While the clinical information system is remarkably robust for supporting patient care, the current capacity for national roll-up of discrete data elements is currently limited. So, while most clinical data and patient records are fully electronic, VA uses an audit program to assess clinical performance. Using VA performance criteria, audits are performed by an independent, external contractor under the External Peer Review Program (EPRP). This provides data to support measurement primarily in the more clinical domains of quality and function. Notably, VA's new health data repository will markedly expand capacity for automated aggregation of national performance data.

In the domain of satisfaction, traditional event-driven surveys of satisfaction with ambulatory care visits, hospitalizations, or other services (e.g., prosthetics, spinal cord injury, pharmacy) have been used. However, with recognition that satisfaction is only one component of the patient experience, a new omnibus Survey of Health Experiences of Patients (SHEP) has been introduced to acquire data about general health-care experiences (e.g., waits) and satisfaction, patient functional status (SF-12V; Jones et al. 2001), health risk behaviors (e.g., nutrition, exercise, tobacco) and link with clinical information acquired through EPRP. The conjunction of these data more richly support improvement, program planning, policy development, and (redacted of all identifying information) health services research. Corporate data from scheduling and fiscal systems (and some survey information) are used to support measurement and improvement in the domains of access, cost, and community health.

VA's approach to both improvement of healthcare delivery and improvement of information systems is reflected well in models identifying the convergence of patients, providers, and the health system for optimal outcomes as articulated by Wagner and colleagues. These models suggest that the most productive interactions occur with the conjunction of prepared, proactive providers and informed, activated patients in the context of a supportive, informed health system (Glasgow et al. 2001). In addition to information for performance management supporting improvement at a system level, VA's clinical information system has been a critical strategy and advantage in supporting providers and is emerging as an equally important vehicle for informing and activating patients.

6. Computerized Patient Record System

VA has had automated information systems providing extensive clinical and administrative capabilities in all of its medical facilities since 1985, beginning with its Decentralized Hospital Computer Program (DHCP). The Veterans Health Information Systems and Technology Architecture (VistA), supporting ambulatory, inpatient, and long-term care, delivered significant enhancements to the original system with the release of the Computerized Patient Record System (CPRS) for clinicians in 1997. CPRS was developed to provide a single, highly graphical interface for healthcare providers to review and update a patient's medical record as well as the ability to place orders for various items including medications, procedures, x-rays and imaging, patient care nursing orders, diets, and laboratory tests. CPRS is flexible enough to be implemented in a wide variety of settings by a broad spectrum of healthcare workers, and provides a consistent, event-driven, windows-style interface.

CPRS organizes and presents all relevant patient data in a way that directly supports clinical decision-making. The comprehensive cover sheet displays timely, patient-centric information, including active problems, allergies, current medications, recent laboratory results, vital signs, hospitalization, and outpatient clinic history. This information can be displayed immediately when a patient is selected and provides an accurate overview of the patient's current status before any clinical interventions are ordered. CPRS is fully operational at all medical centers and most other VA sites of care.

In 2004, VistA Imaging became operational in all of the VA medical centers. It provides a multi-media, online patient record that integrates traditional medical chart information with medical images of all kinds including x-rays, pathology slides, video views, scanned documents, cardiology exam results, dental images, endoscopies, etc. Figure 17.3 shows a sample screen from this system.

Other capabilities in CPRS include:

- A Real-Time Order Checking System alerts clinicians during the ordering session that a possible problem could exist if the order is processed (e.g., drug–drug interactions, duplicate labs, etc.). Notably, 91% of all pharmacy orders throughout VA are now electronically entered directly by the prescriber.
- A Notification System immediately alerts clinicians about clinically significant events such as abnormal test results.

- A Patient Posting System, displayed on every CPRS screen, alerts clinicians to issues related to the patient, including crisis notes, special warnings, adverse reactions, and advance directives.
- Remote Data View functionality allows clinicians to view a veteran's medical information from another VA facility or from Department of Defense medical treatment facilities to ensure the clinician has access to all clinically relevant data.
- The Clinical Reminder System allows caregivers to track and improve preventive health care and disease treatment for patients and to ensure that timely clinical interventions are initiated. It provides context-sensitive (e.g., recognizes that patient has a particular diagnosis, such as diabetes), time-sensitive (e.g., 12 months have elapsed since the service was last provided) clinical decision support. The clinical reminder system is now the preferred mechanism for implementation of clinical practice guidelines, and facilitates linking the evidence with the real-time clinical reminder, with the action (e.g., pneumoccocal vaccination in elderly or chronically ill patient), and with the automatically generated documentation as well as a trail of standardized performance data. Figure 17.4 shows a standard screen from this system.

A more recent addition to CPRS provides a multi-patient tool for follow up on clinical interventions. The list of patients can be based on results in addition to clinic schedule and inpatient ward or team. Using this new care management software, clinicians can manage across a group of patients—seeing and taking action on results, unsigned documents, tasks, and events across the patients. Providers can be more efficient using

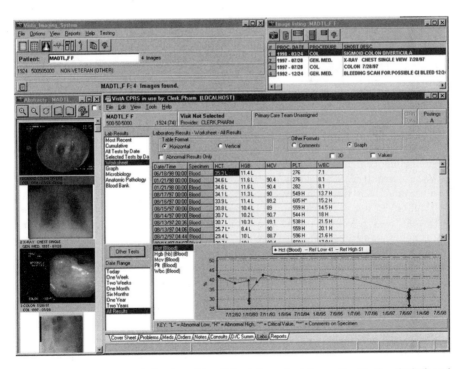

FIGURE 17.3. Actual record of patient (identifying information changed) with diverticulosis and a diverticular hemorrhage, demonstrating graphical data presentation showing endocscopy images and radiographs, including a bleeding scan.

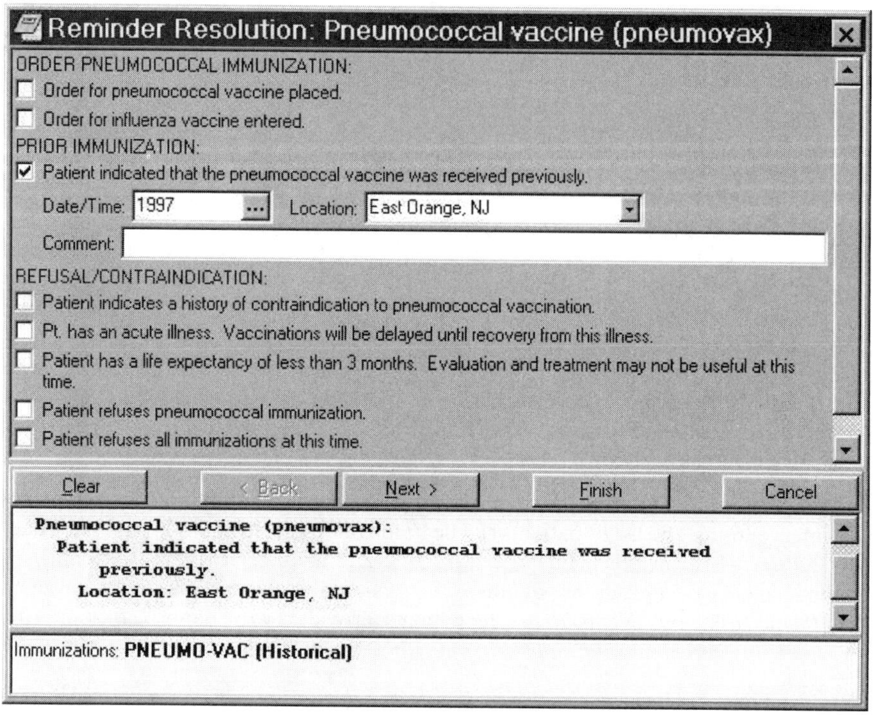

FIGURE 17.4. Clinical reminder for pneumococcal vaccination.

this new environment and have new capabilities such as being able to electronically acknowledge test results, develop and manage tasks and to-do lists, and query across patients using a variety of clinical parameters. The care management software represents an entirely new category of clinician software and will evolve and grow in scope as clinicians gain experience and provide feedback regarding novel applications and desired enhancements.

VA is currently effecting a major transformation in its health information systems to more effectively serve the needs of patients, providers, and the health system. Known as HealtheVet, the new architectural strategy fully integrates a health data repository with registration systems, provider systems, management and financial systems, and information and education systems. The health data repository creates a true longitudinal healthcare record including data from VA and non-VA sources, supporting research and population analyses, improving data quality and security, and facilitating patient access to data and health information.

With an emphasis on e-health, a secure patient portal known as My HealtheVet provides patients access to their personal health record, online health assessment tools, mechanisms for prescription refills and making appointments, and access to high quality consumer health information. The consumer information is evidence based, consistent with the clinician practice guideline recommendations (made proactive through clinical reminders) and, ideally, activating to the patient. A major barrier to the complete deployment of CPRS and e-health extensions at every VA site is the challenge of an inadequate telecommunications infrastructure in the more remote and rural parts of the country.

7. The Results: Outcomes and Value

The active management of quality and value through performance measurement, timely data feedback, and information systems that increasingly support clinicians, managers, and patients in achieving the benefits of evidence-based practice has improved outcomes in each value domain. For example, in the domain of quality, pneumococcal vaccination of at-risk patients is an evidence-based practice that reduces excess morbidity, mortality, and cost (Nichol et al. 1999). Yet in 1995, the rate of pneumococcal vaccination in eligible VA patients was 29%. Today, it is 79%. Figure 17.5 depicts that trend. The trends are identical in each of the preventive services encompassed by the Prevention Index.

Performance improvement and achievement has similarly occurred in the areas of disease treatment encompassed by over 20 clinical practice guidelines such as coronary artery disease, heart failure, diabetes, and major depressive disorder. Increasingly, VA performance compares favorably with the best performers, where performance is, in fact, measured and performance data are available, as shown in Table 17.3.

Veterans are increasingly satisfied by changes in the VA health system. On the American Customer Satisfaction Index (University of Michigan 2000, 2001), VA bested private sector's mean healthcare score of 68 on a 100 point scale, with scores of 79 for ambulatory care, 82 for inpatient care, and 83 for pharmacy services. Similar improvements have been manifest in each domain. It is worth noting that dollars available per patient have decreased over 25%. Returning to the value equation, it would seem evident that the numerator (outputs) have risen while the denominator (resource inputs) have dropped, signifying enhanced value.

In sum, electronic health records have provided critical success to VA's achievement in every value domain. VA's value domains are remarkably consistent with the ideal health system aims spelled out by the IOM in *Crossing the Quality Chasm*, providing evidence for the premise that a more effective healthcare delivery is possible with their adoption (Institute of Medicine 2001).

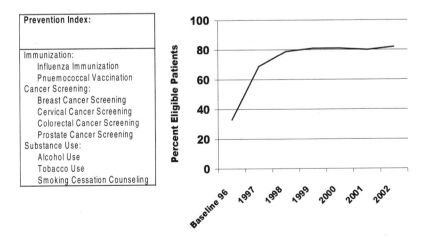

FIGURE 17.5. Components of VA's Prevention Index and performance over time.

TABLE 17.3. VA performance bests best measured non-VA performance for 18 comparable performance quality indicators.

Comparable measure (data are percentage eligible patients)	VA '01	VA '02	Medicaid/ Medicare	Best reported outside VA
Advise smoking cessation annually	93	>95	NA	66[NCQA 2001]
Beta blocker, D/C post-MI	94	97	83/89	94[MMCP 2001]
Breast CA screening	80	80	55/74	75[MMCP 2001]
Cervical CA screening	89	89	60/NA	80[NCQA 2001]
Cholesterol screening, all pts	88	91	44/71	73[BRFSS 2001]
Cholesterol screening, post-MI	89	NA	NA	77[NCQA 2001]
LDL cholesterol <130 post-MI	71	69	NA	59[NCQA 2001]
Colorectal CA screening	60	64	NA	59[BRFSS 1999]
Diabetes: Hgb A1c in past year	93	94	68/82	86[MMCP 2001]
Diabetes: Hgb A1c >9.5 (lower is better)	20	17	55/33	37[NCQA 2001]
Diabetes: LDL measured	91	94	NA	87[MMCP 2001]
Diabetes: LDL controlled <130	68	64	NA	50[NCQA 2001]
Diabetes: eye (retinal) exam	66	72	43/63	69[MMCP 2001]
Diabetes: kidney function assessed	72	78	38/45	46[NCQA 2001]
Immunization: influenza, >65 yrs	73	68	NA	65[BRFSS 2001]
Immunization: pheumococcal, >65 yrs	79	81	NA	60[BRFSS 2001]
Mental health F/U <30 days of inpt D/C	84	NA	55/59	73[NCQA 2001]

All measures are directly comparable, except mental health follow up, as VA accepts telephonic follow up; all data are 2001, published by the sources noted.

Source: NCQA: National Committee for Quality Assurance 2001. The state of managed care quality, industry trends and analysis. Patients are all ages in private managed care programs.

MMCP: Medicare Managed Care Programs, U.S. Department of Health and Human Services, Center for Medicare and Medicaid Services (CMS).

BRFSS; Centers for Disease Control, Behavioral risk factor surveillance system (BRFSS) survey from National Center for Chronic Disease Prevention & Health Promotion. (Rhode Island is benchmark for Influenza Immunization.)

References

Glasgow RE, Orleans CT, Wagner EH. 2001. Does the chronic care model serve also as a template for improving prevention? Milbank Q 79(4):579–612.

Institute of Medicine. 2001. Crossing the quality chasm: a new health system for the 21st century. Washington, DC: National Academy Press.

Jones D, Kazis L, Lee A, Rogers W, Skinner K, Cassar L, Wilson N, Hendricks A. 2001. Health assessments using the Veterans SF-12 and SF-36: methods for evaluating outcomes in the Veterans Health Administration. J Ambulatory Care Manage 24(3):68–86.

Kizer KW. 1995. Vision for change: a plan to restructure the Veterans Health Administration. Washington, DC: Department of Veterans Affairs.

Kizer KW. 1996. Prescription for change: the guiding principles and strategic objectives underlying the transformation of the Veterans Health Administration. Washington, DC: Department of Veterans Affairs.

Nelson EC, Mohr JJ, Batalden PB, Plume SK. 1996. Improving health care, part 1: the clinical value compass. Joint Commission J Qual Improve 22(4):243–258.

Nichol KL, Baken L, Wuorenma J, Nelson A. 1999. The health and economic benefits associated with pneumococcal vaccination of elderly persons with chronic lung disease. Arch Int Med 159(20):2437–2442.

Orion Studios. 1992. Article 99. Hollywood, CA: Orion Studios.

University of Michigan. 2000. American Customer Satisfaction Index. Ann Arbor, MI: University of Michigan School of Business.

University of Michigan. 2001. American Customer Satisfaction Index. Ann Arbor, MI: University of Michigan School of Business.

Index

Health Informatics Series
(formerly Computers in Health Care)

(continued from page ii)

Introduction to Clinical Informatics
P. Degoulet and M. Fieschi

Behavioral Healthcare Informatics
N.A. Dewan, N.M. Lorenzi, R.T. Riley, and S.R. Bhattacharya

Patient Care Information Systems
Successful Design and Implementation
E.L. Drazen, J.B. Metzger, J.L. Ritter, and M.K. Schneider

Introduction to Nursing Informatics, Second Edition
K.J. Hannah, M.J. Ball, and M.J.A. Edwards

Strategic Information Management in Hospitals
An Introduction to Hospital Information Systems
R. Haux, A. Winters, E. Ammenwerth, and B. Brigl

Information Retrieval
A Health and Biomedical Perspective, Second Edition
W.R. Hersh

The Nursing Informatics Implementation Guide
E.C. Hunt, S.B. Sproat, and R.R. Kitzmiller

Information Technology for the Practicing Physician
J.M. Kiel

Computerizing Large Integrated Health Networks
The VA Success
R.M. Kolodner

Medical Data Management
A Practical Guide
F. Leiner, W. Gaus, R. Haux, and P. Knaup-Gregori

Organizational Aspects of Health Informatics
Managing Technological Change
N.M. Lorenzi and R.T. Riley

Transforming Health Care Through Information, Second Edition
N.M. Lorenzi, J.S. Ash, J. Einbinder, W. McPhee, and L. Einbinder

Trauma Informatics
K.I. Maull and J.S. Augenstein

Consumer Informatics
Applications and Strategies in Cyber Health Care
R. Nelson and M.J. Ball

Public Health Informatics and Information Systems
P.W. O' Carroll, W.A. Yasnoff, M.E. Ward, L.H. Ripp,
and E.L. Martin

Advancing Federal Sector Health Care
A Model for Technology Transfer
P. Ramsaroop, M.J. Ball, D. Beaulieu, and J.V. Douglas

Medical Informatics
Computer Applications in Health Care and Biomedicine, Second Edition
E.H. Shortliffe and L.E. Perreault

Filmless Radiology
E.L. Siegel and R.M. Kolodner

Cancer Informatics
Essential Technologies for Clinical Trials
J.S. Silva, M.J. Ball, C.G. Chute, J.V. Douglas, C.P. Langlotz, J.C. Niland,
and W.L. Scherlis

Clinical Information Systems
A Component-Based Approach
R. Van de Velde and P. Degoulet

Knowledge Coupling
New Premises and New Tools for Medical Care and Education
L.L. Weed

Healthcare Information Management Systems
Cases, Strategies, and Solutions, Third Edition
M.J. Ball, C.A. Weaver, and J.M. Kiel

Organizational Aspects of Health Informatics, Second Edition
Managing Technological Change
N.M. Lorenzi and R.T. Riley